Human Nutrition from the Gastroenterologist's Perspective

Enzo Grossi • Fabio Pace

Editors

Human Nutrition from the Gastroenterologist's Perspective

Lessons from Expo Milano 2015

Foreword by Reinhold Stockbrugger

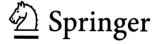 Springer

Editors
Enzo Grossi
Villa Santa Maria
Research & Development
Milan
Italy

Fabio Pace
ASST Bergamo Est
Gastroenterology
Seriate (BG)
Italy

ISBN 978-3-319-30359-8   ISBN 978-3-319-30361-1   (eBook)
DOI 10.1007/978-3-319-30361-1

Library of Congress Control Number: 2016940504

Printed on acid-free paper

This Springer imprint is published by Springer Nature
The registered company is Springer International Publishing AG Switzerland

Foreword

Macro-cosmos, Women and Men, Micro-cosmos: A Preface

The World Exhibition in Milano in the year 2015 has not only been a public, touristic, and economic success for the country, but has also given the opportunity to bring into sharp focus a field not always recognized as the spearhead for Italian epidemiological, medical, and biological research. Certainly, many tourists and travellers visit the country to satisfy their culinary tastes, and there is presently a worldwide boom of Italian and Italian-like restaurants. However, few people can imagine that the pleasure of creating good food and drink in this country is paralleled by a great invention, production, preparation, and the consumption of these products in delightful environments that can increase the sensual pleasure of 'nutrition' (what a poor word for the pleasure of a beautiful evening in a stylish restaurant or a pittoresque terrace).

However, the exhibition has also given the opportunity to demonstrate our role as clinical and/or scientific gastroenterologists in this context under the most varying aspects. This multiauthor publication, very actually designed and edited by my friends Enzo Grossi and Fabio Pace, leads us through the various areas of our professional involvement with 'nutrition' and may in the conclusion allow me some suggestions for an even tighter engagement in the field, not only aiming at a better service for patients and society, but also for a continuing penetration into the above quoted macro- and micro-cosmos and its inhabitants.

When 'Nutrition' Causes Disease

Exactly 100 years ago, lack of food, bad politics, and subsequent global wars have been the most prominent causes of incidence and prevalence of death. Who could imagine that in these days over- and mal-consumption of food have taken the primary places at epidemiological mortality statistics. The landscape of global medicine has changed, and nowadays cardiovascular, oncological, and gastrointestinal disciplines are the most consulted medical players in the game. Not for nothing do five of the 13 articles in this volume reflect this historical change that not only touches the rich – so-called developed – countries, but also increasing segments in countries where exact statistics still are lacking.

I still remember that friends and colleagues laughed at me when I some decennia ago proposed the idea that GERD and obesity seemed to be connected with each other. Nowadays, the global advancement of PPIs is based on this correlation and gastroenterologists are helped by oto-rhino-laryngologists to promote that reality.

Our specialist partners, the hepatologists, can make a good living from the fatty livers and the more or less useful therapeutic measures that can be proposed, from life-long pre-/probiotic prescriptions to increasingly adventurous surgical applications.

And finally, a long and sumptuous life with the wrong hyper-caloric habits and diets claims its toll with malignancies in the esophagus, liver, pancreas, and colon (only to mention our own gastroenterological/oncological territory).

How Nutrition Influences Human and 'Micro-cosmic Biology'

We live in an exiting phase of human redefinition: we are no longer alone with our sorrows, alerts, intelligence, activities, and moods: we have found powerful partners (brothers and sisters?; servants or masters?): the gut microbiome, probably more diversified and stronger and possibly ontogenetic older than we ourselves, that function as their home and feeding company. Previously, the disciplines of 'microbiology' and 'infective diseases' were concerned with them; nowadays, every medical branch, either in research or in clinics, has to learn to know this newly discovered partner and must care about recognition, collaboration, and hopefully friendship with him/her/it/them.

In this volume, three articles deal with the gastrointestinal microbiome – our alter ego – and its influence on obesity, neuro-psychiatry (autism), and the way how we develop to 'tasters' and 'super-tasters'. Will it surprise you that we have got a flood of new scientific findings (but unfortunately still a lack of remedies) in our new daughter-discipline 'neuro-gastroenterology' that hosts 'gut microbiota' research in journals and congresses worldwide? Apropos, in this context: did you know that long-term use of 'PPI's profoundly changes the 'gut microbiome'? If not: on PubMed there are nine hits since 2014!

Nutritional Modifications As Therapy?

This is for the practicing gastroenterologist, internist, and surgeon probably the most asked question by patients and relatives. The answer is 'yes, but …': There are very few diseases that really can be definitely healed by a specific diet; however, dietary interventions can limit and decrease the symptomatic impact in disorders where a biochemical and/or anatomical defect is present and well defined. A peptic stenosis in the esophagus or any subsequent gastrointestinal structure needs a liquid or very well-chewed diet, chronically; the diarrhea of chronic pancreatitis may ask for fat-reduced diet, and – certainly – coeliac disease does not like gluten; however, also after decennia of gluten-free diet, a coeliac will not be healed and can relapse at dietary failure!

Take the new kid on the block – FODMAPs – so well described in this volume: the patient has the choice: either to continue with wrong dietary habits or to diminish/abolish the symptoms with an adequate and not too difficult to keep diet.

Why do I mention all this? Haven't we enough dieticians to advise the patients? It might be, but in many cases a referral costs and also requires a new anamnesis by the dietician. It can also happen that the dietician would not recognize the entire pathogenesis and pathophysiology of the specific patient as well as the referring physician who has already obtained all relevant data.

I advise in this context what I have learned to practice myself: to identify the individual pathology and pathophysiology, to insert into the puzzle the present dietary habits of the patient and his social surroundings, and give a few relevant and clear – sometimes even strict – rules to the patient to be followed and thereafter to see the patient back after a medium-long pilot period. In this way, some referrals to a dietician might have become unnecessary and your own value has risen in the eyes of this patient.

Certainly, it is necessary that we are able to teach students and specialist fellows completely in this matter and that we also discuss such aspects seriously with family practitioners, who are asked by the same patients once more.

And Now the Italian FINALE: Can the Mediterranean Diet and the Mediterranean Wine Save the Mediterranean and Extra-Mediterranean Humanity?

Who will really know? Yes, there are some very suggestive data. But has there really been a valid, large, controlled study on this, putting into the accountancy all positive and negative confounding factors from environment, genetics, and other life modifiers? Wouldn't it be worthwhile to do these experiments (Italian food and wine industry could sponsor them) and to report the results at the opening of the next World Exhibition in Dubai, 2020? This would make people remember the beautiful event in Milan 2015 and might add power to specialists' knowledge and dietary advise.

Maastricht, The Netherlands; Ferrara, Italy   Reinhold Stockbrugger
March 3, 2016

Preface

Gastroenterology and the science of clinical nutrition share many pathophysiological and research interests. From this perspective, the idea of publishing a multiauthor text where both gastroenterologists and dietitians join together is not a surprise. What is new is the stimulus that has made all projects starting, i.e., the Universal Exposition held in Milan, Italy, in 2015 and devoted the theme of nutrition worldwide.

The theme of the 2015 Expo in Milan, "Feeding the Planet, Energy for Life," addresses a crucial issue for all countries of the world and has a double meaning: on the one hand, to try to ensure enough food to those who live in conditions of malnutrition and, on the other hand, to be able to prevent new large-scale illnesses of our time, including obesity and cardiovascular disease, valuing innovations and practices that allow a healthier life.

Will the bacteria become the key to success for a better quality of life? What is really the role of "microbiota" on human health? The view of human beings as a superorganism in which bacteria dominate is revolutionizing the medical knowledge by introducing new concepts of disease and also suggesting possible applications in veterinary and agriculture.

The lifestyles and critical events produce inheritable genetic modification. This is the fundamental of another emerging discipline, epigenetics, which is another real cultural revolution.

The nutraceuticals and their impact on health is another argument in rapid evolution. The targeted use of substances naturally present in foods, taken in forms similar to those commonly used for drugs, can improve the state of health and prevent chronic diseases. Italy is playing a leading role in this new scientific segment. Many of these substances are part of the Mediterranean diet.

The Mediterranean diet is more and more put under the lens to ascertain if it is really relevant and effective. Clarifying this aspect has been crucial for the 2015 Expo since Italy is the most important testimonial of this archetype, described for the free time in the Cilento area, south of Italy.

We can recover in the future a diet and a lifestyle that ensure everything you need at our livelihood in perfect balance with our gene developed by homo sapiens in the last 50,000 years?

Can we use this new science to prevent heart disease and cancer and prolong life far beyond what we ever thought possible? We believe the answer is a resounding yes as long as it recognizes a unique and essential role for specialists of food and nutrition both in the hospital setting for secondary prevention and in the land for primary prevention. Today the theme nutrition sees alternation professionals often do not fully qualified that apart from potential damage increase the confusion among end users. While the change of legislative policies can play an important role, people need more care, education, and appropriate tools to help them increase their personal responsibility for their health with regard to eating habits.

These and many other questions have been answered in scientific events organized by the Italian Pavilion in which gastroenterologists have played a substantial role.

Gastroenterologists should act more and more in front end of this new and exciting scenario to unify the opinions of different experts and give more certainty to the final stakeholders.

Milan, Italy   Enzo Grossi
Seriate (BG), Italy   Fabio Pace

Contents

Advances in the Comprehension of the Diet as a Magic Bullet to Prevent Cancer of the Gastrointestinal System

Franco Bazzoli and Stefano Rabitti

1.1 Introduction

Gastrointestinal cancers are among the most frequent cancers worldwide. According to Globocan [1], colon cancer is the third most commonly diagnosed cancer, after lung and breast cancer, and is fourth for mortality. Gastric cancer ranks fourth for incidence and second for mortality; its incidence seems to be declining [2]; however, even assuming that incidence rate will continue to decline by 2 % per annum, increased longevity and predicted growth in world population will contribute to keep gastric cancer at the top of the list of most frequent cancers [1]. Esophageal adenocarcinoma, although less prevalent than colon and gastric cancers, is characterized, in the recent decades, by a sharp increase in incidence, most likely connected with the increase of gastroesophageal reflux disease and related risk factors.

The role of diet and environmental and lifestyle factors have been proposed to reduce or increase the risk for gastrointestinal cancer [3–5].

This review will deal with some of the nutrients, foods, and dietary patterns which have been associated with either a decreased or increased risk of the most frequent cancers of the digestive tract.

1.2 Meat

Meat intake has been associated with several gastrointestinal cancers, as well as other non-gastrointestinal malignancies such as breast and prostate cancers.

Regarding the association between meat intake and esophageal cancer, an initial consensus report based on studies published up to 2004 stated that available evidence was

F. Bazzoli (✉) • S. Rabitti
Department of Medical and Surgical Sciences, S. Orsola-Malpighi Hospital, University of Bologna, 40138 Bologna, Italy
e-mail: franco.bazzoli@unibo.it

© Springer International Publishing Switzerland 2016   1
E. Grossi, F. Pace (eds.), *Human Nutrition from the Gastroenterologist's Perspective*,
DOI 10.1007/978-3-319-30361-1_1

suggestive but inconclusive for such an association [6]. In 2010, Kubo et al. in a careful review on dietary factors and the risk of esophageal adenocarcinoma and Barrett's esophagus, although confirming the presence of mixed results in the published literature, concluded that the evidence from cohort studies was in favor of an increased risk of developing esophageal adenocarcinoma associated with high meat intake, particularly red and processed meat [7]. In a more recent meta-analysis focusing on the consumption of red and processed meat and esophageal cancer risk, Choi et al. concluded that findings from both case-control studies and prospective cohort studies supported a positive association; results however were less strong for cohort studies [8].

In 2006 the European Prospective Investigation into Cancer and Nutrition (EPIC), a large cohort study, examined the risks of gastric cancer associated with meat consumption. Total, red, and processed meat intakes were associated with an increased risk of noncardia gastric cancer, but not with cardia gastric cancer [9]. Recently, Song et al. performed a meta-analysis of cohort and case-control studies to provide a quantitative assessment of the association of red meat consumption with the risk of gastric cancer. When stratified by study design, significant associations were observed in population-based case-control studies and hospital-based case-control studies; however, no association was observed among cohort studies. Authors concluded that increased intake of red meat might be a risk factor for stomach cancer, but further studies are needed to confirm this association [10].

According to the World Cancer Research Fund/American Institute for Cancer Research, there is convincing evidence that red meat and processed meat increase CRC risk [11]. Furthermore, Chan et al. have performed a meta-analysis of prospective studies evaluating the effect of red and processed meat on colorectal cancer incidence and conducted dose-response analyses. The risk of colorectal cancer was increased by the intake of total, red, and processed meat; there was about a 20 % higher risk per 100 g/day increase in red meat; the risk increases linearly up to 140 g/day of intake and then tends to level off. Associations were more pronounced for distal colon and rectosigmoid adenocarcinoma than other sites. Authors conclude that the provided strong evidence support the recommendation of limiting the consumption of red and processed meat for colorectal cancer prevention [12]. More recently, another meta-analysis provided similar results for colorectal adenomas [13].

Several factors may contribute to the increased risk for gastrointestinal cancers related to meat consumption. Meats cooked at high temperatures, either grilled or fried, for long duration are a source of mutagens such as heterocyclic amines and polycyclic aromatic hydrocarbons [7, 14]. Furthermore, heme iron in red meat can induce oxidative stress and colonocyte proliferation and is responsible for endogenous intestinal N-nitrosation [15, 16].

1.3   Sulfur

As recently reviewed in detail [5], inorganic sulfur contained in food preservatives or wine and sulfur-containing amino acids present in red meat and animal proteins are metabolized to hydrogen sulfide (H_2S) by intestinal bacteria. H_2S has been shown to be associated with factors promoting carcinogenesis such as DNA damage, epithelial hyperproliferation, and increased inflammation. Differently, other sources of sulfur, such as allyl sulfur contained in garlic and sulfur-containing glycosides present in cruciferous vegetables (cabbage, broccoli, etc.), have shown antineoplastic effects related to different protective mechanisms. Authors conclude that sulfur-containing foods may have opposite effects depending on the specific sulfur-containing compounds.

1.4   Salt

As stated by the World Cancer Research Fund/American Institute for Cancer Research, salt and salty foods can cause gastric cancer [17]. It is recognized already for several decades the hypothesis that salt could be involved in the etiology of gastric cancer. Gastric cancer mortality has been shown to correlate with salt excretion in urine in different populations from different geographical areas [18]. In a recent meta-analysis of prospective studies, dietary salt intake was directly associated with risk of gastric cancer in prospective population studies, with progressively increasing risk across consumption levels [19]. A number of possible mechanisms have been provided to explain the causal role of high-salt intake in gastric carcinogenesis. In the animal model, high dietary salt intake has been shown to exacerbate gastric carcinogenesis by inducing more severe gastric inflammation, higher gastric pH, increased parietal cell loss, and increased gastric expression of interleukin 1. All these effects however were present only in $cagA^+$ H. pylori-infected animals, suggesting that a high-salt diet potentates the carcinogenic effects of $cagA^+$ H. pylori infection [20]. In line with this and other observations, the Maastricht IV/Florence Consensus Report stated that "The influence of environmental factors, in particular dietary factors, is subordinate to the effect of H. pylori infection" (evidence level, 1a; grade of recommendation, A) [21].

1.5   Dietary Fibers

Several studies have addressed the issue of dietary fiber in the prevention of gastric cancer [22].

Dietary fiber may act as nitrite scavenger reducing the carcinogenic effects of N-nitrous compounds; furthermore, short-chain fatty acids produced by fermentation may have anticancer effects in the gastrointestinal tract [23]. The effect of dietary fiber in reducing the risk of gastric cancer has been evaluated in a recent meta-analysis. Authors showed that dietary fiber intake was inversely associated with gastric cancer risk. In particular, a 10/day increment in fiber intake was associated with a reduction in gastric cancer risk of 44 %, thus suggesting a potential role of increasing dietary fiber intake as primary prevention to the development of this disease [24].

Several decades ago it was proposed that dietary fiber intake could reduce the risk of colorectal cancer. This hypothesis was based on the observation of low rates of colorectal cancer in African populations on high fiber content diet [25].

To support this hypothesis, factors such as fermentation of fiber to short fatty acid, increased stool bulk, reduced transit time, and dilution of carcinogens in the intestinal lumen have been proposed.

However, in spite of the initial observational suggestions and plausible hypothesis, studies have not been able to provide strong evidence for this association.

In particular, while case-control studies supported a protective role of fiber, cohort studies provided conflicting results. A systematic review and meta-analysis of prospective studies have been recently performed to certify the association of dietary fiber and colorectal cancer risk.

Overall a high intake of dietary fiber was associated with a reduced risk of colorectal cancer; however, after subgrouping by different types of fiber, only cereal fiber maintained a significant protective effect, while no significant association was found with fruit, vegetables, or legume fiber [26].

1.6   Micronutrients, Antioxidants, and Vitamins

It is proven that many carcinogens cause DNA alteration by the production of reactive oxygen species. It is therefore plausible that supplementation with antioxidants as beta-carotene, vitamins C and E, selenium, methionine, and other micronutrients may have a protective role against cancer development.

In fact, several studies have been conducted on this topic, and an inverse association between gastrointestinal malignancies and serum levels of micronutrients and vitamins has been reported [27].

However, many micronutrients and vitamins are contained in foods and drinks so results can be easily confounded by diet and lifestyle. Moreover, most of the data we have come from studies conducted on Chinese population where the prevalence of nutritional deficiencies is high.

Finally, very few well-designed large-scale randomized controlled trials have been performed to date making the evidence on this topic quite poor.

This is underlined by the current guidelines that do not advise large-scale supplementation with vitamins and micronutrients as primary cancer prevention [28].

1.7   Fruit and Vegetables

The association between gastrointestinal malignancies and the consumption of fruit and vegetables has been largely proposed. In particular, a high intake of fruit and vegetables has been inversely associated with gastric and esophageal cancer [6]. In 2014, Li et al. in a meta-analysis of 12 observational studies showed a significant reduction of risk of esophageal adenocarcinoma with high intake of fruits and vegetables [29]. A similar study reported an inverse association between vegetable and fruit intake and squamous cell carcinoma of the esophagus [30]. Interestingly, a recent systematic review reported a statistically significant reduction of gastric cancer risk in association with high intake of fruit but not with high consumption of vegetables [31].

A role against the development of colorectal cancer has been also investigated. However epidemiological studies failed to demonstrate a strong association between vegetables and fruit intake and colorectal neoplasia. A recent meta-analysis of prospective studies found only a nonlinear association between fruit and vegetable intake and the incidence of colorectal cancer. A consumption of about 100 g/day of fruits and 100–200 g/day of vegetable showed the best results [32].

The protective effect of fruit and vegetables may be in relation to the large quantities of anticarcinogenic elements that are contained in these foods like minerals, flavonoids, antioxidants, and fibers as we mentioned before.

1.8 Alcohol

The International Agency for Research on Cancer (IARC) classified alcoholic beverages as class 1 carcinogens. It is estimated that chronic alcohol consumption is responsible for about 3.6 % of all cancers worldwide. Gastrointestinal malignancies, hepatocellular carcinoma, and breast cancer in females have been clearly associated with alcoholic beverages [33].

The development of esophageal squamous cell carcinoma has been strongly related to heavy alcohol consumption [34]. Conversely no significant association has been reported with esophageal adenocarcinoma [35] and gastric cancer [36].

In 2011, a meta-analysis showed a positive association between heavy drinking and colorectal cancer both in case-control and cohort studies [37].

Several experimental studies demonstrate the role of alcohol in provoking cancer in animals [38, 39].

A recent review focused on the molecular mechanism of alcohol-related carcinogenesis showing multiple ways in which alcohol may lead to cancer development.

Acetaldehyde is the first product of alcohol metabolism and is considered a carcinogenic agent that can lead to DNA mutation interfering with DNA repair and methylation proteins.

Furthermore, the ethanol oxidation is responsible for the generation of reactive oxygen species that lead to the increase of oxidative stress but also to the reduction of retinoic acid that has a fundamental role in cell differentiation and growth [40]. As the correlation between alcohol toxic effects and cancer development seems to be a dose-dependent response, it is useful to define the safe amount of alcohol intake per day. European guidelines recommend not to exceed a daily alcohol consumption of 20–30 g in men and 10–15 g in women [41]. Similar indications are provided by the American Departments of Agriculture and Health and Human Services [42].

1.9 Vitamin D

Vitamin D is a lipid-soluble prohormone synthesized by the skin exposed to ultraviolet light. It is also present in little amount in most of foods.

The principal role of vitamin D is to regulate the metabolism of calcium and phosphate being essential for bone mineralization.

In the last decades, large attention has been focused on the potential extra-skeletal effects of this vitamin because of its thought anti-inflammatory and immune-mediatory effect.

The association between gastrointestinal malignancies and vitamin D has been investigated in several studies with mixed results.

In 2007, Chen et al. reported an association between serum 25(OH)-vitamin D concentration and risk of esophageal cancer, but no association with gastric cancer was found [43].

A recent case-control study evaluated the correlation between vitamin D and colorectal cancer according to tumor immunity status. Results showed that high serum levels of 25(OH)-vitamin D were associated with lower risk of colorectal cancer with high count of lymphocytes suggesting a possible role of this hormone in cancer immune prevention [44]. Despite these good results, several RCTs failed to demonstrate a beneficial effect of vitamin D supplementation in reduction of cancer incidence [45, 46].

The potential protective effect of vitamin D against cancers and in particular gastrointestinal malignancies is linked to biologic plausibility and supported by epidemiological studies; anyway literature showed mixed results.

We hope that more data will be provided by a large ongoing study evaluating the effect of vitamin D and omega-3 supplementation on colorectal cancer incidence [47].

1.10   Calcium and Dairy Products

Calcium is a mineral essential for healthy bones and teeth. A possible beneficial effect of calcium on carcinogenesis may be related to several mechanisms as the inhibition of cell proliferation and the promotion of cell differentiation and apoptosis or the reduction of oxidative stress and DNA damage [48].

A pooled analysis of ten cohort studies showed a 10–15 % reduction in incidence of colorectal cancer in association with high intake of calcium [49].

Furthermore calcium supplementation resulted to be effective in decreasing polyp recurrence [50].

However, some small trials and a large RCT did not find any significant reduction of incidence in CRC after a mean of 7 years of supplementation with calcium and vitamin D [45].

In consideration of the high content of calcium and other micronutrients, dairy products have been investigated as protective factors against gastrointestinal tumors.

However, studies reported conflicting results.

A recent meta-analysis reported a protective role of milk in the reduction of CRC risk with a consumption of at least 200 g per day. Best results were associated with an intake of 500–800 per day [51]. Unfortunately, these results were not confirmed in other epidemiological studies [52].

It has been proposed that the anticarcinogenic activity of dairy products may be associated to calcium-related and calcium-unrelated factors.

Conjugated linoleic acid, butyric acid, and SCFA have been investigated as calcium-unrelated factors, and good results emerged from animal models [53].

In summary, milk consumption may have a protective role against the development of colorectal cancer; meanwhile, even if some evidence suggests that a calcium intake lower than 700/1,000 mg per day increases CRC risk, data remains inconsistent, and routinely calcium supplementation is not advisable in primary cancer prevention.

1.11   Dietary Patterns

In the last decades, growing interest has been addressed to the possible relationship between dietary patterns and cancer development.

Dietary patterns represent a complex integration of nutrients and food in a certain population better reflecting real everyday life. People do not eat nutrients, people do eat meals.

Furthermore, interesting data showed that dietary patterns, rather than specific nutrients or foods, may demonstrate stronger association with chronic disease and cancer [54].

Two main dietary patterns have been identified: the Western pattern composed by unhealthy foods (red and processed meat, high-fat dairy foods, starchy foods and sweets, refined grains) and the prudent pattern characterized mainly by high consumption of fruits and vegetables, fish, poultry, and whole-grain products.

Several studies evaluated the association between dietary patterns and gastrointestinal cancer risk.

In 2014, Liu et al. performed a systematic review and meta-analysis showing that a healthy pattern based on high intake of fruit and vegetables was associated with a significantly decreased risk of esophageal squamous cell carcinoma. Conversely, drinker/alcohol pattern was significantly associated with an increased risk. No association was found between Western pattern and esophageal squamous cell carcinoma [55].

A large multicenter, European, prospective study conducted on 485,000 subjects reported that Mediterranean diet based on high consumption of fruit, vegetables, olive oil, fish and seafood, legumes, nuts, and seed and low presence of red and processed meat and dairy products with a moderate intake of alcohol (red wine) was protective against the development of gastric cancer [56].

It is known that many lifestyle factors (diet, alcohol consumption, smoke, and weight) are independently associated with gastric cancer.

Starting from this consideration, recently, a lifestyle score, the "healthy lifestyle index," based on healthy behavior related to smoking status, alcohol consumption, Mediterranean diet quality, and body mass index, has been proposed with the aim of analyzing the overlapping risk factors.

The EPIC cohort study performed on 461,550 participants followed up for a mean of 11.4 years showed that about 18 % of all gastric cancers and 62 % of cardia gastric cancer cases could have been prevented if participants had followed healthy lifestyle behaviors [57].

The correlation between dietary patterns and colorectal cancer has been also investigated.

Vegetarian dietary pattern and especially pesco-vegetarian diet were associated with an overall lower incidence of colorectal cancer; meanwhile a higher risk of recurrence and mortality among patients with stage III colon cancer treated with surgery and adjuvant chemotherapy was found in association with Western/unhealthy dietary pattern [58].

Finally, dietary pattern was also analyzed during adolescence.

Interesting results showed that, independently of adult dietary pattern, prudent pattern during adolescence was associated with lower risk of rectal adenomas, whereas a Western pattern was associated with higher risk [59].

1.12 Obesity

Obesity and waist circumference have been correlated with gastrointestinal malignancies. Hyperlipidemia and insulin resistance together with the production of adipokines could lead to a pro-inflammatory condition that stimulates tumor cell growth and neo-angiogenesis and reduces apoptosis [60].

This is confirmed by an analysis evaluating the correlation between body mass index and incidence of all cancers worldwide.

A significant association between increased BMI and gastrointestinal tumors was found especially in men with esophageal adenocarcinoma and colorectal cancer [61].

Conclusion

In conclusion, several evidences show a strong association between gastrointestinal cancers and red and processed meat, salt and salty foods, and heavy alcohol consumption. Western/unhealthy dietary patterns have been related to increased risk of gastrointestinal cancers, while a protective role has been observed for prudent/healthy dietary pattern such as the so-called Mediterranean diet.

Obesity is a crucial risk factor for esophageal adenocarcinoma and colorectal cancer.

Better understanding of the effects of different dietary patterns on disease outcomes may help to provide the public with suggestions for wise eating habits.

References

1. Ferlay J, Soerjomataram I, Ervik M, Dikshit R, Eser S, Mathers C, Rebelo M, Parkin DM, Forman D, Bray F (2013) GLOBOCAN 2012 v1.0. Cancer Incidence and Mortality Worldwide: IARC CancerBase No. 11 [Internet]. International Agency for Research on Cancer, Lyon. http://globocan.iarc.fr
2. IARC Helicobacter pylori Working Group (2014) Helicobacter pylori eradication as a strategy for preventing gastric cancer. International Agency for Research on Cancer (IARC Working Group Reports, No. 8), Lyon. Available from: http://www.iarc.fr/en/publications/pdfsonline/wrk/wrk8/index.php

3. Center MM, Jemal A, Smith RA, Ward E (2009) Worldwide variations in colorectal cancer. CA Cancer J Clin 59(6):366–378
4. Abnet CC, Corley DA, Freedman ND, Kamangar F (2015) Diet and upper gastrointestinal malignancies. Gastroenterology 148(6):1234–1243
5. Song M, Garrett WS, Chan AT (2015) Nutrients, foods, and colorectal cancer prevention. Gastroenterology 148(6):1244–1260
6. World Cancer Research Fund/American Institute for Cancer Research (2007) Food, nutrition, physical activity, and the prevention of cancer: a global perspective. AICR, Washington, DC
7. Kubo A, Corley AD, Jensen CD, Kaur R (2010) Dietary factors and the risks of Esophageal adenocarcinoma and Barrett's esophagus. Nutr Res Rev 23(2):230–246
8. Choi Y, Song S, Song Y, Leet JE (2013) Consumption of red and processed meat and esophageal cancer risk: meta-analysis. World J Gastroenterol 19(7):1020–1029
9. González CA, Jakszyn P, Pera G et al (2006) Meat intake and risk of stomach and esophageal adenocarcinoma within the European Prospective Investigation Into Cancer and Nutrition (EPIC). J Natl Cancer Inst 98(5):345–354
10. Song P, Lu M, Yin Q et al (2014) Red meat consumption and stomach cancer risk: a meta-analysis. J Cancer Res Clin Oncol 140(6):979–992
11. World Cancer Research Fund/American Institute for Cancer Research (2011) Continuous update project: keeping the science current. Report: food, nutrition, physical activity, and the prevention of colorectal cancer. Colorectal Cancer. http://www.dietandcancerreport.org/cancer_resource_center/downloads/cu/Colorectal-Cancer-2011-Report.pdf
12. Chan DS, Lau R, Aune D et al (2011) Red and processed meat and colorectal cancer incidence: meta-analysis of prospective studies. PLoS One 6(6):e20456
13. Xu X, Yu E, Gao X et al (2013) Red and processed meat intake and risk of colorectal adenomas: a meta-analysis of observational studies. Int J Cancer 132:437–448
14. Zheng W, Lee SA (2009) Well-done meat intake, heterocyclic amine exposure, and cancer risk. Nutr Cancer 61(4):437–446
15. Cross AJ, Pollock JRA, Bingham SA (2003) Haem, not protein or inorganic iron, is responsible for endogenous intestinal N-nitrosation arising from red meat. Cancer Res 63:2358–2360
16. Bastide NM, Chenni F, Audebert M et al (2015) A central role for heme iron in colon carcinogenesis associated with red meat intake. Cancer Res 75(5):870–879
17. Wiseman M (2008) The second World Cancer Research Fund/American Institute for Cancer Research expert report. Food, nutrition, physical activity, and the prevention of cancer: a global perspective. Proc Nutr Soc 67:253–256
18. Joossens JV, Hill MJ, Elliott P et al (1996) Dietary salt, nitrate and stomach cancer mortality in 24 countries. European Cancer Prevention (ECP) and the INTERSALT Cooperative Research Group. Int J Epidemiol 25:494–504
19. D'Elia L, Rossi G, Ippolito R et al (2012) Habitual salt intake and risk of gastric cancer: a meta-analysis of prospective studies. Clin Nutr 31:489–498
20. Gaddy JA, Radin JN, Loh JT et al (2013) High dietary salt intake exacerbates Helicobacter pylori-induced gastric carcinogenesis. Infect Immun 81:2258–2267
21. Malfertheiner P, Megraud F, O'Morain CA et al (2012) Management of Helicobacter pylori infection the Maastricht IV/Florence Consensus Report. Gut 61:646–664
22. Gonzalez CA, Riboli E (2010) Diet and cancer prevention: contributions from the European Prospective Investigation into Cancer and Nutrition (EPIC) study. Eur J Cancer 46:2555–2562
23. Augenlicht LH, Anthony GM, Church TL et al (1999) Short-chain fatty acid metabolism, apoptosis, and Apc-initiated tumorigenesis in the mouse gastrointestinal mucosa. Cancer Res 59(23):6005–6009
24. Zhang Z, Xu G, Ma M, Yang J, Xinfeng Y (2013) Dietary fiber intake reduces risk for gastric cancer: a meta-analysis. Gastroenterology 145:113–120
25. Burkitt DP (1971) Epidemiology of cancer of the colon and rectum. Cancer 28:3–13
26. Aune D, Lau R, Vieira R et al (2011) Dietary fibre, whole grains, and risk of colorectal cancer: systematic review and dose-response meta-analysis of prospective studies. BMJ 343:d6617

27. Taylor PR, Qiao YL, Abnet CC et al (2003) Prospective study of serum vitamin E levels and esophageal and gastric cancers. J Natl Cancer Inst 95:1414–1416
28. Moyer VA (2014) Vitamin, mineral, and multivitamin supplements for the primary prevention of cardiovascular disease and cancer: U.S. preventive services task force recommendation statement. Ann Intern Med 160:558–564
29. Li B, Jiang G, Zhang G et al (2014) Intake of vegetables and fruit and risk of esophageal adenocarcinoma: a meta-analysis of observational studies. Eur J Nutr 53:1511–1521
30. Navarro Silvera SA, Mayne ST, Risch H et al (2008) Food group intake and risk of subtypes of esophageal and gastric cancer. Int J Cancer 123:852–860
31. Wang Q, Chen Y, Wang X et al (2014) Consumption of fruit, but not vegetables, may reduce risk of gastric cancer: results from a meta-analysis of cohort studies. Eur J Cancer 50:1498–1509
32. Aune D, Lau R, Chan DS et al (2011) Nonlinear reduction in risk for colorectal cancer by fruit and vegetable intake based on meta-analysis of prospective studies. Gastroenterology 141:106–118
33. Rehm J et al (2004) In: Ezzati M, Murray C, Lopez AD, Rodgers A (eds) Comparative quantification of health risks: global and regional burden of disease attributable to selected major risk factors. World Health Organization, Geneva, pp 959–1108
34. Engel LS, Chow WH, Vaughan TL et al (2003) Population attributable risks of esophageal and gastric cancers. J Natl Cancer Inst 95:1404–1413
35. Freedman ND, Murray LJ, Kamangar F et al (2011) Alcohol intake and risk of oesophageal adenocarcinoma: a pooled analysis from the BEACON Consortium. Gut 60:1029–1037
36. Freedman ND, Abnet CC, Leitzmann MF et al (2007) A prospective study of tobacco, alcohol, and the risk of esophageal and gastric cancer subtypes. Am J Epidemiol 165:1424–1433
37. Fedirko V, Tramacere I, Bagnardi V et al (2011) Alcohol drinking and colorectal cancer risk: an overall and dose-response meta-analysis of published studies. Ann Oncol 22(9):1958–1972
38. Beland FA et al (2005) Effect of ethanol on the tumorigenicity of urethane (ethyl carbamate) in B6C3F mice. Food Chem Toxicol 43:1–19
39. Baan R et al (2007) Carcinogenicity of alcoholic beverages. Lancet Oncol 8:292–293. Most recent and precise summary of the IARC Working Group on Alcohol and Cancer
40. Seitz HK, Stickel F (2007) Molecular mechanisms of alcohol mediated carcinogenesis. Nat Rev Cancer 7(8):599–612
41. Boyle P et al (2003) European code against cancer and scientific justification: third version. Ann Oncol 14:973–1005
42. International Center for Alcohol Policies. International Drinking Guidelines (2007) ICAP [online]. http://www.icap.org/PolicyIssues/DrinkingGuidelines/GuidelinesTable/tabid/204/Default.aspx
43. Chen W, Dawsey SM, Qiao YL et al (2007) Prospective study of serum 25(OH)-vitamin D concentration and risk of oesophageal and gastric cancers. Br J Cancer 97:123–128
44. Song M, Nishihara R, Wang M, Chan AT (2006) Plasma 25-hydroxyvitamin D and colorectal cancer risk according to tumour immunity status. Gut 65(2):296–304
45. Wactawski-Wende J, Kotchen JM, Anderson GL et al (2006) Calcium plus vitamin D supplementation and the risk of colorectal cancer. N Engl J Med 354:684–696
46. Avenell A, MacLennan GS, Jenkinson DJ et al (2012) Long-term follow-up for mortality and cancer in a randomized placebo-controlled trial of vitamin D(3) and/or calcium (RECORD trial). J Clin Endocrinol Metab 97:614–622
47. Manson JE, Bassuk SS, Lee IM et al (2012) The VITamin D and OmegA-3 TriaL (VITAL): rationale and design of a large randomized controlled trial of vitamin D and marine omega-3 fatty acid supplements for the primary prevention of cancer and cardiovascular disease. Contemp Clin Trials 33:159–171
48. Lamprecht SA, Lipkin M (2001) Cellular mechanisms of calcium and vitamin D in the inhibition of colorectal carcinogenesis. Ann N Y Acad Sci 952:73–87

49. Cho E, Smith-Warner SA, Spiegelman D et al (2004) Dairy foods, calcium, and colorectal cancer: a pooled analysis of 10 cohort studies. J Natl Cancer Inst 96:1015–1022
50. Bonithon-Kopp C, Kronborg O, Giacosa A et al (2000) Calcium and fibre supplementation in prevention of colorectal adenoma recurrence: a randomised intervention trial. European Cancer Prevention Organisation Study Group. Lancet 356:1300–1306
51. Aune D, Lau R, Chan DS et al (2012) Dairy products and colorectal cancer risk: a systematic review and meta-analysis of cohort studies. Ann Oncol 23:37–45
52. McCullough ML, Robertson AS, Rodriguez C et al (2003) Calcium, vitamin D, dairy products, and risk of colorectal cancer in the cancer prevention study II nutrition cohort (United States). Cancer Causes Control 14:1–12
53. Evans NP, Misyak SA, Schmelz EM et al (2010) Conjugated linoleic acid ameliorates inflammation-induced colorectal cancer in mice through activation of PPARgamma. J Nutr 140:515–521
54. Hu F (2002) Dietary pattern analysis: a new direction in nutritional epidemiology. Curr Opin Lipidol 13(1):3–9
55. Liu X, Wang X, Lin S, Yuan J, Yu IT (2014) Dietary patterns and oesophageal squamous cell carcinoma: a systematic review and meta-analysis. Br J Cancer 110(11):2785–2795
56. Buckland G et al (2010) Adherence to a Mediterranean diet and risk of gastric adenocarcinoma within the European Prospective Investigation into Cancer and Nutrition (EPIC) cohort study 1–3. Am J Clin Nutr 91:381–390
57. Buckland G, Travier N, Huerta JM (2015) Healthy lifestyle index and risk of gastric adenocarcinoma in the EPIC cohort study. Int J Cancer 137:598–606
58. Orlich MJ, Fraser GE (2015) Diet and colorectal cancer incidence-reply. JAMA Intern Med 175(10):1727
59. Nimptsch K, Malik VS, Fung TT, Pischon T (2014) Dietary patterns during high school and risk of colorectal adenoma in a cohort of middle-aged women. Int J Cancer 134(10):2458–2467
60. Alemán JO, Eusebi LH, Ricciardiello L (2014) Mechanisms of obesity-induced gastrointestinal neoplasia. Gastroenterology 146(2):357–373
61. Renehan AG, Tyson M, Egger M, Heller RF, Zwahlen M (2008) Body-mass index and incidence of cancer: a systematic review and meta-analysis of prospective observational studies. Lancet 371(9612):569–578

How a Gastroenterologist Interprets the Mediterranean Diet

Gioacchino Leandro, A. Giliberti, A.M. Cisternino, R. Inguaggiato, R. Reddavide, and M.G. Caruso

2.1 Origins and Definition of the Mediterranean Diet

Mediterranean diet has become a popular expression that is widely used by expert and lay people, even though actually not always appropriately.

The Mediterranean diet is not a vegetarian diet, although plant foods have their relevance; not the diet of bread and pasta, even if the consumption of cereals represents an important component; not a diet of "poor nutrients" but rather a genuine diet based on the so-called functional foods; not the grandmother's soup, since it is also a rich culinary heritage of recipes, smells, and tastes; not a trendy diet, because of its historical roots and evidence-based benefits; and not the diet that allows one to lose or gain weight as it relates to food's quality and not to its energy content.

The traditional Mediterranean diet is the diet consumed by the people living in the Mediterranean area in the 1950s and 1960s, immediately after World War II. Rather than being simply a way of eating, it is a body of knowledge, social customs and cultural traditions historically handed down by populations bordering the *Mare Nostrum*. Then, more than a restrictive or limiting regime, we should define it as a "lifestyle" whose importance has been recognized worldwide by UNESCO, which in November 2010 recognized the Mediterranean diet as "intangible heritage

G. Leandro (✉)
Department of Gastroenterology, Scientific Institute for Digestive Disease "Saverio de Bellis" Hospital, Via Turi 27, Castellana Grotte, Bari 70013, Italy

Department of Liver and Digestive Health, University College of London, London, UK

AIGO, Italian Association of Hospital Gastroenterologists and Endoscopists, Milan, Italy
e-mail: gioacchino.leandro@irccsdebellis.it

A. Giliberti • A.M. Cisternino • R. Inguaggiato • R. Reddavide • M.G. Caruso
Department of Gastroenterology, Scientific Institute for Digestive Disease "Saverio de Bellis" Hospital, Via Turi 27, Castellana Grotte, Bari 70013, Italy

© Springer International Publishing Switzerland 2016
E. Grossi, F. Pace (eds.), *Human Nutrition from the Gastroenterologist's Perspective*,
DOI 10.1007/978-3-319-30361-1_2

of humanity." The decision is based on the recognition that "this simple and frugal way to have meals favored over time intercultural contacts and conviviality, creating a formidable corpus of knowledge, social customs and traditional celebrations of many populations of the Mediterranean."

A single definition of the Mediterranean diet is not easy because of the coexistence of many countries, different cultural backgrounds, ethnic and religious roots, social and economic status, as well as agricultural productions involving different food choices in the area. In other words, there is no single "Mediterranean diet," but a common "Mediterranean dietary pattern" characterized by the following main features [1, 2]:

- High intake of plant foods (vegetables, fresh and dried fruits, legumes, bread and pasta from not reconstituted whole-wheat flour, and other cereals such as barley, spelt, and oats which assure both a low glycemic index and a stabilizing and filling role).
- Main consumption of fresh and seasonal products, mostly locally produced.
- The use of olive oil as the main source of dietary fat.
- Moderate intake of fish, poultry, and free-range eggs, eaten few times a week.
- Daily but moderate consumption of cheese and yogurt produced with milk from grazing animals, rich in omega-3 fatty acids and antioxidant vitamins.
- Low intake of red and processed meats which were eaten only on Sundays in the wealthiest families and occasionally in the less affluent families.
- Regular use of aromatic herbs determining good taste and palatability and reducing the excessive use of salt and fat ingredients.
- Wine in moderation, consumed with meals.
- Low intake of sweets, which were prepared only during family and religious celebrations.

The nutrients contained in foods are therefore:

- Few proteins, mainly of vegetable origin.
- Carbohydrates with low glycemic index and glycemic load and simple sugars almost absent.
- High monounsaturated-to-saturated fatty acid ratio.
- Much greater amount and ratio between omega-3 and omega-6 than in our current alimentation which is close to 1:1.
- Abundant use of beta-carotene, tocopherols, and vitamin C.
- High polyphenols (which make the Mediterranean diet as a *functional diet*).
- High calcium, magnesium, and potassium.
- Low sodium.

The Mediterranean diet is also a predominantly "raw food" diet: almost all dishes are cooked at low temperatures for a long time, while many foods and seasonings, in particular olive oil, are added raw to dishes, becoming also a diet low in AGEs (advanced glycation end products) [3]. An extensive literature indicates that AGEs are dangerous molecules for our organism because their effects, being related to inflammation and aging, are involved in the pathogenesis of many degenerative diseases [4]. AGEs are the products of the later stages of the nonenzymatic glycation of proteins. This phenomenon occurs in the organism as well as in foods subjected to special physicochemical treatments (e.g., high temperatures and low humidity). Then, the total amount of AGEs has both an endogenous and a dietary origin that contributes to the progressive accumulation of AGEs in tissues. Almost all food produced through industrial processes are very rich in AGEs not only for the high temperature but also for the manufacturing methodologies used, capable of altering the chemical nature of the substances involved. Even in the home environment, it is possible to treat foods so that they contain a greater or lesser amount of glycation products: scorching, roasting, or toasting leads to the production of AGEs.

2.2   The Origins of Research

The authorship of the research on the Mediterranean diet can be attributed to the nutritionist Lorenzo Piroddi (1911–1999), who in 1939 suggested the connection between diet and onset of metabolic diseases. To treat his patients, Piroddi developed a first version of the Mediterranean diet, limiting the consumption of animal fats in favor of vegetable fats.

Nevertheless the first researcher who brought the concept of the "Mediterranean diet" to the attention of the scientific world was Ancel Keys (1904–2004), expert in epidemiology and nutritionist at the School of Public Health, University of Minnesota, who coincidentally realized the health benefits of this food style during World War II.

In the 1940s, Keys was in Crete in the wake of the allied troops and noted that the incidence of cardiovascular diseases in that island was considerably lower than in the United States. In 1944, landed at Paestum in the wake of the Fifth Army, he was struck by the eating habits of the population living in the Cilento region and developed the intuition that the low incidence of cardiovascular diseases in the two populations was due to the food type that they adopted for secular tradition. He was so convinced of the goodness of the dietary traditions and way of life of southern Italy and other Mediterranean countries that he moved with his family to Pioppi, a small town of the Cilento region.

During his stay he observed that the usual food of the farmers living in the small countries of southern Italy was low in fats of animal origin (as they rarely ate meat, unlike rich people that consumed it almost every day) and rich mainly of bread, different types of pasta often consumed with vegetables, legumes used for soups, seasonal fruits and vegetables available in their gardens, extra virgin olive oil, and often also cheese and dried fruit when available, integrated with wine. Food choices were dictated by poverty, frugality, and parsimony, but the farmers from Cilento and Crete lived longer and had a low prevalence of cardiovascular diseases compared to the citizens of northern Europe and the United States and even their own relatives emigrated in previous years, despite the high consumption of olive oil (vegetable fats) giving not less than 40 % of total daily energy.

These observations led Keys to start the famous "Seven Countries Study," an epidemiological study involving the following seven countries: Finland, Japan, Greece, Italy, the Netherlands, the United States, and Yugoslavia. The survey compared lifestyle and diets adopted by the different populations, and Italy was represented by the small towns of Nicotera (Calabria), Crevalcore (Emilia), Montegiorgio (Marche), and Pioppi (Cilento) [5]. The results confirmed the relationship between diet and incidence of some diseases, clarifying in particular that the type and not the quantity of fat used had a major influence on cardiovascular diseases. Among the populations of the Mediterranean area, the mortality rate from ischemic heart disease was much lower than in countries such as Finland and the United States where the daily diet included a lot of saturated animal fats (butter, lard, milk, cheese, red meat).

The conclusion of this research led Ancel Keys to define the Mediterranean diet as the best "*life style*" allowing a better and longer life and making it popular worldwide.

In his 1975 book *How to Eat Well and Stay Well the Mediterranean Way* and more recently in a presentation at the first Congress on the Mediterranean Diet held in Boston in 1993, under the patronage of two famous devotees of the Mediterranean diet, Dimitrios Trichopoulos and his wife Antonia Trichopoulou, Ancel Keys described the Mediterranean diet as follows [6]:

> "The heart of what we now consider the Mediterranean diet is mainly vegetarian: pasta in many forms, leaves sprinkled with olive oil, all kinds of vegetables in season, and often cheese, all finished off with fruit, and frequently washed down with wine. No main meal in the Mediterranean countries is replete without lots of verdure (greens). Mangiafoglia is the Italian word for "to eat leaves" and that is a key part of the good Mediterranean diet. In fact, the best Mediterranean we associate with health is almost vegetarian (or lactovegetarian) because cheese is and always has been a part of this diet."

The Mediterranean diet is quantitatively defined in different ways, especially through the techniques of the food pyramid and the Mediterranean adequacy indexes.

The most representative food pyramids of the Mediterranean diet are the American pyramid [7], developed by Walter Willett at the Harvard Medical School of Public Health in collaboration with Oldways, and the Greek pyramid influenced by the leadership of Antonia Trichopoulou and her husband Dimitrios, respectively, professor in Athens and professor of epidemiology at Harvard.

The Harvard pyramid recommends:

- Daily: derivatives of whole grains, vegetables, legumes, fruits, nuts, olive oil, cheese, and yogurt.
- Weekly: fish, eggs, poultry, and sweets.
- Monthly: red meat.
- Wine in moderation with meals and plenty of water.
- Daily physical activity.

This pyramid was built from the data and research available at that time on nutrition and food traditions and based on the Cretan, Greek, and Italian food traditions, populations in which the rate of chronic diseases recorded in the 1960s was the lowest in the world.

The Greek pyramid recommends the same feeding even though legumes and nuts are not provided daily but weekly.

In January 2003, Walter C. Willett and Meir J. Stampfer, professors of epidemiology and nutrition at the Harvard School of Public Health, reviewed the American food pyramid and introduced a food guide incorporating improvements designed to address many of the problems in the old pyramid [8].

They adopted an innovative approach related to the consumption of fat presumably derived from the information collected by the authors who coordinated from many years three large epidemiological cohort studies – the Nurses' Health Study, the Health Professionals Follow-Up Study, and the Physicians' Health Study – which provided a huge amount of information to evaluate the association between specific nutritional aspects and risk factors for cardiovascular events.

Willett and Stampfer sustained that total fat intake alone was not associated with heart disease risk, asserting that unsaturated fats have positive health benefits, whereas *trans* and saturated fats have opposite effects.

In particular, the Nurses' Health Study, characterized by the higher follow-up period, showed that an increased consumption of monounsaturated fatty acids, and especially polyunsaturated fats, was inversely associated with coronary heart disease risk [9]. In fact, the quintile of the population with the higher consumption of polyunsaturated fats had a risk of cardiovascular events reduced by 25 % compared to the quintile of the population with the lowest intake of the same fatty acids (RR, 0.75; 95 % confidence interval (CI), 0.60–0.92; p (trend) 0.004). On the other hand, *trans* fat intake was associated with an elevated risk of coronary heart disease (RR, 1.33; 95 % CI, 1.07–1.66; p (trend) 0.01).

Their pyramid thus recommended to include generous servings of unsaturated fats, including liquid vegetable oils, especially olive and fish oils. On the other hand, saturated fats, as butter, were maintained at the top, while *trans* fats, as margarines, did not appear at all in the pyramid, because they have no place in a healthy diet. Margarines are produced converting vegetable oils from liquids to solids by the hydrogenation reaction. During the hydrogenation process, the fatty acid structure undergoes to a geometric molecular conversion from *cis* configuration to *trans* configuration which modifies the functions and metabolism within the human body [10].

Compared to saturated fatty acids or to liquid *cis*-unsaturated fats, consumption of *trans* fats has shown to increase even more the risk of coronary heart disease, in part by raising levels of low-density lipoproteins (LDLs, the so-called "bad cholesterol"), lowering levels of high-density lipoproteins (HDLs, "good cholesterol"), increasing triglycerides in the bloodstream, and promoting systemic inflammation. Therefore, replacing lipids from animals with margarines should not be considered a correct food choice.

Willett and Stampfer also moved refined carbohydrates as white rice, white bread, white pasta, and potatoes from the base of the pyramid up to the top with a "use sparingly" recommendation. On the other hand, they still recommended eating daily healthy carbohydrates at meals in the form of whole-grain foods, such as whole-wheat bread, oatmeal, and brown rice. The difference between whole and refined grains seems to be related to their different glycemic indexes which measure how fast and how much a food raises blood glucose levels. In fact, evidence from the Nurses' Health cohort suggested that the preferential consumption of foods with a low glycemic index is associated with a better cardiovascular prevention. Low glycemic index foods are associated to higher levels of antiatherogenic HDL cholesterol and lower plasma inflammatory markers and plasma triglyceride levels [11].

More recently, Mediterranean scientific experts and international research institutions developed the new food pyramid for the Mediterranean diet during the Third International Conference of CIISCAM (University Centre for International Studies on Mediterranean Food Cultures), held in Parma in 2009 [12]. The new pyramid, based upon the latest research in the field of nutrition and health promotion, is addressed to a healthy adult population and considers the nutritional, economic, and sociocultural changes occurred in the Mediterranean region.

To acquire all the benefits from the Mediterranean diet, the new pyramid incorporates lifestyle and cultural elements, including:

1. Physical activity: regular physical activity offers many health benefits as the balance on energy intake and healthy body weight maintenance (peasants and workers of the last decades worked manually all day long and moved mostly on foot or using nonmotorized forms of transportation).
2. Socialization: beyond nutritional aspects, the conviviality is important for the social and cultural value of the meal. Cooking and sitting around the table and sharing food with family and friends offer a sense of community.
3. Sustainability: experts suggest to prefer the consumption of seasonal and local foods promoting the short food chain and the local agriculture.

The new pyramid follows the previous pattern of foods that should sustain the diet at the base and foods to be eaten in moderate amounts or left for special occasions at the upper levels. The proportion and frequency consumption of each food group are fundamental for defining a diet as healthy or harmful. The pyramid establishes dietary daily, weekly, and occasional guidelines aimed at following a healthy and balanced diet. At every meal, a healthy adult would need to consume cereals, fruits, and vegetables (finally suggested in greater quantities than fruits) paying close attention to vary colors and textures in order to obtain the right intake of antioxidants which protect the body against free radical damage.

A daily supply of water including 1.5–2.0 l to ensure a proper hydration and to maintain a good balance of body water is strongly suggested. The new pyramid also reports two important indications: frugality, which should inspire the quantitative amount of servings, and moderation in the consumption of wine, respecting religious and social beliefs. The Mediterranean diet appears revisited in a modern key without neglecting the different cultural and religious traditions and the different national identities.

2.3   Healthy Foods from the Mediterranean Diet

Each food has beneficial effects on health when its consumption is qualitatively and quantitatively appropriate to satisfy the energetic and nutritional needs of the organism. It is to be highlighted that all meals, including breakfast, lunch, dinner, and snacks, should be balanced and contain all the nutrients we need, a goal that can be reached easily with a diet as varied as possible.

As stated, the Mediterranean diet is based on dishes where the protagonists are the following Mediterranean foodstuffs: olive oil, whole grains, fresh fruits, vegetables, fish, legumes, moderate amounts of dairy products and meat, and red wine.

2.3.1   Olive Oil

The olive oil, heart of the Mediterranean diet, is rich in monounsaturated fatty acids, in particular oleic acid (70–86 %), becoming one of the best condiments to keep under control the serum concentrations of very low-density lipoprotein rich in LDL cholesterol that tends to remain in the blood and to deposit in the arteries' walls. Furthermore, the relatively high concentration of oleic acid in the phospholipids of cell membranes makes the cell less susceptible to oxidation, reducing the formation of pro-inflammatory molecules.

In 2011, the European Food Safety Authority recommended the daily ingestion of olive oil rich in phenolic compounds, such as virgin olive oil [13]. Some of these compounds, in particular flavonoids and secoiridoid, showed significant effects in the prevention of chronic diseases such as cardiovascular diseases, certain types of cancer, premature aging, and degenerative diseases of the central nervous system, explaining the health benefits of virgin olive oil in addition to the oleic acid content. Olive oil is not only important for its intrinsic properties but also because it replaces other fats used in the extra-Mediterranean kitchen, such as those of animal origin (lard or butter) or from vegetable oils of lower quality. However, it is noteworthy that it still remains a fat and that all fats, irrespective of other nutritional characteristics, have the same caloric intake.

2.3.2   Cereals

Cereals are a vital element of the Mediterranean diet and occupy the base of the food pyramid together with vegetables and fruit. Cereals include corn, barley, rice, wheat (soft and hard wheat), and spelt. They are an important source of food energy provided as starch, a polysaccharide which yields glucose after digestive process. They are also a good source of proteins. According to the Whole Grains Council, bran, germ, and endosperm must be present to qualify grains as whole grains which are rich in vitamins, minerals, dietary fiber, and other bioactive compounds.

Whole grains may be eaten whole, cracked, split, flaked, or ground. Most often, they are milled into flour and used to make breads, cereals, pasta, and other grain-based foods.

Until the last century grains were commonly eaten as whole grains. Advances in the milling and processing of grains allowed large-scale separation and removal of the bran and germ, resulting in refined flour that consists only of the endosperm or in recombined flour which may be composed of white flour and bran originating from different batches of the grain. However, current dietary recommendations suggest to substitute refined grains with whole grains, because many of the beneficial bioactive components intrinsic to whole grains are lost during the refining process.

Current epidemiological evidence indicates that whole grains have a beneficial effect on health; foods from whole grains substantially reduce the risk of cardiovascular disease, diabetes, and cancer and play a role in weight management and digestive health. The essential macro- and micronutrients and the phytonutrients found in grains synergistically contribute to their beneficial effects.

The inverse association between intake of whole grains and cardiovascular disease has been demonstrated in a meta-analysis that evaluated seven cohort studies and found that higher intake of whole grains (2.5 compared to 0.2 servings per day) was associated with a risk lower than 21 % of cardiovascular events. In contrast, there was no association with the intake of refined grains [14]. In another recent meta-analysis, the whole-grain consumption did not show any effect on body weight change and a small effect on the percentage of fat mass [15].

A recent meta-analysis of 25 prospective studies confirmed a lower colorectal cancer risk, for an increase of three servings a day of whole grains [16]. The nutritional components of whole grains, which improve the health status and prevent chronic degenerative diseases, include tocotrienols, lignans, and phenolic compounds, as well as anti-nutrients such as phytic acid, tannins, and enzyme inhibitors.

2.3.3 Fresh Fruits and Vegetables

They are low energy density foods with a high content of fiber, water, vitamins, and minerals. Dietary fiber found in fruits and vegetables increase the distension of the stomach and consequently the sense of satiety which leads to not exceed in the consumption of other types of foods with higher calorific value. The portions of fruits and vegetables consumed per day should be five. The habit to eat regularly seasonal fruits and vegetables reduces the risk to take them with the harmful substances used in agriculture and preserves the biodiversity, ensuring higher organoleptic qualities.

2.3.4 Fish

Fish consumption has shaped and determined the history of the countries bordering the Mediterranean Sea. It is an excellent source of proteins, vitamin D, long-chain omega-3 polyunsaturated fatty acids, and some mineral salts such as selenium, phosphorus, and potassium that regulate the exchange of substances through the cell membranes. In particular, fishes contain the docosahexaenoic acid and the eicosa-pentaenoic acid, defined as essential fatty acids because our body is not able to produce them, and they must necessarily be included in the diet. Omega-3 fatty acid consumption has been shown to decrease the risk of coronary heart disease, hypertension, atherosclerosis, and thrombosis because of their antithrombotic effects that inhibit platelet aggregation: omega-3 fatty acids substitute the arachidonic acid that leads to the production of thromboxane A3 which has anti-aggregant and weak vasoconstrictor effects. Omega-3 fatty acids also play an antidyslipidemic effect due to the reduced expression of ApoB100 present in LDL.

2.3.5 Legumes

Often defined as the "meat of poor people", legumes have a dual function for the presence of carbohydrates slowly absorbed and for their high content in proteins. The association of cereals and legumes is complete from the viewpoint of the protein consumption as it provides all the essential amino acids required. Legumes contain discrete quantities of minerals, some vitamins, and dietary fiber, which help to achieve the sense of satiety. They also help to modulate the glycemic response to meals.

2.3.6 Dairy Products and Meat

Milk is an excellent source of proteins, minerals, and vitamins. White meat is to be preferred to red and processed meat that should be consumed in smaller quantity and frequency. Meat is rich in proteins, fats (whose quantity depends on the type and origin of the animal breeding), vitamins, and mineral salts.

2.3.7 Wine

Wine consumption came to scientific attention because of the presence of antioxidant compounds such as resveratrol and quercetin which are able to protect cellular proteins, lipids, and nucleic acids from free radicals. Epidemiological and clinical studies have pointed out that regular and moderate wine consumption during meals (one glass per day for women and two glasses per day for men) reduces the cardiovascular risk and improves lipid profile, hemostatic balance, blood pressure, insulin sensitivity, and HDL cholesterol level [17].

2.4 Adherence to the Mediterranean Diet

Diet quality indexes have been formulated to assess and quantify adherence to dietary patterns (food groups, foods, and/or nutrients) [18]. The most used Mediterranean diet indexes are reported as follows: (a) The Mediterranean Adequacy Index (MAI) was developed by the investigators of the Seven Countries Study and used the

Italian-Mediterranean diet from the Nicotera population in 1960 as reference. The MAI is the quotient between the sum of energy provided by Mediterranean and non-Mediterranean products [19]. The median value of MAI among men aged 40–59 from Nicotera in 1960 was 7.2, whereas in 1996 it decreased to 2.8, thus clearly showing how these Italian groups have changed their diet over the last four decades, gradually abandoning the reference dietary pattern. (b) The Mediterranean Diet Score (MDS) was developed by Trichopoulou et al. and measures the adherence to the Greek-Mediterranean diet [20]. The MDS assigned a score from 0 to 1 according to the daily intake of eight components: high ratio of monounsaturated to saturated fat, moderate alcohol intake, high legume intake, high intake of grains, high fruit intake, high vegetable intake, low intake of meat and meat products, and moderate intake of milk and dairy products. The MDS ranges from 0 (minimal adherence) to 8 (maximum adherence). (c) The MedDietScore was developed by Panagiotakos and assesses the consumption of 11 main components of the Mediterranean diet [21]: non-refined cereals, fruit, vegetables, legumes, potatoes, fish, meat and meat products, poultry, full-fat dairy products, olive oil, and alcohol intake. Each item is scored 0–5 according to rare, frequent, very frequent, weekly, and daily consumption.

Anyway, individual still close to the Mediterranean style are significantly protected. A comprehensive meta-analysis including European and American prospective cohort studies analyzed the relationship between adherence to a Mediterranean diet and mortality and incidence of chronic diseases in a primary prevention setting [22]. Greater adherence to a Mediterranean diet significantly reduced overall mortality (9 %), mortality from cardiovascular diseases (9 %), incidence of cancer or mortality from cancer (6 %), and incidence of Parkinson's disease and Alzheimer's disease (13 %).

Since the Mediterranean dietary pattern improves the global health status by protecting not only against cardiovascular diseases but also against chronic diseases, the World Health Organization strongly supports dietary modification in the direction of a Mediterranean style to prevent chronic diseases [23].

However, evidence from dietary intake surveys [19, 24–29] indicate that the dietary patterns of the so-called Mediterranean diet have changed among the populations bordering the *Mare Nostrum* in the last decades.

Dietary pattern had evolved toward a diet with a high content of saturated fats, high animal proteins, refined grains, and low dietary fiber (the so-called Western diet) [30, 31] due to the lower consumption of home food and high diffusion of ready-cooked food and fast-food restaurants. The caloric intake also increased by 30–40 % (from 2,500 to 3,300 kcal per day), with a progressive depletion of vegetable fats and proteins and complex carbohydrates.

Unhealthy dietary patterns and physical inactivity resulted in a constant and worrying increased prevalence of overweight and obesity that led the World Health Organization to recognize the "obesity epidemic" as a major public health concern worldwide [23]. Nearly 30 % of the world's adult population is obese or overweight, with a significant impact on public health and socioeconomic costs [32]. According to the McKinsey Global Institute report, the global economic impact from obesity is $2.0 trillion, roughly equivalent to the global impact from smoking or armed violence, war, and terrorism [33].

Moreover, the changes in dietary habits with the adoption of sedentary lifestyle are a big concern especially for the younger generations [34]. Overweight and obese children are more likely to become obese adults and to develop nutrition-related diseases, such as type 2 diabetes, cardiovascular diseases, and certain types of cancers [35, 36].

Healthy diet, weight control, and physical activity are the main strategies of the primary prevention against obesity [37].

These recommendations should lead to rediscover and propose daily on our tables the Mediterranean diet because the adequate qualitative and quantitative combination of its typical foods allows to prevent nutritional inadequacies, by excess or by defect, and to provide protection against degenerative and chronic diseases, thanks to their antioxidant and anti-inflammatory properties [38].

The Mediterranean dietary pattern is properly considered the world's healthiest way of eating and living.

2.5   Summary and Conclusions

Healthy diet, weight control, and physical activity are the main strategies of the primary prevention against chronic illnesses.

The Mediterranean dietary pattern, considered the world's healthiest way of eating and living, should be rediscovered and proposed daily on our tables.

The traditional Mediterranean diet – that is, the diet consumed by the people living in the Mediterranean area in the 1950s–1960s after World War II – is not only a way of eating but a body of knowledge, social customs, and cultural traditions historically handed down by populations bordering the *Mare Nostrum*.

The Mediterranean lifestyle includes high intake of whole cereals, legumes, extra virgin olive oil, fruits, and vegetables, moderate to high consumption of fish, moderate consumption of dairy products (mostly as cheese and yogurt), moderate wine consumption, and low consumption of red and processed meats.

The adequate qualitative and quantitative combination of these traditional foods allows to prevent nutritional inadequacies, by excess or by defect, and to provide protection against degenerative and chronic diseases, thanks to their antioxidant and anti-inflammatory properties.

References

1. Nestle M (1995) Mediterranean diets: historical and research overview. Am J Clin Nutr 61(6):1313S–1320S
2. Davis C, Bryan J, Hodgson J, Murphy K (2015) Definition of the Mediterranean diet; a literature review. Nutrients 7(11):9139–9153
3. Rodríguez JM, Leiva Balich L, Concha MJ, Mizón C, Bunout Barnett D, Barrera Acevedo G, Hirsch Birn S, Jiménez Jaime T, Henríquez S, Uribarri J, de la Maza Cave MP (2015) Reduction of serum advanced glycation end-products with a low calorie Mediterranean diet. Nutr Hosp 31(6):2511–2517

4. Uribarri J, Woodruff S, Goodman S, Cai W, Chen X, Pyzik R, Yong A, Striker GE, Vlassara H (2010) Advanced glycation end products in foods and a practical guide to their reduction in the diet. J Am Diet Assoc 110(6):911–916, e12
5. Keys A, Blackburn H, Menotti A et al (1970) Coronary heart disease in seven countries. Circulation 41(suppl 1):1–211
6. Ancel and Margaret Keys (1959) Eat well and stay well. Publisher: Doubleday
7. US Department of Agriculture (1992) Food guide pyramid (1992). Human Nutrition Information Service (Publication HG252), Hyattsville
8. Willett WC, Stampfer MJ (2003) Rebuilding the food pyramid. Sci Am 288(1):64–71
9. Oh K, Hu FB, Manson JE, Stampfer MJ, Willett WC (2005) Dietary fat intake and risk of coronary heart disease in women: 20 years of follow-up of the nurses' health study. Am J Epidemiol 161(7):672–679
10. Mozaffarian D, Katan MB, Ascherio A, Stampfer MJ, Willett WC (2006) Trans fatty acids and cardiovascular disease. N Engl J Med 354(15):1601–1613
11. Slavin J (2003) Why whole grains are protective: biological mechanisms. Proc Nutr Soc 62(1):129–134
12. Bach-Faig A, Berry EM, Lairon D, Reguant J, Trichopoulou A, Dernini S, Medina FX, Battino M, Belahsen R, Miranda G, Serra-Majem L, Mediterranean Diet Foundation Expert Group (2011) Mediterranean diet pyramid today. Science and cultural updates. Public Health Nutr 14(12A):2274–2284
13. Covas MI, de la Torre R, Fitó M (2015) Virgin olive oil: a key food for cardiovascular risk protection. Br J Nutr 113(Suppl 2):S19–S28
14. Mellen PB, Walsh TF, Herrington DM (2008) Whole grain intake and cardiovascular disease: a meta-analysis. Nutr Metab Cardiovasc Dis 18(4):283–290
15. Pol K, Christensen R, Bartels EM, Raben A, Tetens I, Kristensen M (2013) Whole grain and body weight changes in apparently healthy adults: a systematic review and meta-analysis of randomized controlled studies. Am J Clin Nutr 98(4):872–884
16. Aune D, Chan DS, Lau R, Vieira R, Greenwood DC, Kampman E, Norat T (2011) Dietary fibre, whole grains, and risk of colorectal cancer: systematic review and dose-response meta-analysis of prospective studies. BMJ 343:d6617
17. Arranz S, Chiva-Blanch G, Valderas-Martínez P, Medina-Remón A, Lamuela-Raventós RM, Estruch R (2012) Wine, beer, alcohol and polyphenols on cardiovascular disease and cancer. Nutrients 4(7):759–781
18. Bach A, Serra-Majem L, Carrasco JL, Roman B, Ngo J, Bertomeu I, Obrador B (2006) The use of indexes evaluating the adherence to the Mediterranean diet in epidemiological studies: a review. Public Health Nutr 9(1A):132–146
19. Alberti-Fidanza A, Fidanza F (2004) Mediterranean adequacy index of Italian diets. Public Health Nutr 7(7):937–941
20. Trichopoulou A, Kouris-Blazos A, Wahlquivist M, Gnardellis D, Lagiou P, Polychronopoulos E et al (1995) Diet and overall survival in elderly people. Br Med J 311:1457–1460
21. Panagiotakos DB, Pitsavos C, Stefanadis C (2006) Dietary patterns: a Mediterranean diet score and its relation to clinical and biological markers of cardiovascular disease risk. Nutr Metab Cardiovasc Dis 16(8):559–568
22. Sofi F, Cesari F, Abbate R, Gensini GF, Casini A (2008) Adherence to Mediterranean diet and health status: meta-analysis. BMJ 337:a1344
23. World Health Organization (2003) Diet, nutrition and the prevention of chronic diseases. Report of a joint WHO/FAO expert consultation, World Health Organisation technical report series 916. World Health Organization, Geneva
24. Vareiro D, Bach-Faig A, Raidó Quintana B, Bertomeu I, Buckland G, Vaz de Almeida MD et al (2009) Availability of Mediterranean and non-Mediterranean foods during the last four decades: comparison of several geographical areas. Public Health Nutr 12(9A):1667–1675
25. Trichopoulou A, Costacou T, Bamia C, Trichopoulos D (2003) Adherence to a Mediterranean diet and survival in a Greek population. N Engl J Med 348(26):2599–2608

26. Garcia-Closas R, Berenguer A, Gonzalez C (2006) Changes in food supply in Mediterranean countries from 1961 to 2001. Public Health Nutr 9(1):53–60
27. Da Silva R, Bach-Faig A, Raido Quintana B, Buckland G, Vaz de Almeida MD, Serra-Majem L (2009) World variation of adherence to the Mediterranean diet, in 1961–1965 and 2000–2003. Public Health Nutr 12(9A):1676–1684
28. León-Muñoz LM, Guallar-Castillón P, Graciani A, López-García E, Mesas AE, Aguilera MT et al (2012) Adherence to the Mediterranean diet pattern has declined in Spanish adults. J Nutr 142(10):1843–1850
29. Roccaldo R, Censi L, D'Addezio L, Toti E, Martone D, D'Addesa D et al (2014) Adherence to the Mediterranean diet in Italian school children (The ZOOM8 Study). Int J Food Sci Nutr 65(5):621–628
30. Strazzullo P, Ferro-Luzzi A, Siani A, Scaccini C, Sette S, Catasta G, Mancini M (1986) Changing the Mediterranean diet: effects on blood pressure. J Hypertens 4(4):407–412
31. Ferro-Luzzi A, Strazzullo P, Scaccini C, Siani A, Sette S, Mariani MA, Mastranzo P, Dougherty RM, Iacono JM, Mancini M (1984) Changing the Mediterranean diet: effects on blood lipids. Am J Clin Nutr 40(5):1027–1037
32. Ng M, Fleming T, Robinson M, Thomson B, Graetz N, Margono C, Mullany EC, Biryukov S, Abbafati C, Abera SF et al (2014) Global, regional, and national prevalence of overweight and obesity in children and adults during 1980–2013: a systematic analysis for the Global Burden of Disease Study 2013. Lancet 384(9945):766–781
33. Dobbs R, Sawers C, Thompson F, Manyika J, Woetzel J, Child P, McKenna S, Spatharou A (2014) Overcoming obesity: an initial economic analysis. McKinsey Global Institute. Available at www.mckinsey.com/mgi
34. Lobstein T, Baur L, Uauy R, IASO International Obesity TaskForce (2004) Obesity in children and young people: a crisis in public health. Obes Rev 5(S1):S4–S104
35. Leon BM, Maddox TM (2015) Diabetes and cardiovascular disease: epidemiology, biological mechanisms, treatment recommendations and future research. World J Diabetes 6(13):1246–1258
36. World Cancer Research Fund/American Institute for Cancer Research (2007) Food, nutrition, physical activity, and the prevention of cancer: a global perspective. AICR, Washington, DC
37. Kar SS, Dube R, Kar SS (2014) Childhood obesity-an insight into preventive strategies. Avicenna J Med 4(4):88–93
38. Assmann G, Buono P, Daniele A, Della Valle E, Farinaro E, Ferns G, Krogh V, Kromhout D, Masana L, Merino J, Misciagna G, Panico S, Riccardi G, Rivellese AA, Rozza F, Salvatore F, Salvatore V, Stranges S, Trevisan M, Trimarco B, Vetrani C (2014) Functional foods and cardiometabolic diseases*. International Task Force for Prevention of Cardiometabolic Diseases. Nutr Metab Cardiovasc Dis 24(12):1272–1300

The Gut Microbiota and Obesity in Humans

3

Konstantinos Efthymakis, Rocco Leonello,
Fabio Pace, and Matteo Neri

3.1   Introduction

Based on animal studies, the gut microbiome has been put forth as an effector of
host metabolic disease, with various possible mechanisms regulating its metabolic
effect on energy balance and fat storage. Intestinal microbiota could directly regulate energy harvesting by increasing the fermentation of indigestible dietary polysaccharides and by favoring the primary short-chain fatty acid (SCFA) production
in the gut, thus increasing lipogenesis in the liver [1]. It could also modulate fat
tissue activity by suppressing the fasting-induced adipocyte factor (FIAF) in the gut,
thus increasing lipoprotein lipase (LPL) activity in adipocytes [1]. Fatty acid oxidation could be also indirectly modulated by suppression of adenosine monophos-
phate-activated protein kinase (AMPK) [2]. Lastly, altered gut permeability has
been linked to increased metabolic endotoxemia; increased lipopolysaccharide
(LPS) plasma levels seem to be a herald of metabolic disease and chronic low-grade
inflammation, potentially leading to insulin resistance, diabetes, obesity, metabolic
syndrome, steatosis, and atherogenesis [3]. Endotoxemia has been shown to increase
fat consumption in humans [4]. For the purpose of this review, in order to overcome
the transferability limitations of animal studies to humans, we have decided to con-
centrate only on human studies aimed at revealing the role of gut microbiota as a
major determinant of obesity.

K. Efthymakis, MD • M. Neri, MD (✉)
Department of Medicine and Aging Sciences and Ce.S.I., G. D'Annunzio University,
Chieti, Italy
e-mail: mneri@unich.it

R. Leonello, MD • F. Pace, MD
Complex Operating Unit of Gastroenterology, Seriate Hospital, Bergamo, Italy

© Springer International Publishing Switzerland 2016   27
E. Grossi, F. Pace (eds.), *Human Nutrition from the Gastroenterologist's Perspective*,
DOI 10.1007/978-3-319-30361-1_3

3.2   Normative Studies

Already by 1996, polymerase chain reaction (PCR) based methods for studying fecal microbiota were shown to have an advantage over classical culture-based techniques, confirming the basic structure of the human gut microbiome as comprising mostly of two major phyla: Firmicutes (60 % of total bacterial 16S rDNA clones) and Bacteroidetes (30 %) [5]. Additionally, PCR was capable of characterizing previously undescribed organisms, which at that time amounted up to 76 % of total signatures [6]. An early 2002 study further confirmed these results on colonic biopsy samples, demonstrating intersubject variability [7]. A 2005 report that examined 13,355 prokaryotic 16S ribosomal RNA gene sequences, obtained from colon biopsy and fecal sampling in healthy subjects, revealed that most of the bacterial sequences corresponded to novel or uncultivated species, with a significant intersubject variability in microbiota composition. Some differences were observed also regarding bacterial abundance and structure when comparing mucosal and fecal samples of the same individuals, possibly reflecting differences between adherent and luminal populations. Intersubject variations with a "patchy" distribution were observed but did not display a clear pattern reflecting the anatomy of the colon [8].

This complex gut ecosystem is not well established at birth but undergoes evolutionary phases, from initial postpartum colonization [9] to diversification and differential growth influenced by infant physiology, lactation, solid diet composition, hygienic conditions and human contact, as well as antibiotic treatments. Early gut microbiota are highly idiosyncratic; they show lower total microbe counts, being dominated by the *Bifidobacterium* group and to a lesser extent by *E. coli* (Proteobacteria) and *Bacteroides* (Bacteroidetes) (bacterial phylum in parenthesis). Convergence to adult type gradually increases total counts and primarily Clostridia (*C. leptum* and *C. coccoides* – Firmicutes) and reduces *Bifidobacterium* and *E. coli*; populations of *Bacteroides* and *Lactobacillus* remain stable. This heavily modifies the Firmicutes/Bacteroidetes ratio from 0.4 to 10.9. Interestingly, although in the elderly total bacterial counts are conserved, Firmicutes are reduced again, with a return of the F/B ratio to low values (0.6). *Escherichia coli* concentrations reprise, while *Bifidobacterium* remains stable [10]. Convergence from infant- to adult-type microbiome is thought to occur by the first year of age, although with important intersubject variations [11]. The specific outcome and metabolic impact of this maturation process can lead to acquisition of specific "pro-inflammatory" or "obesogenic" adult enterotypes; modulation of gut microbiota during this maturation period could represent a potential therapeutic target for the prevention of metabolic pathology including obesity.

After numerous early animal studies, some data on the relation between obesity and microbiome composition on humans began to emerge. Rey et al., back in 2006, showed that human colonic microbiota was prevalently dominated by the Firmicutes and Bacteroidetes phyla, with most (70 %) of the 4,074 identified species-level signatures being unique to each person [12]. The Bacteroidetes and Firmicutes phyla were found to dominate the ecosystem (92.6 % of all 16S rRNA sequences), although there were marked interpersonal differences in species-level diversity.

Remarkably, microbiota composition was fairly stable within subjects, fecal samples being generally more similar to one another than to those from other people over time. The authors found that, considering the percentage of total sequences, obese subjects (BMI, >30) showed fewer Bacteroidetes ($P<0.001$) and more Firmicutes ($P=0.002$) than lean controls. Fecal microbiota composition was responsive to restrictive dietary intervention, toward a lean-type relative abundance for both the prominent bacterial phyla, being division-wide and not attributable to any specific species (see "Dietary Intervention Studies" section).

3.2.1 Children

Kalliomäki et al. in 2008 sought to explore gut microbiota composition in overweight/obese and healthy children, matched for gestational age and body mass index at birth, mode of delivery, probiotic supplementation, duration of breastfeeding, and use of antibiotics during infancy, by fluorescent in situ hybridization (FISH) with flow cytometry and quantitative real-time polymerase chain reaction (qRT-PCR), at 6 and 12 months of age. They found significantly lower numbers of *Bifidobacterium* (Actinobacteria) in children who afterward became overweight/obese, with higher counts of *Staphylococcus aureus* (Firmicutes), thus possibly predicting future weight gain [13].

A more direct approach was undertaken by Turnbaugh et al. exploring gut microbiome diversities between obese and lean mono- and dizygotic female twins and their mothers, based on fecal sampling and 16S rRNA qPCR [14]. They found that individuals from the same family, being generally concordant for metabolic status, had a more similar microbiome structure compared to unrelated individuals. Differences were less evident between twins (regardless of them being mono- or dizygotic) than between twins and their mothers, with no observable effects due to geographical separation of the subjects. Furthermore, they showed that the similarities in microbial composition were independent from metabolic status (obese vs. lean), as related concordant individuals were significantly less distant from each other than from unrelated concordant individuals, measured by UniFrac distance (lean-related vs. lean-unrelated and obese-related vs. obese-unrelated, $p<0.001$). Overall, obesity was associated with a significant decrease in microbiota population diversity. Significantly less Bacteroidetes, more Actinobacteria ($p<0.005$), but no significant difference in Firmicutes were observed in obese versus lean individuals. Metabolic clustering based on carbohydrate-active enzyme (CAZyme) DNA sequences showed two distinct metabolic clusters, corresponding to prevalent abundance of Firmicutes/Actinobacteria or Bacteroidetes. Similarities in the metabolic profiles of bacterial communities were more prominent between related individuals. Interestingly, functional diversity in each cluster was significantly linked to the relative abundance of the Bacteroidetes. Regarding the metabolically functional groups, 26–53 % were shared across all microbiomes, defined as the "core microbiome," being also highly abundant (over 90 % of sequences) and consistent across samples. Variable functional groups showed marked differences in abundance between lean and obese individuals, paralleling taxonomic differences at the phylum level: 75 % of the obesity-enriched genes were from Actinobacteria (compared with 0 % of lean-enriched genes; the other 25 % were from Firmicutes), whereas 42 % of the lean-enriched genes were from Bacteroidetes (compared with 0 % of the obesity-enriched genes). The authors concluded that shared microbial genes reflecting metabolic function, rather than actual species, are principally related to host metabolic status and these seem to be more influenced by nurture than actual genetic similarity.

De Filippo et al. in a 2010 retrospective study evaluated the impact of diet in shaping the gut microbiome, by comparing fecal samples of healthy children from Burkina Faso ($n = 14$) and from Florence, Italy ($n = 15$) [15]. The respective dietary habits differed principally in the ratio of fiber to animal fat and protein content, being higher in the former group, thought to be representative of a neolithic-type diet, and lower in the latter, as is generally in the Western world. Bacteroidetes and Actinobacteria were more represented in African than in European children's microbiome. Firmicutes and Proteobacteria followed an inverse trend. In fact, Firmicutes were twice as abundant in Western children further affecting differences in ratio between Firmicutes and Bacteroidetes (F/B ratio $\pm$ SD, 2.8 $\pm$ 0.06 in EU and 0.47 $\pm$ 0.05 in BF). Biodiversity was also highly increased in Africans, with some genera being exclusive to each population. The African exclusive bacterial community was highly productive of anti-inflammatory SCFAs. Other SCFA-producing bacteria, such as *Bacteroides* and *Faecalibacterium* species, particularly *F. prausnitzii*, were found in both populations. However, a significantly higher total SCFA concentration was observed in the fecal samples of Burkina Faso children compared with Europeans, particularly so for propionic and butyric acids which were four times more abundant. Notably, not only total fiber content differed in the diets of the subject groups; total daily calories were almost half among African children, and this alone could account for a selective shift toward a more efficient microbiome in terms of energy harvesting and SCFA production. Interestingly, clustering of the European and African samples according to their bacterial genera defined a clear separation of the respective populations. However, the subcluster that joined the two major clusters contained samples taken from the three youngest African children (1–2 years old) and two European 1-year-olds. Breastfeeding duration in these populations differs significantly, with Africans being breastfed until the second year of age compared to 1 year in Europeans, suggesting a possible effect of lactation duration. The study does not compare to another unrelated Western population to establish any degree of similarity in microbiota composition between subjects, thus not accounting for some profoundly different genealogies between populations.

3.2.2 Women

Santacruz et al. evaluated differences in microbiome composition, by fecal sampling, in pregnant women at 24 weeks of gestation, considered normal or overweight based on BMI (>25) and of normal or excessive weight gain during pregnancy (>16 kg for normal-weight and >11.5 kg for overweight subjects) [16]. They found that *Bifidobacterium* and *Bacteroides* numbers were significantly higher ($p < 0.001$ and $p = 0.035$, respectively) in normal-weight than in overweight women, whereas Enterobacteriaceae ($p = 0.001$), *E. coli* ($p = 0.005$), and tentatively *Staphylococcus* ($p = 0.006$) numbers were lower in normal-weight than in overweight women. *Bifidobacterium* and *Bacteroides* numbers correlated with normal-weight women (R, -0.56; $p < 0.001$; and R, -0.34; $p = 0.02$, respectively); inverse was the case for *Staphylococcus* (R, 0.67; $p = 0.003$), Enterobacteriaceae (R, 0.46; $p < 0.001$), and *E. coli* (R, 0.4; $p = 0.004$). Considering weight gain during pregnancy, *E. coli* numbers were significantly higher ($p = 0.045$) in women with excessive weight gain. On the contrary, *A. muciniphila* numbers were higher in subjects with normal weight gain ($p = 0.02$). Increased numbers of *Bifidobacterium*, *Bacteroides*, and *A. mucinophila* correlated weakly but significantly with normal weight gain (R, -0.31; $p = 0.029$; R, -0.36; $p = 0.019$; R, -0.34; $p = 0.017$, respectively). The opposite was found for increased numbers of *E. coli* (R, 0.42; $p = 0.002$) and Enterobacteriaceae (R, 0.28; $p = 0.05$). A very similar earlier study however, applying the same criteria for overweight and severity of weight gain, with fecal sampling at 10–15 weeks and at 30–35 weeks of gestation, had shown similar results for *Staphylococcus*, but noted an association of higher *Bacteroides* numbers to overweight status [17].

Another study investigated the microbiome composition in overweight and obese women, with or without signs of metabolic dysfunction, namely, impairment of glucose and lipid metabolism, and normal-weight women [18]. Gut microbiota was profiled from fecal samples in 85 premenopausal women. Body composition was measured by bioimpedance, and dietary intakes were collected via food diaries. Results showed that the *Eubacterium rectale-Clostridium coccoides* group (Firmicutes) was significantly more represented in the metabolic disorder group while independently correlating with greater body weight, BMI, fat mass, and fat mass percentage, higher serum triglycerides, and lower HDL levels ($p < 0.05$). The inverse was true for *Bacteroides* abundance. This study did not find differences in the relative amounts of *Bifidobacterium*, *Bacteroides*, and *F. prausnitzii*. The calculated F/B ratio was higher in the metabolic disorder group compared to the non-metabolic disorder and normal weight groups, but after adjustment for body weight, the significance in the F/B ratio between groups disappeared. Regarding inflammatory status, no difference in PCR concentrations between groups was observed, although Il-6 was significantly higher in patients with metabolic dysfunction. No other pro-inflammatory cytokines were measured. An association to a positive diagnosis of metabolic syndrome, and not individual components of metabolic dysfunction, is lacking. Lastly, F/B ratio was only roughly estimated, as it was calculated but not directly measured.

A recent study in women with normal, impaired, and diabetic glucose control sought to characterize both composition and function of the gut microbiome by fecal sampling and to develop a model predictor of a diabetes-like metabolism [19]. Increases in the abundance of four *Lactobacillus* species and decreases of five *Clostridium* species in the diabetes group ($p < 0.05$) were observed. *Lactobacillus* species correlated positively with fasting glucose and HbA1c ($P < 0.05$), while *Clostridium* species correlated negatively with fasting glucose, HbA1c, insulin,

C-peptide, and plasma triglycerides and positively with adiponectin and HDL. These *Lactobacillus* and *Clostridium* species did not correlate with BMI, waist circumference (WC), or waist-to-hip ratio (WHR). Composition of the microbiota was determined by means of metagenomic clusters (MGCs, clustered sets of genes with high correlation between them), with a fair correlation at the species (36 %) or order level (30 %). MGC-based microbiota composition correlates better with type 2 diabetes mellitus than with individual risk factors (BMI, WC, WHR). Some MGCs showed an inverse significant correlation with BMI and WC, namely, several Clostridiales (including Lachnospiraceae) ($p < 0.05$). Notably, WC inversely correlated also to *Bacteroides intestinalis*. One species, *L. gasseri*, had the highest score for the identification of diabetic women; *Roseburia*, several Clostridiales, *B. intestinalis*, *C. clostridioforme*, and Coriobacteriaceae were among the ten most important clusters in the model based on MGCs. Thus, the MGC model was better than species model in predicting type 2 diabetes. However, metagenomic markers differ between the European and Chinese cohorts; age and geographical location of the populations studied should be taken into account. The study also does not address causality as diabetic status is known to alter microbiota composition on other mucosal microenvironments, notably the vaginal flora in diabetic women. Poor blood glucose control could be an independent factor leading to dysbiosis: an increase in Lactobacillales, mainly *Streptococcus* species, and a decrease in species belonging to *Bacteroides*, *Eubacterium*, and *Clostridium* in women with high HbA1c were detected. Furthermore, certain drugs seemed to correlate with certain microbes, for instance, metformin, and increased counts of Enterobacteriaceae (i.e., *Escherichia*, *Shigella*, *Klebsiella*, and *Salmonella*) and decreased levels of *Clostridium* and *Eubacterium*.

3.2.3   Mixed Populations

Le Chatelier et al. [20], assessing the abundance of bacterial genes in a population of obese and nonobese subjects, observed a bimodal distribution of gene counts across individuals. Defining "low gene count" (LGC) and "high gene count" (HGC) based on a threshold of 480,000 gene counts, subjects fell broadly in two groups, the latter being more populous. *Bacteroides*, *Parabacteroides*, *Porphyromonas* (Bacteroidetes), *Ruminococcus*, *Dialister*, *Staphylococcus*, *Anaerostipes* (Firmicutes), and *Campylobacter* (Proteobacteria) were more dominant in LGC; *Faecalibacterium*, *Lactobacillus*, *Butyrivibrio*, *Coprococcus* (Firmicutes), *Bifidobacterium* (Actinobacteria), *Alistipes* (Bacteroidetes), *Akkermansia* (Verrucomicrobia), and *Methanobrevibacter* (Euryarchaeota) were significantly associated with HGC. At the phylum level, they noted a higher abundance of Proteobacteria and Bacteroidetes in LGC individuals, with increased populations of Verrucomicrobia, Actinobacteria, and Euryarchaeota in HGC. Their analyses highlight the contrast between the distribution of anti-inflammatory species, such as *Faecalibacterium prausnitzii*, which are more prevalent in HGC individuals, and potentially pro-inflammatory *Bacteroides* and *R. gnavus*, found to be more frequent in LGC individuals. Microbiota composition was less different between obese and nonobese individuals, than between LGC and HGC subjects, indicating the presence of underlying factors that independently confer a risk toward weight status. Furthermore, higher BMI, weight, and whole body fat were significantly more associated with LGC status ($p=0.035$, $p=0.019$, and $p=0.0069$, respectively). Such results shifted the focus from composition to function, putting forth a paradigm in which microbiota metabolic function, strongly associated to enriched gene diversity in the gut flora populations, influenced host metabolism and disease more than specific bacterial phyla or species.

However, the initial results showing that changes in the proportion and/or level of predominant bacterial phyla (a decrease in Bacteroidetes and/or an increase in Firmicutes) occur in obese individuals and may be reversed by dieting and weight loss were challenged. Already in 2008 a study [21] examining the microbiota composition in obese patients and lean controls by fluorescent in situ hybridization (FISH) showed no difference regarding the proportion of Bacteroidetes; furthermore, they found no significant change in the percentage of Bacteroidetes after weight loss induced by caloric restriction, independently of carbohydrate intake. However, among the Firmicutes, the *Roseburia/Eubacterium rectale* group of butyrate-producing bacteria showed a striking reduction ($P<0.001$). Interestingly, as the *Roseburia/E. rectale* group declined, other bacteria within the same cluster (*C. coccoides* cluster) tended to increase, thus lending support to the idea that diet composition and specifically carbohydrate availability primarily affect the balance between various groups. Armougom et al. also reported a reduced abundance of Bacteroidetes between obese and lean subjects, while among the Firmicutes only the *Lactobacillus* increased [22]. Schwiertz et al., considering initial reports on the Firmicutes and Bacteroidetes abundance, found the opposite to be the case when comparing gut microbiome composition between healthy lean, overweight, and obese subjects, by 16S rRNA qPCR [23]: Firmicutes were less abundant, while Bacteroidetes increased proportionally, the F/B ratio decreasing from a 3.3 in lean individuals to as low as 1.1 and 1.2 in overweight and obese, respectively. That difference remained largely unaffected by BMI, as no change was noted between the dysmetabolic groups. In addition, they found that some Bacteroidetes subgroups exhibited lower cell numbers, such as *Ruminococcus flavefaciens*. Interestingly, SCFA content was significantly increased by 20% in obese individuals versus lean individuals ($p=0.024$), with propionate showing the highest increase (41%).

Others have found no association between obesity and the Bacteroidetes/Firmicutes ratio [24–26]. The decreased Bacteroidetes component was in at least one case shown to associate with decreased Firmicutes, although determined in this case by culture-based methods [27].

Finucane et al. [28] examined gut microbial signature datasets from the Human Microbiome Project (HMP) [29] and MetaHIT [30] surveys for possible associations to subject BMI. Both surveys included both lean and obese but otherwise healthy individuals. They found no difference between obese and lean individuals regarding the relative abundance of Bacteroidetes or Firmicutes ($p=0.30$ and 0.86, respectively). Similarly, the BMI variable showed no association to the Bacteroidetes/Firmicutes ratio or to the taxonomic composition at the phylum or the genus level.

Furthermore, the authors examined the relationship between gut microbiome diversity and an obese phenotype (BMI, >30), using the approach of Turnbaugh et al. [14]. Again, no relationship between richness and obesity was observed. When the relationship between stool microbiome composition and BMI across two previous studies was examined [12, 14], the apparent variability between studies far exceeded differences in composition between individuals within each study. Although some limitation could arise from population selection (e.g., absence of obese subjects with BMI >35 among the HMP samples), the study had the advantage regarding sample size, depth of compositional profiling, and strength of statistical analysis. The authors point to possible substantial inter-study variability due to unmeasured clinical factors such as dietary habits and caloric input or due to technical factors such as DNA extraction technique, region of the 16 S locus targeted, or sequencing platform.

More recently, Suzuki et al. [31] observed a significant positive correlation between Firmicutes abundance and increasing latitude ($r=0.857$, $p<0.0001$), while the opposite was true for Bacteroidetes ($r=-0.637$, $p=0.001$). These correlations did not seem to be influenced by age, sex, method of detection (FISH vs. 16S sequencing), or ancestry. Possible dietary differences owing to different cultural backgrounds were not accounted for; another possible factor could be attributed to differences in pathogen distribution. The observed patterns parallel the Bergmann's rule of differences in physiology across latitudes [32]. If such a pattern should be confirmed, we would need to change our current understanding of the concept of "healthy microbiome" to account for such differences.

3.2.4 Pathophysiological Mechanisms

Two principal mechanisms have been proposed for how the gut microbiota can contribute to host adiposity: (1) increased energy extraction efficiency from the diet and (2) altered host-microbial interactions that promote metabolic inflammation. A recent study [33] tracking gut microbiota changes in pregnant women suggests that although some shifts in compositional patterns are common both in pregnancy and obesity, the second mechanism seems primarily to drive dysbiosis in the former. In fact, microbiota during the final trimester are similar to those of the obesity-associated microbiome shown to have enhanced energy extraction efficiency and low taxonomic richness. However, excess energy intake, shown to favor Firmicutes over Bacteroidetes in obesity [34], was not a factor at all in the pregnant population of the study. The relative abundances of Bacteroidetes and Firmicutes remained largely unchanged between trimesters, and no shift occurred regarding specific gene function or metabolic pathway abundance. On the contrary, low-grade inflammation markers (specifically cytokines) seemed prevalently affected, implying a primarily pro-inflammatory feedback loop between hormonal/immune changes during pregnancy and gut microbiota composition. Late-pregnancy microbiome transplantation from otherwise healthy women in a murine model however triggered a rapid increase in adiposity. This suggests that altered host hormonal/immune states can drive pro-obesogenic shifts in the microbiome composition, partially linking adiposity in the obese with potential primary or secondary hormonal/immune dysfunctions.

Differences in the techniques used could account for some of the observed differences between reported data in some studies. For example, FISH-based methods had higher Firmicutes and lower Bacteroidetes values compared with 16S sequencing-based methods in some studies [29]. It is possible that, in FISH-based studies, Bacteroidales populations in human fecal samples have been underestimated [35]. Methodological differences in DNA extraction protocols as well as primer design may have caused additional variation. Body exercise (see "Dietary Intervention Studies") and smoking have been shown to relate to changes in intestinal flora composition. When comparing individuals during a 9-week smoking cessation period to smoking or nonsmoking controls, Biedermann L. et al. observed a shift to higher abundances of Firmicutes and lower counts of Bacteroidetes already at 4 weeks, the pattern remaining stable at 2 months [36]. During this time no significant changes had been observed in the control groups. In both cases, however, causality has not been addressed and whether or not these differences reflect a primary effect on gut microbiota composition or are secondary to changes in dietary patterns or caloric intake remains to be elucidated.

3.3   Dietary Intervention Studies

Diet-induced effects on microbiota populations have been extensively documented in published literature as previously discussed in this review. Numerous intervention studies have explored the effects of weight loss regimens, regarding both composition and function of the gut microbiome. It is generally the case however that such studies suggest diet modification as the effector of both weight loss and microbiome shifts. The opposite hypothesis, that diet-induced modifications of the microbiota could independently drive weight loss, is much more difficult to prove, although direct metabolic effects on the host have been widely confirmed by observation. In addition, weight-reducing hypocaloric dietary regimens are generally hypolipidic, hypoglucidic, or both, almost always being moderately or highly hyperproteic, with an increased total fiber intake. As such, it is difficult to explore any individual effects associated with those features; it is known, for instance, that fiber intake increase alone could result in some weight loss and selective bacterial flora modifications, almost certainly due to its prebiotic properties [37–39].

Rey et al. back in 2006 showed that human colonic microbiota was prevalently dominated by the Firmicutes and Bacteroidetes phyla [12]. In that study, 12 obese people (BMI, >30) were randomly assigned to either a fat-restricted (FAT-R) or to a carbohydrate-restricted (CARB-R) low-calorie diet. Gut microbiota composition was monitored over the course of 12 months by 16S ribosomal RNA gene sequencing from stool samples. Before diet, obese subjects showed fewer Bacteroidetes ($P<0.001$) and more Firmicutes ($P=0.002$) than lean controls. Over time, the relative abundance of Bacteroidetes increased ($P<0.001$), while the abundance of Firmicutes decreased ($P=0.002$), irrespective of diet composition. Evolution toward a lean-type composition for both the prominent bacterial phyla was division-wide and not attributable to the bloom of any specific species. An increased abundance of Bacteroidetes correlated with percentage loss of body weight (R2 was 0.8 for the CARB-R diet and 0.5 for the FAT-R diet, $P<0.05$), and not with changes in dietary calorie content over time (R2 was 0.06 for the CARB-R diet and 0.09 for the FAT-R diet). The change in relative abundance of Firmicutes and Bacteroidetes was small but evident by the 12th week of the dietary intervention; the correlation of Bacteroidetes abundance to weight loss held only after subjects had lost at least 6% of their body weight on the FAT-R diet and at least 2% on the CARB-R diet. Taken together these two facts seem to be pointing at an adaptive response of the microbiome to a new low-energy environment, rather than a bacterial drive on host metabolism. Despite the small number of recruits, this was essentially the first interventional study on the subject that confirmed the possibility of gut microbiota composition modulation by dietary means.

Subsequently, Nadal et al. evaluated changes in fecal microbiota composition in overweight and obese adolescents undergoing caloric restriction and increased physical activity [40]. The *E. rectale-C. coccoides* group (Firmicutes) dropped significantly, whereas those of the *Bacteroides-Prevotella* group (Bacteroidetes) increased in those subjects who lost more than 4 kg, confirming the reversibility although not the causality of the correlation.

Exercise and physical activity, a prominent modulator of metabolic balance in humans, has been shown to relate to microbiota composition. When examining fecal samples of elite athletes and obese or lean controls, principal component analysis based on unweighted UniFrac distances of 16S rRNA sequences showed that microbial populations fall in distinct clusters [41]. Furthermore, the diversity of the athlete microbiota was significantly higher than that of the groups, irrespective of BMI. Interestingly, athletes exhibited significantly less Bacteroidetes and more Firmicutes than high BMI controls, although not than lean controls, maybe reflecting in part caloric input differences and food preferences. Very little differences were observed between high and low BMI controls.

3.4   Antibiotic Intervention Studies

Antibiotic treatments have been known to increase body weight in animal models; they have in fact been utilized in livestock farming as growth promoters for decades [42], and their use has been proposed for the treatment of malnutrition in childhood [43]. Their anabolic properties, at least in humans, seem closely related to infection control, as improved hygiene reduces the efficacy of such malnutrition treatments; however, a small independent effect on growth promotion has been observed, with data remaining inconclusive [43]. Numerous studies have provided data on the post-antibiotic treatment modifications of human microbiome, both in diversity and metabolic function [44–47].

A 2010 study retrospectively evaluated weight gain in patients undergoing antibiotic treatment for infective endocarditis [48]. A total of 28 patients received a 4–6-week amoxicillin treatment, while 11 patients received vancomycin treatment of the same duration; both groups received also a variable duration of gentamicin treatment. Nine patients received other antibiotics, namely, oxacillin or alternate courses of both vancomycin and amoxicillin. A population of consecutive patients initially suspected for infected endocarditis, but later dismissed, was defined as the control group. Over a 12-month period, the authors found that BMI increased significantly in the antibiotic group (mean [±SE] kg/m^2, +1.1 [±0.5]; $p=0.02$) but not in the controls (mean [±SE] kg/m^2, −0.2 [±0.2]; $p=0.38$). Within the antibiotic group, BMI significantly increased only after treatment with vancomycin (mean [±SE] kg/m^2, +2.3 [±0.9]; $p=0.03$), but not after amoxicillin or the other antibiotics. After multivariable analysis, treatment with vancomycin remained the only predictor of a major increase in BMI ($\geq 10\%$) (adjusted OR, 6.7; 95 % CI, 1.37–33.0; $p=0.02$), with an adjusted odds ratio of 6.7. The authors hypothesize that a differential vancomycin sensitivity within Firmicutes results in an altered gut flora composition which drives obesogenic metabolism. Specifically, they invoke the notable resistance of lactobacilli to vancomycin, within the generally sensitive Firmicutes, as the possible cause of a selective growth of this bacterial genus, known for its probiotic properties and possible effects on weight gain. However, different species of *Lactobacillus* have been linked to either weight gain (notably *L. reuteri* and *L. acidophilus*) or weight loss (*L. gasseri, L. plantarum*) [49]. The study does not include direct characterization of gut microbiota composition by fecal or biopsy sampling; as such it remains only speculative about the true effects of antibiotic treatment on patient metabolic status.

In a recent (2013) single-blinded, randomized, controlled trial, 20 male obese subjects with metabolic syndrome were randomized to 7 days of amoxicillin 500 mg t.i.d. or 7 days of vancomycin 500 mg t.i.d. to assess the effect on fecal microbiota composition, bile acid, and glucose metabolism [50]. Although such a short-term treatment did not have a measurable effect on the total number of bacteria in the two groups, vancomycin significantly decreased microbial diversity and the total number of gram-positive bacteria, namely, Firmicutes (*Clostridium* cluster IV and XIVa, *Lactobacillus plantarum* and various butyrate-producing species including *Faecalibacterium prausnitzii* and *Eubacterium hallii*, as well as pathogens from the Proteobacteria phylum (*Escherichia coli, Haemophilus*, and *Serratia*), with a compensatory boost in gram-negatives. Furthermore, vancomycin affected bile acid metabolism, increasing primary bile acid fecal excretion and postprandial plasma concentrations, while having the opposite effect on secondary bile acids; peripheral insulin sensitivity was decreased after vancomycin treatment ($p<0.05$), but was unchanged after amoxicillin. Probably owing to the short treatment duration, the authors did not observe any effects on body weight or BMI.

3.5 Pre-/Probiotic Intervention Studies

Available observational data show a correlation between fiber intake, microbial population diversity, and bacterial metabolic signatures [16]. A 2013 interventional study performed on 30 obese women treated with prebiotic inulin-type fructans (inulin/oligofructose 50/50 mix) or placebo for 3 months, showed a statistically significant increase in *Bifidobacterium* (Actinobacteria) and *Faecalibacterium prausnitzii* (Firmicutes). Both bacteria negatively correlated with serum lipopolysaccharide levels. Furthermore, *Bacteroides* species (Bacteroidetes) and *Propionibacterium* (Actinobacteria) decreased. This was associated with a mild decrease in fat mass, although not statistically significant; BMI and waist-hip ratio remained unchanged [37]. The treatment did not have any significant effect on metabolic parameters such as fasting glucose, insulin, cholesterol, triglycerides, and plasma CRP; post oral glucose tolerance test glycemia showed some improvement in the prebiotic group. Treatment period could be too short for accurately reflecting changes in body composition and mass.

The anti-obesity effects of probiotic preparations have been studied in humans in some extent. A randomized, double-blind, crossover trial examined the effects on satiety of a dairy beverage containing propionic acid obtained by fermentation, in a population of healthy, lean women [51]. The beverage was fermented with *Lactobacillus acidophilus* (Firmicutes) and *Propionibacterium freudenreichii* (Actinobacteria), the latter being a propionate-producing species. Each subject consumed the fermented beverage, a non-fermented placebo, and a non-fermented beverage with addition of 0.6 % calcium propionate (positive control) once a week in a randomized order; 25 min later a standardized meal was provided and appetite profile measurements were performed before, during, and after lunch. While food consumption was similar irrespective of the type of beverage, subjects reported higher satiety and less hunger and had less desire to eat after consuming the fermented dairy beverage or the positive control propionate-rich beverage compared with the placebo. These effects seemed attributable to the propionate content of such preparations and thus to the metabolites of *P. freudenreichii*; whether the effects were mediated by sensory or metabolic mechanisms (or mixed), they seemed to occur within 2 min from consumption and persisted for over 20 min.

In another double-blind, randomized, placebo-controlled intervention trial, Kadooka et al. administered fermented milk containing *Lactobacillus gasseri* SBT2055 (vs. normal fermented milk) to otherwise healthy overweight individuals (BMI between 25 and 30) [52]. At 12 weeks a small but significant decrease in body weight, BMI, waist circumference, and importantly abdominal visceral and subcutaneous fat (-1.4%, -1.5%, -1.8%, -5.8%, and -3.3%, respectively; $p < 0.01$) was observed. This small but measurable effect could suggest a microbiota-driven modulation of adipose tissue metabolism, independently of caloric intake or dietary preference. Despite this, the authors observed an increase in serum high-molecular-weight adiponectin levels in both groups; this suggests a possible effect of fermented milk independently of *L. gasseri*.

In a randomized control trial, *Lactobacillus* was administered daily postoperatively after Roux-en-Y gastric bypass (RNYGB) surgery [53]. Patients were instructed to take 2.4 billion live cells of *Lactobacillus* (species not specified) daily. During follow-up, the probiotic group not only showed a significant reduction in small intestinal bacterial overgrowth (SIBO) but yielded a higher percent excess weight loss than that of the control group: at 3 months excess weight loss was 10 %

higher in the probiotic group (47 % vs. 38 %, respectively). This trend continued but did not maintain statistical significance at 6 months; the 6-month follow-up period is probably too short to permit the long-term effects of such treatments on adiposity. Furthermore, it is possible that the combined antibiotic (cefazolin 2 g) and probiotic treatment primarily influenced the SIBO severity and prevalence in the treated group; SIBO has been correlated to increased intestinal permeability and endotoxemia with cytokine release, contributing to systemic inflammation and insulin resistance, thus influencing lipid metabolism and weight loss [54].

A very recent randomized placebo control trial on obese postmenopausal women that primarily evaluated the short-term (6 weeks) effects of probiotic (*L. paracasei* F19) or prebiotic (flaxseed mucilage) formulations on metabolic status and gut microbiota serves to illustrate further this point. In this trial, comparison of microbiota composition at baseline and at 6 weeks of intervention with *L. paracasei F19* showed an increased abundance for *Eubacterium rectale* and *Ruminococcus torques* (Firmicutes). On the other hand, intervention with flaxseed mucilage showed even richer overall effects on bacterial populations, with decrease in the relative abundance of multiple *F. prausnitzii* strains and *Ruminococcus lactaris* (Firmicutes) but increases in other Clostridia (Firmicutes), *Bilophila* (Proteobacteria), and *Parabacteroides* (Bacteroidetes). In the placebo group also some changes in abundance were seen: *Roseburia hominis* and two Clostridiales (Firmicutes) decreased, while relative abundance of *Eubacterium ventriosum* (Firmicutes) increased. Bacterial gene counts decreased in the prebiotic group, though not significantly over placebo; they remained constant in the probiotic group. While some beneficial metabolic effects were seen, notably on insulin sensitivity, those were limited to the prebiotic intervention group. These results seem to suggest some very early modulating effects on gut microbiome following pro-/prebiotic administration, not always accompanied by metabolic host response. However, considering the observed changes in gut microbiota composition in the placebo group also, the brief intervention time, the swift metabolic response limited to the prebiotic group, and the previously known properties of mucilage (delayed gastric emptying, inhibition of nutrient absorption, improvement on metabolic markers), the authors concluded that any effects were not likely correlated to changes in abundance of microbial species [55].

3.6 Surgical Intervention Studies

Bariatric surgery has been shown to be moderately effective in inducing long-term weight loss in severely obese patients, primarily by reducing intake volumes, accelerating GI transit times, and inducing a "malabsorptive" status. Some data are available on the modifications of the gut microbiome following bariatric surgery.

Roux-en-Y gastric bypass (RYGB) procedure performed on 30 obese subjects (27 women and three men), with a BMI ≥ 40 kg/m^2 and at least two comorbidities (hypertension, type 2 diabetes, dyslipidemia, or obstructive sleep apnea syndrome), has been shown to affect profoundly the composition of fecal microbiota [56]. When compared to healthy lean controls, obese subjects before surgery showed lower Bacteroidetes concentrations, mainly due to lower counts of the *Bacteroides/Prevotella* group ($p < 0.05$), while other phyla and groups were similarly represented (Firmicutes were marginally more abundant but not significantly so). Only in the subgroup of obese diabetics did *Faecalibacterium prausnitzii* show significantly lower counts ($p < 0.05$). Significant decrease in body weight, fat mass, BMI, and adipocyte cell diameter at 3 and 6 months from surgery was paralleled by changes in the bacterial community, both at the phylum and at the species level. The *Bacteroides/Prevotella* group promptly increased at 3 months and remained at 6 months close to levels similar to those of lean subjects; it was negatively correlated to BMI, body weight, fat mass, and leptin serum levels, probably reflecting an adaptation to a lower caloric intake in post-surgery. An inverse pattern emerged in the case of *Escherichia coli* (Proteobacteria) during follow-up, with this species reaching higher counts than in controls, maybe due to increased transit and lack of an efficient acid barrier; however, it showed a negative correlation to leptin serum levels (Rs, -0.53; $P < 0.001$) and no correlation to caloric intake. *Bifidobacterium* abundance, while similar between groups at baseline, decreased after surgery, positively correlating to weight, fat mass, and leptin serum levels. *Faecalibacterium prausnitzii* increased and was negatively correlated to inflammatory markers in all groups, independently of caloric intake or BMI. Among the Firmicutes, the *Lactob acillus/Leuconostoc/Pediococcus* group showed some reduction, but this attained significance only in the obese/nondiabetic group. No antibiotics were taken before surgery or during the post-surgery period. Proton pump inhibitors (PPI) were administered during the first trimester. Antidiabetic drugs were stopped after the first trimester in all diabetic subjects due to the observed amelioration of blood glucose control. Importantly, though BMI significantly decreased, subjects remained obese at 6 months. Furthermore, changes in bacterial populations were promptly established by the third month, remaining stable at 6 months, while anthropometric parameters continued to improve throughout the entire follow-up period. This strengthens the hypothesis that shifts in microbiota composition reflect primarily an adaptive response to reduced energy intake, as one would expect from caloric restriction alone during dietary intervention in obesity [12]. However, some difference was independent of caloric intake and could have specific roles in metabolic or inflammatory status modulation. The study did account for caloric intake; however, it failed to take into account dietary data as prebiotic and probiotic properties of some functional foods could influence microbiota composition. PPI treatment in the first trimester, as well as overall reduction of acid flux in the gut, could drive some adaptive response on the intestinal flora. Also, the short-term 6-month follow-up is not very informative on the long-term stability of the observed shifting patterns and their effect on host metabolism.

A later study from the same group on the same population of patients and controls used pyrosequencing techniques to improve methodology and examine additional effects, also including potential associations to white adipose tissue (WAT) gene expression [57]. A total of 58 genera, undetectable before RYGB, were detected during follow-up in all patients. Of these, 37 % belonged to the phylum Proteobacteria with several species being initially isolated from the periodontal environment (*Aggregatibacter*, *Filifactor*, and *Pyramidobacter*), from the oral cavity (*Leptotrichia*), and from the oropharynx (*Cardiobacterium*, *Cryptobacterium*, *Kingella*), enhancing gut microbiota richness already at 3 months after RYGB. This is likely due to the absence of an acid barrier and a rapid GI transit. Principal component analysis showed that the bacterial profiles before RYGB significantly differed from those at 3 and 6 months of follow-up, with 8.1 % of the variance being explained by the procedure effects. A total of 14 bacterial genera significantly changed after RYGB, 7 of which were considered dominant ($\geq$1 % of obtained gut microbiota sequences). Firmicutes, such as *Lactobacillus*, *Dorea*, and *Blautia*, as well as *Bifidobacterium* (Actinobacteria), decreased; *Bacteroides* and *Alistipes* (Bacteroidetes), as well as *Escherichia* (Proteobacteria) increased. The remaining seven were subdominant genera, namely, *Turicibacter*, *Filifactor*, *Gemella*, *Peptostreptococcus* (Firmicutes), *Neisseria*, *Phenylobacterium*, and *Campylobacter* (Proteobacteria). No significant difference in overall composition was found between 3 and 6 months, although some genera returned to baseline values by 6 months. Variations in 13 of those bacterial genera were correlated with changes in total caloric intake and at least one marker related to body composition; after adjusting for energy input, half of those correlations (from eight genera) remained significant. Notably a positive association to body weight and/or BMI and/or fat mass remained significant for *Bifidobacterium* (Actinobacteria) and *Dorea* (Firmicutes), while a negative one for *Bacteroides* and *Alistipes* (Bacteroidetes). The previously reported *E. coli* correlation to leptin serum levels was not confirmed after adjustment for energy input, although this time it was associated to WAT gene activation. Before RYGB, only 8 WAT genes correlated to 28 bacterial genera, whereas at 3 months from surgery, 562 WAT genes correlated to 102 bacterial genera. Each bacterial genus correlated with no less than 28 WAT genes. Most gene correlations were attributed to *Lactobacillus*, which correlated with 71 WAT genes, followed by *Escherichia* (66 genes), *Blautia* (64 genes), *Alistipes* (61 genes), *Turicibacter* (52 genes), *Phenylobacterium* (50 genes), *Dorea* (38 genes), *Bacteroides* (36 genes), *Filifactor* (33 genes), *Peptostreptococcus* (33 genes), *Bifidobacterium* (30 genes), *Campylobacter* (30 genes), *Gemella* (28 genes), and *Neisseria* (28 genes). After adjustment for caloric intake, 51.8 % (320/620) of these correlations remained significant. The increased periodontal bacterial genera were not correlated with WAT genes. Upregulated genes belonged to transforming growth factor-b (TGF-b) signaling pathway, while most downregulated genes belonged to metabolic pathways (such as 24-dehydrocholesterol reductase). Although the less detailed RT-PCR technique was replaced by the more powerful pyrosequencing in this later study, the shortcomings of such a short follow-up period remain.

However, another team [58] analyzing fecal samples from six morbidly obese patients (BMI, $\geq$40 kg/m^2), five of them affected by type 2 diabetes mellitus, taken before and 3 months after RYGB, reached somewhat different conclusions. They found that in the postoperative period, both Firmicutes and Bacteroidetes diminished significantly, the ratio between them increasing, as shown in previous studies; Actinobacteria (containing *Bifidobacterium*) also decreased. Proteobacteria (containing *Escherichia* and *Klebsiella*) and Verrucomicrobia (containing *Akkermansia*), on the other hand, increased substantially. *Faecalibacterium prausnitzii* decreased substantially (70%, $p=0.013$), being directly correlated to inflammatory markers. Mainly associated with BMI and C-reactive protein reduction were increased numbers of *Enterobacter cancerogenus* (Proteobacteria) and decreased *Faecalibacterium prausnitzii* and *Coprococcus comes* (Firmicutes). Notably, most species and genera reported to significantly change after surgery differed from those reported by Furet et al., thus highlighting possible effects of concomitant treatments (PPI, antibiotics), methodology, or technology used.

Possible confounders of the previous studies could include the prominent use of antidiabetic medications that could interfere with some bacterial species or genera; for instance, an association between metformin and *Clostridium botulinum* has been previously reported [20].

3.7   Fecal Transplant Intervention Studies

Currently, fecal transplant treatments are clinically indicated solely for the treatment of relapsing or severe *Clostridium difficile* colitis [59]. It has also been proposed as a treatment for severe or relapsing forms of ulcerative colitis [60]. A single 2012 brief report, exploring insulin sensitivity modification by fecal microbiota transplant (FMT) from lean donors to metabolic syndrome patients ($n=9$) vs. autologous transplant ($n=9$), found an improvement of peripheral insulin resistance 6 weeks after allogeneic gut microbiota infusion. Gut microbial diversity increased after FMT, boosting butyrate-producing *Roseburia intestinalis* and other Firmicutes. On the other hand, fecal butyrate and other SCFA concentrations, recognized as important for energy and signaling purposes in both the enteric and the colonic epithelium, significantly decreased. However, no differences in weight, BMI, body fat mass, or resting energy expenditure were observed [61].

In a recent report [62], a mildly overweight woman diagnosed with *Clostridium difficile* infection resistant to multiple antibiotic courses became obese (BMI = 34.5), 36 months after successful FMT. The donor was the patient's daughter, aged 16, herself overweight at the time of FMT and subsequently obese (BMI = 33) but otherwise healthy. The recipient was previously treated multiple times with metronidazole and vancomycin; she also received triple and quadruple therapy for *H. pylori* infection (outcome not reported). Weight gain could be at least partially attributed to CDI resolution, multiple antibiotic treatments, and presumable *H. pylori* eradication; however, both donor and recipient experienced weight gain almost simultaneously, the patient furthermore reporting scarce effectiveness of adopted dietary and exercise regimens. Unfortunately, microbiota compositions were not determined.

Conclusion

The gut microbiota is involved in the development of obesity through energy harvest and communication with both inflammatory and metabolic cascades via microbial metabolites and by interaction with the brain-gut axis. The most prominent issue in the context of the studies of the gut microbiome and its interactions with health and disease is to infer causality: resident bacterial populations are complex ecosystems that establish intricate and often fragile relationships within their members and the environment. Thus, any change in metabolic, immune, hormonal, pharmacological, or dietary status, among others, could in principle drive microbiota adaptation. It is not always as clear, however, whether and to which degree the gut microbiota can trigger disease or if its observed changes are merely a consequence.

In the specific case of obesity and adipose tissue modulation, what seems better established is that at least a subset of obese subjects show specific signatures in relative abundances of bacterial phyla and that the microbial metabolic functions affected have been correlated to systemic metabolic effects on inflammatory response and lipid and glucose metabolism. Moreover, microbial populations rapidly respond even to short-term dietary interventions, probably adapting to the new energy and substrate environment available. Whether these responses have specific metabolic outcomes is still the subject of research. Short-term trial protocols are intrinsically hardly able to detect adipose tissue changes; thus, long-term trials are needed. This is also the case for antibiotic intervention studies. Probiotics and prebiotics are promising; however, the direct effects of such treatments on gastric emptying, intestinal motility, absorption, mucosal inflammation, and modulation of satiety are not to be underestimated as possible confounding factors. Similarly, bariatric intervention studies suffer mainly from the inevitable concomitant changes in dietary habits that render questionable causal interpretations.

Although crucial information on the structure and balance of microbial populations in obese and lean individuals are to some extent well established, studies are characterized by significant variability of results. Differences in the fecal sampling techniques used, methodological differences in DNA extraction and primer design, and differences in individuals' habits, including body exercise and smoking, could account for some of the observed differences between reported results. The main source of information for the putative connection between obesity and the gut microbiome in humans is observational studies, especially those involving lean subjects as controls; intervention studies evaluating the long-term effects on microbiota modulation are needed.

Advances in methodology, increasing quality of established protocols, and technique availability are promising in widening the possibilities for original research and possible development of therapeutic tools for a wide range of metabolic disturbances by simple and safe targeted modulation of the human gut microbiome.

References

1. Bäckhed F, Ding H, Wang T, Hooper LV, Koh GY, Nagy A, Semenkovich CF, Gordon JI (2004) The gut microbiota as an environmental factor that regulates fat storage. Proc Natl Acad Sci U S A 101(44):15718–15723
2. Bäckhed F, Manchester JK, Semenkovich CF, Gordon JI (2007) Mechanisms underlying the resistance to diet-induced obesity in germ-free mice. Proc Natl Acad Sci U S A 104(3): 979–984

3. Cani PD, Amar J, Iglesias MA, Poggi M, Knauf C, Bastelica D, Neyrinck AM, Fava F, Tuohy KM, Chabo C, Waget A, Delmée E, Cousin B, Sulpice T, Chamontin B, Ferrières J, Tanti JF, Gibson GR, Casteilla L, Delzenne NM, Alessi MC, Burcelin R (2007) Metabolic endotoxemia initiates obesity and insulin resistance. Diabetes 56(7):1761–1772
4. Amar J, Burcelin R, Ruidavets JB, Cani PD, Fauvel J, Alessi MC, Chamontin B, Ferriéres J (2008) Energy intake is associated with endotoxemia in apparently healthy men. Am J Clin Nutr 87(5):1219–1223
5. Wilson KH, Blitchington RB (1996) Human colonic biota studied by ribosomal DNA sequence analysis. Appl Environ Microbiol 62(7):2273–2278
6. Suau A, Bonnet R, Sutren M, Godon JJ, Gibson GR, Collins MD, Doré J (1999) Direct analysis of genes encoding 16S rRNA from complex communities reveals many novel molecular species within the human gut. Appl Environ Microbiol 65(11):4799–4807
7. Hold GL, Pryde SE, Russell VJ, Furrie E, Flint HJ (2002) Assessment of microbial diversity in human colonic samples by 16S rDNA sequence analysis. FEMS Microbiol Ecol 39(1):33–39
8. Eckburg PB, Bik EM, Bernstein CN, Purdom E, Dethlefsen L, Sargent M, Gill SR, Nelson KE, Relman DA (2005) Diversity of the human intestinal microbial flora. Science 308(5728):1635–1638
9. Musilova S, Rada V, Vlkova E, Bunesova V, Nevoral J (2015) Colonisation of the gut by bifidobacteria is much more common in vaginal deliveries than caesarean sections. Acta Paediatr 104(4):e184–6
10. Mariat D, Firmesse O, Levenez F, Guimaräes V, Sokol H, Doré J, Corthier G, Furet JP (2009) The Firmicutes/Bacteroidetes ratio of the human microbiota changes with age. BMC Microbiol 9:123
11. Palmer C, Bik EM, DiGiulio DB, Relman DA, Brown PO (2007) Development of the human infant intestinal microbiota. PLoS Biol 5(7):e177
12. Ley RE, Turnbaugh PJ, Klein S, Gordon JI (2006) Microbial ecology: human gut microbes associated with obesity. Nature 444(7122):1022–1023
13. Kalliomäki M, Collado MC, Salminen S, Isolauri E (2008) Early differences in fecal microbiota composition in children may predict overweight. Am J Clin Nutr 87(3):534–538
14. Turnbaugh PJ, Hamady M, Yatsunenko T, Cantarel BL, Duncan A, Ley RE, Sogin ML, Jones WJ, Roe BA, Affourtit JP, Egholm M, Henrissat B, Heath AC, Knight R, Gordon JI (2009) A core gut microbiome in obese and lean twins. Nature 457(7228):480–484
15. De Filippo C, Cavalieri D, Di Paola M, Ramazzotti M, Poullet JB, Massart S, Collini S, Pieraccini G, Lionetti P (2010) Impact of diet in shaping gut microbiota revealed by a comparative study in children from Europe and rural Africa. Proc Natl Acad Sci U S A 107(33):14691–14696
16. Santacruz A, Collado MC, García-Valdés L, Segura MT, Martín-Lagos JA, Anjos T, Martí-Romero M, Lopez RM, Florido J, Campoy C, Sanz Y (2010) Gut microbiota composition is associated with body weight, weight gain and biochemical parameters in pregnant women. Br J Nutr 104(1):83–92
17. Collado MC, Isolauri E, Laitinen K, Salminen S (2008) Distinct composition of gut microbiota during pregnancy in overweight and normal-weight women. Am J Clin Nutr 88(4):894–899
18. Munukka E, Wiklund P, Pekkala S, Völgyi E, Xu L, Cheng S, Lyytikäinen A, Marjomäki V, Alen M, Vaahtovuo J, Keinänen-Kiukaanniemi S, Cheng S (2012) Women with and without metabolic disorder differ in their gut microbiota composition. Obesity (Silver Spring) 20(5):1082–1087
19. Karlsson FH, Tremaroli V, Nookaew I, Bergström G, Behre CJ, Fagerberg B, Nielsen J, Bäckhed F (2013) Gut metagenome in European women with normal, impaired and diabetic glucose control. Nature 498(7452):99–103
20. Le Chatelier E, Nielsen T, Qin J, Prifti E, Hildebrand F, Falony G, Almeida M, Arumugam M, Batto JM, Kennedy S, Leonard P, Li J, Burgdorf K, Grarup N, Jørgensen T, Brandslund I, Nielsen HB, Juncker AS, Bertalan M, Levenez F, Pons N, Rasmussen S, Sunagawa S, Tap J, Tims S, Zoetendal EG, Brunak S, Clément K, Doré J, Kleerebezem M, Kristiansen K, Renault P, Sicheritz-Ponten T, de Vos WM, Zucker JD, Raes J, Hansen T, MetaHIT consortium, Bork

P, Wang J, Ehrlich SD, Pedersen O (2013) Richness of human gut microbiome correlates with metabolic markers. Nature 500(7464):541–546

21. Duncan SH, Lobley GE, Holtrop G, Ince J, Johnstone AM, Louis P, Flint HJ (2008) Human colonic microbiota associated with diet, obesity and weight loss. Int J Obes (Lond) 32(11):1720–1724

22. Armougom F, Henry M, Vialettes B, Raccah D, Raoult D (2009) Monitoring bacterial community of human gut microbiota reveals an increase in Lactobacillus in obese patients and Methanogens in anorexic patients. PLoS One 4(9):e7125

23. Schwiertz A, Taras D, Schäfer K, Beijer S, Bos NA, Donus C, Hardt PD (2010) Microbiota and SCFA in lean and overweight healthy subjects. Obesity (Silver Spring) 18(1):190–195

24. Arumugam M, Raes J, Pelletier E, Le Paslier D, Yamada T, Mende DR, Fernandes GR, Tap J, Bruls T, Batto JM, Bertalan M, Borruel N, Casellas F, Fernandez L, Gautier L, Hansen T, Hattori M, Hayashi T, Kleerebezem M, Kurokawa K, Leclerc M, Levenez F, Manichanh C, Nielsen HB, Nielsen T, Pons N, Poulain J, Qin J, Sicheritz-Ponten T, Tims S, Torrents D, Ugarte E, Zoetendal EG, Wang J, Guarner F, Pedersen O, de Vos WM, Brunak S, Doré J, MetaHIT Consortium, Antolín M, Artiguenave F, Blottiere HM, Almeida M, Brechot C, Cara C, Chervaux C, Cultrone A, Delorme C, Denariaz G, Dervyn R, Foerstner KU, Friss C, van de Guchte M, Guedon E, Haimet F, Huber W, van Hylckama-Vlieg J, Jamet A, Juste C, Kaci G, Knol J, Lakhdari O, Layec S, Le Roux K, Maguin E, Mérieux A, Melo Minardi R, M'rini C, Muller J, Oozeer R, Parkhill J, Renault P, Rescigno M, Sanchez N, Sunagawa S, Torrejon A, Turner K, Vandemeulebrouck G, Varela E, Winogradsky Y, Zeller G, Weissenbach J, Ehrlich SD, Bork P (2011) Enterotypes of the human gut microbiome. Nature 473(7346):174–180

25. Human Microbiome Project Consortium (2012) Structure, function and diversity of the healthy human microbiome. Nature 486(7402):207–214

26. Million M, Maraninchi M, Henry M, Armougom F, Richet H, Carrieri P, Valero R, Raccah D, Vialettes B, Raoult D (2012) Obesity-associated gut microbiota is enriched in Lactobacillus reuteri and depleted in Bifidobacterium animalis and Methanobrevibacter smithii. Int J Obes (Lond) 36(6):817–825

27. Zuo HJ, Xie ZM, Zhang WW, Li YR, Wang W, Ding XB, Pei XF (2011) Gut bacteria alteration in obese people and its relationship with gene polymorphism. World J Gastroenterol 17(8):1076–1081

28. Finucane MM, Sharpton TJ, Laurent TJ, Pollard KS (2014) A taxonomic signature of obesity in the microbiome? Getting to the guts of the matter. PLoS One 9(1):e84689

29. Human Microbiome Project Consortium (2012) A framework for human microbiome research. Nature 486(7402):215–221

30. Qin J, Li R, Raes J, Arumugam M, Burgdorf KS, Manichanh C, Nielsen T, Pons N, Levenez F, Yamada T, Mende DR, Li J, Xu J, Li S, Li D, Cao J, Wang B, Liang H, Zheng H, Xie Y, Tap J, Lepage P, Bertalan M, Batto JM, Hansen T, Le Paslier D, Linneberg A, Nielsen HB, Pelletier E, Renault P, Sicheritz-Ponten T, Turner K, Zhu H, Yu C, Li S, Jian M, Zhou Y, Li Y, Zhang X, Li S, Qin N, Yang H, Wang J, Brunak S, Doré J, Guarner F, Kristiansen K, Pedersen O, Parkhill J, Weissenbach J, MetaHIT Consortium, Bork P, Ehrlich SD, Wang J (2010) A human gut microbial gene catalogue established by metagenomic sequencing. Nature 464(7285):59–65

31. Suzuki TA, Worobey M (2014) Geographical variation of human gut microbial composition. Biol Lett 10(2):20131037

32. Roberts DF (1953) Body weight, race and climate. Am J Phys Anthropol 11:533–558

33. Koren O, Goodrich JK, Cullender TC, Spor A, Laitinen K, Bäckhed HK, Gonzalez A, Werner JJ, Angenent LT, Knight R, Bäckhed F, Isolauri E, Salminen S, Ley RE (2012) Host remodeling of the gut microbiome and metabolic changes during pregnancy. Cell 150(3):470–480. doi:10.1016/j.cell.2012.07.008

34. Jumpertz R, Le DS, Turnbaugh PJ, Trinidad C, Bogardus C, Gordon JI, Krakoff J (2011) Energy-balance studies reveal associations between gut microbes, caloric load, and nutrient absorption in humans. Am J Clin Nutr 94(1):58–65. doi:10.3945/ajcn.110.010132

35. Hoyles L, McCartney AL (2009) What do we mean when we refer to Bacteroidetes populations in the human gastrointestinal microbiota? FEMS Microbiol Lett 299(2):175–183
36. Biedermann L, Zeitz J, Mwinyi J, Sutter-Minder E, Rehman A, Ott SJ, Steurer-Stey C, Frei A, Frei P, Scharl M, Loessner MJ, Vavricka SR, Fried M, Schreiber S, Schuppler M, Rogler G (2013) Smoking cessation induces profound changes in the composition of the intestinal microbiota in humans. PLoS One 8(3):e59260
37. Dewulf EM, Cani PD, Claus SP, Fuentes S, Puylaert PG, Neyrinck AM, Bindels LB, de Vos WM, Gibson GR, Thissen JP, Delzenne NM (2013) Insight into the prebiotic concept: lessons from an exploratory, double blind intervention study with inulin-type fructans in obese women. Gut 62(8):1112–1121
38. Lattimer JM, Haub MD (2010) Effects of dietary fiber and its components on metabolic health. Nutrients 2(12):1266–1289
39. Wu GD, Chen J, Hoffmann C, Bittinger K, Chen YY, Keilbaugh SA, Bewtra M, Knights D, Walters WA, Knight R, Sinha R, Gilroy E, Gupta K, Baldassano R, Nessel L, Li H, Bushman FD, Lewis JD (2011) Linking long-term dietary patterns with gut microbial enterotypes. Science 334(6052):105–108
40. Nadal I, Santacruz A, Marcos A, Warnberg J, Garagorri JM, Moreno LA, Martin-Matillas M, Campoy C, Martí A, Moleres A, Delgado M, Veiga OL, García-Fuentes M, Redondo CG, Sanz Y (2009) Shifts in clostridia, bacteroides and immunoglobulin-coating fecal bacteria associated with weight loss in obese adolescents. Int J Obes (Lond) 33(7):758–767
41. Clarke SF, Murphy EF, O'Sullivan O, Lucey AJ, Humphreys M, Hogan A, Hayes P, O'Reilly M, Jeffery IB, Wood-Martin R, Kerins DM, Quigley E, Ross RP, O'Toole PW, Molloy MG, Falvey E, Shanahan F, Cotter PD (2014) Exercise and associated dietary extremes impact on gut microbial diversity. Gut 63(12):1913–1920
42. Hao H, Cheng G, Iqbal Z, Ai X, Hussain HI, Huang L, Dai M, Wang Y, Liu Z, Yuan Z (2014) Benefits and risks of antimicrobial use in food-producing animals. Front Microbiol 5:288
43. Brüssow H (2015) Growth promotion and gut microbiota: insights from antibiotic use. Environ Microbiol 17(7):2216–2227
44. De La Cochetière MF, Durand T, Lepage P, Bourreille A, Galmiche JP, Doré J (2005) Resilience of the dominant human fecal microbiota upon short-course antibiotic challenge. J Clin Microbiol 43(11):5588–5592
45. Jakobsson HE, Jernberg C, Andersson AF, Sjölund-Karlsson M, Jansson JK, Engstrand L (2010) Short-term antibiotic treatment has differing long-term impacts on the human throat and gut microbiome. PLoS One 5(3):e9836
46. Dethlefsen L, Relman DA (2011) Incomplete recovery and individualized responses of the human distal gut microbiota to repeated antibiotic perturbation. Proc Natl Acad Sci U S A 108(Suppl 1):4554–4561
47. Pérez-Cobas AE, Gosalbes MJ, Friedrichs A, Knecht H, Artacho A, Eismann K, Otto W, Rojo D, Bargiela R, von Bergen M, Neulinger SC, Däumer C, Heinsen FA, Latorre A, Barbas C, Seifert J, dos Santos VM, Ott SJ, Ferrer M, Moya A (2013) Gut microbiota disturbance during antibiotic therapy: a multi-omic approach. Gut 62(11):1591–1601
48. Thuny F, Richet H, Casalta JP, Angelakis E, Habib G, Raoult D (2010) Vancomycin treatment of infective endocarditis is linked with recently acquired obesity. PLoS One 5(2):e9074
49. Million M, Angelakis E, Paul M, Armougom F, Leibovici L, Raoult D (2012) Comparative meta-analysis of the effect of Lactobacillus species on weight gain in humans and animals. Microb Pathog 53(2):100–108
50. Vrieze A, Out C, Fuentes S, Jonker L, Reuling I, Kootte RS, van Nood E, Holleman F, Knaapen M, Romijn JA, Soeters MR, Blaak EE, Dallinga-Thie GM, Reijnders D, Ackermans MT, Serlie MJ, Knop FK, Holst JJ, van der Ley C, Kema IP, Zoetendal EG, de Vos WM, Hoekstra JB, Stroes ES, Groen AK, Nieuwdorp M (2014) Impact of oral vancomycin on gut microbiota, bile acid metabolism, and insulin sensitivity. J Hepatol 60(4):824–831
51. Ruijschop RMAJ, Boelrijk AEM, te Giffel MC (2008) Satiety effects of a dairy beverage fermented with propionic acid bacteria. Int Dairy J 18(9):945–950

52. Kadooka Y, Sato M, Imaizumi K, Ogawa A, Ikuyama K, Akai Y, Okano M, Kagoshima M, Tsuchida T (2010) Regulation of abdominal adiposity by probiotics (Lactobacillus gasseri SBT2055) in adults with obese tendencies in a randomized controlled trial. Eur J Clin Nutr 64(6):636–643

53. Woodard GA, Encarnacion B, Downey JR, Peraza J, Chong K, Hernandez-Boussard T, Morton JM (2009) Probiotics improve outcomes after Roux-en-Y gastric bypass surgery: a prospective randomized trial. J Gastrointest Surg 13(7):1198–1204

54. Ferolla SM, Armiliato GN, Couto CA, Ferrari TC (2014) The role of intestinal bacteria overgrowth in obesity-related nonalcoholic fatty liver disease. Nutrients 6(12):5583–5599

55. Brahe LK, Le Chatelier E, Prifti E, Pons N, Kennedy S, Blædel T, Håkansson J, Dalsgaard TK, Hansen T, Pedersen O, Astrup A, Ehrlich SD, Larsen LH (2015) Dietary modulation of the gut microbiota: a randomised controlled trial in obese postmenopausal women. Br J Nutr 114(3):406–417

56. Furet JP, Kong LC, Tap J, Poitou C, Basdevant A, Bouillot JL, Mariat D, Corthier G, Doré J, Henegar C, Rizkalla S, Clément K (2010) Differential adaptation of human gut microbiota to bariatric surgery–induced weight loss: links with metabolic and low-grade inflammation markers. Diabetes 59(12):3049–3057

57. Kong LC, Tap J, Aron-Wisnewsky J, Pelloux V, Basdevant A, Bouillot JL, Zucker JD, Doré J, Clément K (2013) Gut microbiota after gastric bypass in human obesity: increased richness and associations of bacterial genera with adipose tissue genes. Am J Clin Nutr 98(1):16–24

58. Graessler J, Qin Y, Zhong H, Zhang J, Licinio J, Wong ML, Xu A, Chavakis T, Bornstein AB, Ehrhart-Bornstein M, Lamounier-Zepter V, Lohmann T, Wolf T, Bornstein SR (2013) Metagenomic sequencing of the human gut microbiome before and after bariatric surgery in obese patients with type 2 diabetes: correlation with inflammatory and metabolic parameters. Pharmacogenomics J 13(6):514–522

59. Kassam Z, Lee CH, Yuan Y, Hunt RH (2013) Fecal microbiota transplantation for Clostridium difficile infection: systematic review and meta-analysis. Am J Gastroenterol 108(4):500–508

60. Sha S, Liang J, Chen M, Xu B, Liang C, Wei N, Wu K (2014) Systematic review: faecal microbiota transplantation therapy for digestive and nondigestive disorders in adults and children. Aliment Pharmacol Ther 39(10):1003–1032

61. Vrieze A, Van Nood E, Holleman F, Salojärvi J, Kootte RS, Bartelsman JF, Dallinga-Thie GM, Ackermans MT, Serlie MJ, Oozeer R, Derrien M, Druesne A, Van Hylckama Vlieg JE, Bloks VW, Groen AK, Heilig HG, Zoetendal EG, Stroes ES, de Vos WM, Hoekstra JB, Nieuwdorp M (2012) Transfer of intestinal microbiota from lean donors increases insulin sensitivity in individuals with metabolic syndrome. Gastroenterology 143(4):913–916.e7

62. Alang N, Kelly CR (2015) Weight gain after fecal microbiota transplantation. Open Forum Infect Dis 4;2(1):ofv004

Gut–Brain Axis: A New Revolution to Understand the Pathogenesis of Autism and Other Severe Neurological Diseases

4

Laura de Magistris, Dario Siniscalco, Carmela Bravaccio, and Carmelina Loguercio

The gut–brain axis (GBA) is a complex communication network interfacing the gut and the brain of a single individual. The central (CNS) and enteric (ENS) nervous systems are, of course, communicating; however, other pathways are involved in GBA, among which are immune activation, intestinal barrier function, and entero-endocrine signaling. All these communication lines are bidirectional and involve neuro-immuno-endocrine mediators [1]. The reason for the development of such a complex network is to maintain gastrointestinal homeostasis keeping in mind its links with cognitive and affective functions [2]. Recently, the role of enteric flora, or microbiota, has been recognized as a part of the gut–brain axis [1, 3]. The gut microbiota can modulate brain function, forming a crucial link in the bidirectional interactions between the intestine and the nervous system [4] (Figs. 4.1 and 4.2).

Recognition of GBA implies that the GI tract and, of course, the ingested food [5] are most probably involved – either primarily or as secondary effect – in neuro-logical/neuropsychiatric disorders [6], among which are autism [7, 8], schizophrenia [9], and Parkinson's disease [10, 11]. On the other hand, it is well recognized that almost all gastrointestinal diseases may have neurological comorbidities/complications. Untreated celiac disease is associated to autistic and psychotic behaviors and neurologic complications [12] besides intestinal mucosal inflammation, increased intestinal permeability, increased absorption, and urinary excretion of neuroactive dietary peptides. Non-celiac gluten sensitivity (NCGS), besides GI symptoms, is characterized by extra-gastrointestinal and neurological symptoms

L. de Magistris (✉) • C. Loguercio
Department of Magrassi-Lanzara, Second University of Naples – SUN, Naples, Italy
e-mail: aura.demagistris@unina2.it

D. Siniscalco
Department of Experimental Medicine, Second University of Naples – SUN, Naples, Italy

C. Bravaccio
Department of Translational Medical Sciences, Federico II University of Naples, Naples, Italy

© Springer International Publishing Switzerland 2016   49
E. Grossi, F. Pace (eds.), *Human Nutrition from the Gastroenterologist's Perspective*,
DOI 10.1007/978-3-319-30361-1_4

such as migraine/headache, clouded mind, fatigue, and fainting [12, 13]. The precise mechanism(s) of central nervous system damage is not yet known; however, toxicity from the gut and immune activation are pathogenetic forerunners [14]. Hepatic encephalopathy – a variable impairment of cerebral functioning in patients with acute or chronic liver disease – is the result of multiple biochemical influences on central neurotransmitter systems, such as the neurotoxic effects of ammonia, derangements in the gamma-aminobutyric acidergic and serotoninergic systems [15], thus representing a prototypic afferent gut–brain interaction. Another typical example is irritable bowel syndrome (IBS) that is a functional syndrome characterized by chronic abdominal pain accompanied by altered bowel habits. There is a

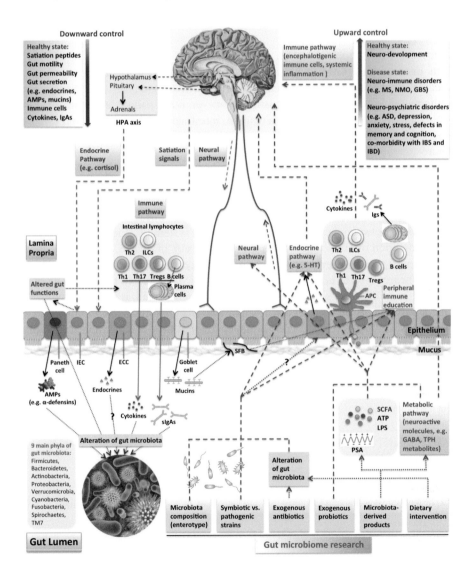

strong interaction between psychiatric disorders – including generalized anxiety disorder, panic disorder, major depressive disorder, bipolar disorder, and schizophrenia – and IBS [16]. Moreover, neuroimaging studies documented changes in the prefrontal cortex, ventrolateral and posterior parietal cortex, and thalami and implicate alteration of brain circuits involved in attention, emotion, and pain modulation [16]. Alterations in the bidirectional interactions between the intestine and the nervous system seem to have important roles in the pathogenesis of irritable bowel syndrome (IBS), and preclinical evidence suggests that the gut microbiota can modulate these interactions. Among other mechanisms, the microbiota could have a role in the dietary habits/restrictions of IBS patients, such as FODMAPs (fermentable oligo-, di-, and monosaccharides and polyols) and GFD (gluten-restricted diets) [4]. The basic hypothetical mechanism underling all these conditions is that neuroactive compounds derived from the intestinal lumen permeate the mucosa, cross the blood–brain barrier, and cause psychiatric, cognitive, and behavioral disturbances. This is supported, for example, by the GI effects of some oral medication administered for psychopathologic conditions, such as selective serotonin reuptake inhibitors (SSRI) and tricyclic antidepressant (TCAs).

4.1 The Second Brain and Enteroendocrine Signaling Pathways

In 1998, Michael Gershon published his most important and worldwide known book [17]; in it the existence of a new scientific branch, namely, *neurogastroenterology*, is ratified.

Fig. 4.1 Microbiota–gut–brain axis in relation to CNS disorders. Multiple pathways guide the downward and upward directions of the microbiota–gut–brain axis in the contexts of health and disease. On the left (*blue arrows*): downwardly, CNS controls gut microbiota composition through satiation signaling peptides that affect nutrient availability and endocrines that affect gut functions and neural pathways. HPA axis release of cortisol regulates gut movement and integrity. Immune (cells, cytokines, and IgAs) pathways can be turned on in response to altered gut functions. Endocrine and neural pathways can also regulate the secretion from specialized gut epithelial cells, including paneth cells, enteroendocrine cells (ECC), and goblet cells. Their secretory products affect the survival and the resident environment of microbiota. On the right (*red arrows*): Upwardly, gut microbiota controls CNS activities through neural (direct activation of neurons by microbiota), endocrine (e.g. ECC release of 5-HT), metabolic (microbiota synthesis of neuroactive molecules), and immune (CNS infiltrating immune cells and systemic inflammation) pathways. Microbiota influences CNS at healthy (neurodevelopment) and disease (a range of neuro-immune and neuro-psychiatric disorders) states. Gut luminal microbiota, their products sampled by APCs, and epithelium-attaching SFBs mediate peripheral immune education. *Abbreviations*: *AMPs* antimicrobial peptides, *TPH* tryptophan, *5-HT* 5-hydroxytryptamine, *SFB* segmented filamentous bacteria, *PSA* polysaccharide A from *B. fragilis*, *ATP* adenosine-5′-triphosphate, *SCFA* short-chain fatty acid, *IEC* intestinal epithelial cell, *ILCs* innate lymphoid cells, *APC* antigen-presenting cell, *MS* multiple sclerosis, *NMO* neuromyelitis optica, *GBS* Guillain-Barré syndrome, *ASD* autism spectrum disorder, *IBS* irritable bowel syndrome, *IBD* inflammatory bowel disease (Source: Wang and Kasper [34]; with permission)

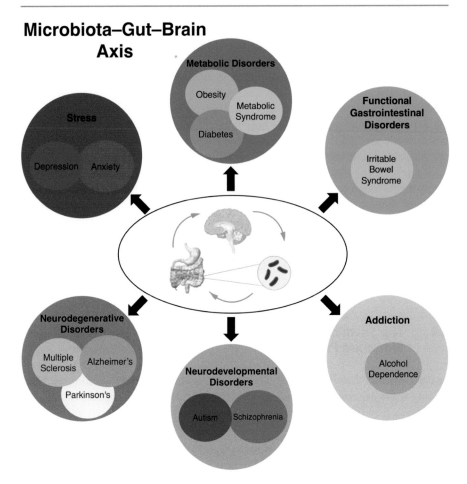

Fig. 4.2 Disorders of the microbiota–gut–brain axis. The microbiota–gut–brain axis plays an important role in maintaining homeostasis, and its dysfunction has been linked to various psychiatric and nonpsychiatric disorders (Source: Burokas et al. [3]; with permission)

Second brain is named the network constituting the autonomous nervous system (ANS), the peripheral nervous system embedded in the walls of the gut which contains something like 100 million neurons, far more than the CNS and spinal cord. This is in strict connection with the "first" brain contributing to determine the mental state and playing key roles in a number of diseases. Gut behavior can in fact be controlled independently by the brain. In the vagus, about 90 % of the fibers constituting the primary visceral nerve carry information from the gut to the brain and much less the other way round. It seems that a big part of our emotions are influenced by the nerves in the gut, like "butterflies in the stomach," as a part of physiological stress response. Both CNS and ANS use a large number of neurotransmitters mostly shared, as, for example, serotonin: more than 90 % of it is found in the bowels. If we use medications like SSRIs or TCAs, besides the antidepressant effects, we will have GI side effects (nausea, altered motility, constipation). In the same way, other treatments thought for mind disorders can unintentionally impact the gut.

Several signaling molecules used for neuronal and neuroendocrine signaling (e.g., catecholamines, serotonin, dynorphin, and cytokines) are also secreted into the gut lumen by neurons, immune cells, and enterochromaffin cells, where the CNS has an important role in the release of these molecules. Also, both norepinephrine and dynorphins are released into the gut lumen during perturbation of homeostasis [1].

Both sympathetic and parasympathetic nervous systems, which are part of the ANS, have a prominent role in the modulation of gut functions, such as motility, secretion of acid, bicarbonates and mucus, intestinal fluids, and mucosal immune response. The ANS also affects epithelial mechanisms involved in immune activation of the gut, either directly, through modulation of the response of the gut immune cells (e.g., macrophages and mast cells) to luminal bacteria, or indirectly, through alteration of the access of luminal bacteria to gut immunocytes [1].

Information coming from the luminal environment (e.g., hyperosmolarity, carbohydrate levels, mechanical distortion of the mucosa, and the presence of cytostatic drugs and bacterial products) is transmitted to the CNS by the vagus nerve. Nerve terminals of vagal afferents are located in close proximity to enterochromaffin cells, and these terminals express the serotonin-specific receptor 5-HT$_3$R. Enterochromaffin cells – present along the gut in large number – are important bidirectional transducers that regulate communication between the gut lumen and the nervous system. Vagal, afferent innervation of enterochromaffin cells provides a direct pathway for enterochromaffin cell signaling to neuronal circuits, which may have an important role in pain and immune response modulation, control of background emotions, and other homeostatic functions. Moreover, the disruption of the bidirectional interactions between the enteric microbiota and the nervous system may be involved in the pathophysiology of acute and chronic gastrointestinal disease states, including functional and inflammatory bowel disorders [17].

The second brain should as well mediate the body's immune response, given that at least 70 % of our immune system is localized in the gut (GALT) and it is in strict contact with autonomous (vagal) nerve fibers. Peripheral outputs of the stress response, in particular glucocorticoids (GCs) and catecholamines, have profound effects on cytokine networks in the gut mucosa. Via its peripheral mediators, stress influences the production of key regulatory type 1 and type 2 cytokines, T helper (Th) 1 and Th2 functions, and components of cellular and humoral immunity. In the healthy organism, both GCs and catecholamines suppress Th1 responses and cellular immunity and shift the immune response toward Th2 responses and humoral immunity [18].

Certain stressful life events have been associated with the onset or symptom exacerbation in some of the most common chronic disorders of the digestive system, including functional gastrointestinal disorders, inflammatory bowel disease, gastroesophageal reflux, and peptic ulcer [18]. Inflammatory cytokines – tumor necrosis factor (TNF-alfa), interleukin IL-1, and IL-6 – cause acute stimulation of the hypothalamic–pituitary–adrenal (HPA) axis alone or in synergy. The cytokine release is mediated through stimulation of corticotropin-releasing hormone (CRH; or corticotropin factor, CRF) and arginine/vasopressin release from hypothalamic neurons and by direct effects at the pituitary and adrenocortical levels. Different mechanisms, including cytokine stimulation of vagal afferents, have been proposed by which the cytokine signal crosses the blood–brain barrier. The ultimate output of peripheral cytokine-stimulated HPA axis activation, plasma cortisol, is the principal negative feedback mediator to shut off both the inflammatory response and HPA axis activation [18].

4.2   Intestinal Barrier

The intestinal luminal mucosa is human's largest surface of contact with the external environment. It acts like a filtering barrier toward food and other substances transiting the gut, preventing them from entering the blood "just like they are." Intestinal barrier is a complex network of epithelial and secretory mechanisms aimed to regulate the crossover of intestinal mucosa. In this contest, the protecting mucous layer, secretion of defensins and mucosal IgA, cell-to-cell junctions (i.e., tight junction), and the resident microbiota have relevant roles [19]. Gut microbiota provides its host with a physical barrier to incoming pathogens by competitive exclusion, consumption of nutrient sources, and production of antimicrobial substances [20].

The various cellular species lining the mucosal surface (epithelium) contribute in different ways to build up such an "intestinal barrier." Among them, enterocytes are the main doors through which the products of hydrolysis of food components enter into the blood (co-transport, diffusion); M cells contribute to transport antigens and microorganisms from the lumen to the inner layers of mucosa, deactivating the dangerous substances during the intracellular transport [19].

The structure of intestinal epithelium resembles that of a polymeric impermeable membrane; it is maintained by positioning its components (cells) in a very precise way [21]; to do this, the junctional complexes linking the cells to their neighbors have a central role. The most apical (toward the lumen) are the tight junctions, often indicated as TJs. These complex structures are constituted by over 50 proteins, some (claudins, occludins, tricellulin) showing extracellular domains – connecting to the corresponding neighbor cell – able to keep close or open the intercellular passage with a sort of zipper mechanism. This intercellular passage is, however, very restricted in physiological conditions of mammals and finely regulated [22]: it is a solvent drug-based absorption site limited to water, ions, and some small molecules (oligopeptides, oligosaccharides) along an electro-chemical gradient, though TJs can open to let vital cells (lymphocytes) cross the mucosa. TJs are dynamic structures sealing paracellular spaces and constantly remodeling under the influence of external and intercellular stimuli, coming from the crosstalk among intestinal epithelial cells, gut content, and commensal microbiota; to do this, signaling proteins, protein phosphorylation, toll-like receptors, etc. are utilized [22].

If one or more components of the polymeric membrane (mucosa) are chronically compromised, damaged, or deregulated, the "leaky gut" condition will be faced. It means that either food components (even indigested) or microorganisms (or part of them) – i.e., any kind of antigenic substances – can unrestrictedly cross the intestinal barrier, enter the inner layer of mucosa, initiate immune reactions, and permit systemic absorption of substances that could adversely affect systemic and/or brain function [19]. A chronic leaky gut condition, interfacing with the individual genetic predisposition, is able to trigger an immune-mediated reaction, as it happens in celiac disease [23] or it was hypothesized in diabetes mellitus type 1 [24].

Evaluation of the state of health of intestinal barrier function plays a critical role in the conditions where a gut-originated "pollution" of the body is suspected, such as NCGS, other alimentary intolerances, or even autism and other neurological disorders. The most common, easy, noninvasive, and harmless way to investigate in vivo the "state of health" of paracellular absorption and TJs is the permeability test. Measuring urinary excretion of orally administered test substances (probes) assesses intestinal permeability [25]. Intestinal permeability resulted in increased presence of intestinal inflammation, as in Crohn disease and celiac disease [26] and in ASDs with and without GI symptoms [27–29].

Intestinal epithelial cells (their functions) are regulated by hormones and cytokines and by external substances, including food components. Food, besides being a supplier of nutrients, is a modulator of the physiological functions of the gut and the body; on this basis, the concept of "functional food" was established. A recent hypothesis puts forward that modern food additives (such as sugars, salt, organic solvents, emulsifiers, gluten, microbial TG, and nanoparticles) increasingly used in the food and beverage industries are a major environmental factor for induction of autoimmune diseases, through a provoked "leaky gut." Such food additives abrogate human epithelial barrier function and increase intestinal permeability through the opening of TJs, resulting in entry of foreign immunogenic antigens and activation of the autoimmune cascade [30].

4.3   Microbiota: Who Is the Host?

The human adult gastrointestinal (GI) tract hosts about 10^{14} microorganisms, that is, ten times more than the cells of the human body. This collectivity is named microbiota. The 500–1,000 different species vary among human populations, alimentary habits, and lifestyles and are also changing during development. The enteric microbiota is distributed in the gut with major quantitative differences along the various tracts (maximal abundance in the colon); in healthy individuals, the two more prominent phyla are *Firmicutes* and *Bacteroides*; it is said that each person's microbiota profile is different, something like a fingerprint. The microbiome (the collective genomes of the microbiota) is 150-folds richer than human genome. A healthy and well-developed microbiota is essential to life as we have learned from experimental studies on germ-free animals. The human microbiota can be looked at "as the interface between genes and individual history of environmental exposures, thus providing new insights into the neurodevelopment and the behavioral phenotypes." Human individuals can thus be considered superorganisms [3, 31].

This microbial community has important metabolic and physiological functions for the host and contributes to its homeostasis during life. Different components of GI microbiota contribute to many aspects of the normal host physiology such as break-down of dietary constituents, development of mucosal immunity, and modulation of the gastrointestinal development. In healthy individuals, the host's immune system maintains homeostasis with the resident microbiota and mycobiota: the resident eukaryotes are mutualistic or commensal important components. Disturbance of the network of competitive commensal bacteria, named dysbiosis, can lead to increased susceptibility to pathogens and, for example, to *Candida* spp. infections [32].

Gut microbiota contributes to nearly every aspect of the host's growth and development, not confined to the gastrointestinal tract; a large number of diseases and dysfunctions have been tentatively associated with an imbalance in the composition, numbers, or habitat of the gut microbiota [20]. Besides the more or less obvious implications in the GI tract (inflammation, malignancies, etc.), dysbiosis has been described/hypothesized in other body districts so far from the gut as the brain [33].

The brain can influence commensal organisms either indirectly, via changes in gastrointestinal motility and secretion and intestinal permeability, or directly, via signaling molecules released into the gut lumen from cells in the lamina propria (enterochromaffin cells, neurons, immune cells). On the other hand, communication from enteric microbiota to the host can occur via epithelial cell, receptor-mediated signaling and, when intestinal permeability is increased, through direct stimulation of host cells in the lamina propria. Metabolic products of intestinal bacteria, such as short-chain fatty acids or chemotactic peptides (e.g., N-formylmethionyl–leucyl–phenylalanine), are able to stimulate the enteric nervous system and influence the rate of gut transit [1].

Similarly to eukaryotes, prokaryotes communicate with each other through hormones and hormone-like compounds. The signaling molecules used for communication by vertebrates, invertebrates, and microbes share structural similarities. Microorganisms can communicate with mammalian cells via the so-called inter-kingdom signaling, which uses various hormones and hormone-like compounds: peptides and monoamines, such as the epidermal growth factor and insulin, and small, diffusible signaling molecules called autoinducers. Signaling molecules are released by the host into the lumen of the gastrointestinal tract during stress; however, receptors and intercellular signaling mechanisms for these same molecules are present on certain luminal microbes; this strongly suggests that the nervous system can also directly modulate microbial behavior [1].

Diet patterns may modulate gut microbiota via alteration of nutrient availability, and dietary intervention can impact gut microbial gene richness. Lower microbiome richness was identified as less healthy and associated with metabolic dysfunction and low-grade inflammation. Dietary formula with high-fiber contents can improve microbiome richness. Western-style diet could negatively affect anxiety-like behavior and memory, depending on immune status. Supplementation with high levels of PUFAs could alleviate depression. These and other experimental findings indicate saturated fat as a risk factor for both neuro-immune and neuropsychiatric disorders [34].

Table 4.1 PubMed analysis of current literature limited to keywords "microbiota" and "autism spectrum disorder"

First author	Year	Journal	Manuscript type
Kantarcioglu AS	2016	Mycopathologia	Research
Son JS	2015	PLoS One	Research
MacFabe DF	2015	Microb Ecol Health Dis	Research
Frye RE	2015	Microb Ecol Health Dis	Review
Rosenfeld CS	2015	Drug Metab Dispos	Review
De Angelis M	2015	Gut Microbes	Review
Reddy BL	2015	J Mol Microbiol Biotechnol	Review
Krajmalnik-Brown R	2015	Microb Ecol Health Dis	Review
McDonald D	2015	Microb Ecol Health Dis	Review
Tomova A	2015	Physiol Behav	Research
Buie T	2015	Clin Therapeutics	Review
Mezzelani A	2015	Nutr Neurosci	Hypothesis
Weston B	2015	Med Hypotheses	Research
Toh MC	2015	Microb Ecol Health Dis	Review
Mayer EA	2014	Bioessays	Review
Wang L	2014	Biomark Med	Review
Goyal DK	2014	Front Endocrinol	Review
de Theije CG	2014	Brain Behav Immun	Research
Hsiao EY	2013	Cell	Research
De Angelis M	2013	PLoS One	Research
Wang L	2013	Mol Autism	Research
Kang DW	2013	PLoS One	Research
Gondalia SV	2012	Autism Res	Research
Williams BL	2012	MBio	Research
Martirosian G	2011	Anaerobe	Research
Critchfield JW	2011	Gastroenterol Res Pract	Review
Finegold SM	2011	Anaerobe	Review
Adams JB	2011	BMC Gastroenterol	Research
Parracho HM	2005	J Med Microbiol	Research
Song Y	2004	Appl Environ Microbiol	Research

The articles published before 2012 were added on the basis of our personal knowledge. 30 articles were found: 16 research papers and 14 review/hypotheses. The publication year highlights that the target "microbiota" is a rather young and increasing field of research

There is a range of indications that alterations of microbiota in the gut might contribute to the pathogenesis of various diseases [20, 34]. It was hypothesized that the principal contributor to the gastrointestinal disturbances among autistic individuals is an abnormal composition of gut microbiota [35]. Several groups have studied the intestinal microbiota of autistic populations and found different composition of many microbial species compared to healthy controls (Table 4.1). These ASD-related microbial species variations mainly include *Clostridium* spp. (various strains), *Ruminococcus*, *Bacteroidetes*, *Bacteroides*, *Firmicutes*, and *Desulfovibrio* species. Various recent studies demonstrated that autistic children with gastrointestinal symptoms show major fecal microbiota alterations. The presence of *C. perfringens* was also reported frequently in ASD with the meaning of a repeated antibiotic therapy that disturbs the balance of physiological microflora and may change its composition, producing colonization by pathogenic bacteria, including those producing toxins. Massive presence of *Clostridia* spp. was shown in autistic children with a history of gastrointestinal issues. The bacteria-produced endotoxins trigger immune cell activation and infiltration into the mucosa, as well as upregulation of pro-inflammatory cytokines, such as TNF-α and Il-1β, which in turn further increases barrier permeability, thereby perpetuating an inflammatory cycle [36]. Interestingly, antibiotic treatment of ASD children did not only lead to gastrointestinal improvements but also improvements in cognitive skills [37].

Less studies were focalized on fungal/yeast infections in ASDs until a very recent retrospective study [38]; several clinicians report the presence of *Candida*-related symptoms in autistic children, and various hypotheses on the biochemical cascade following such an infection have been formulated [39].

The more the research reveals, the greater the effects gut microbiota appears to have, at nearly all systems and levels of the human body. In the absence or dysfunction of normal gut flora, a multitude of diseases may occur, shedding light on the important role maintained by the gut–brain axis [40].

4.4   Autism Spectrum Disorders (ASD)

In addition to frequent gastrointestinal symptoms, children with autism often manifest complex biochemical, metabolic, and immunologic abnormalities that a primary genetic cause cannot readily account for. The gut–brain axis is central to certain encephalopathies of extracranial origin, hepatic encephalopathy being the best characterized. Certain commonalties between the clinical characteristics of hepatic encephalopathy and an increasingly common autistic phenotype (developmental regression in a previously normal child accompanied by immune-mediated gastrointestinal pathology) have led to the hypothesis that an analogous mechanism of toxic encephalopathy may exist in patients with liver failure and some children with autism [14]. Aberrations in opioid biochemistry are common to these two conditions, and evidence suggests that opioid peptides may be among the central mediators of the respective syndromes. In ASD, these mechanisms result into the opioid-excess theory of autism, related to the leaky gut hypothesis, gluten/casein, and gut–brain connection [41]. Accordingly, dietary-derived peptides with opioid activity (exorphins) could sustain autism. Several peptides of dietary origin have been found increased in urine of autistic children [42], and it is well known that gluten and casein are linked to opioid-like peptides (i.e., gliadinomorphin, β-casomorphin, deltorphin 1, and deltorphin 2). Indeed, it was demonstrated that these hydrolytic digestion derivatives are proline-rich opioid peptides able to modulate cysteine uptake in cultured human neuronal and gastrointestinal epithelial cells via activation of opioid receptors [43]. Interestingly, decreases in cysteine uptake were associated with changes in the intracellular levels of the potent antioxidant sulfhydryl tripeptide glutathione. Redox-dependent cellular processes are regulated by the glutathione/glutathione disulfide (GSH/GSSG) redox pair. This GSH/GSSG ratio is considered a marker of cellular toxicity and used as a clinical test to assess the presence of oxidative stress-related autism [41, 44].

Recently, non-celiac gluten sensitivity (NCGS) has been related to autism [28, 45]. NCGS is a syndrome diagnosed in patients with symptoms responding to removal of gluten from the diet, after celiac disease and wheat allergy had been excluded. The peptides originated from dietary components are also neuroactive compounds. They are able to freely permeate the mucosa, through an altered permeability of the intestinal membrane (leaky gut), and cross the blood–brain barrier (BBB) as well, entering the central nervous system. Being neuroactive molecules, they are able to affect the neurotransmission system and disrupt the neuro-regulatory mechanisms required for the normal brain development, causing psychiatric, cognitive, and behavioral disturbances [46]. In addition, in the intestinal lamina propria of autistic children, the dietary-derived peptides are able to trigger an altered immune response with involvement of several cell subtypes, i.e., monocytes, macrophages, antigen-presenting cells, and T and B cells. Monocytes result strongly dysregulated in autism [47, 48], and they could be responsible to further carry pro-inflammatory signals to the higher centers in the nervous system, through a permeable BBB. A further possible mechanism has been proposed: gluten peptides could trigger an innate immune response in the brain similar to that described in the gut mucosa of celiac patients, causing the exposure from neuronal cells of a specific transglutaminase primarily expressed in the brain [45].

Generating biologically plausible and testable hypotheses in this area may help to identify new treatment options in encephalopathies of extracranial origin [14]. Indeed, this axis is critical, for example, in oral medication for psychopathology. Awareness is growing, particularly within the field of childhood developmental disorders, that in a substantial proportion of affected children, gut–brain interactions may be central to abnormal neural development and the subsequent expression of aberrant behaviors [14].

Gut–brain axis disruption has gained a lot of attention in ASD. Serotonin (5-HT) functions as a key neurotransmitter at both terminals of bidirectional communication system between the central nervous system and the gastrointestinal tract [49]. Serotonin might play a role in autism, given its elevated blood levels, which could be related to GI motor abnormalities. In an experimental model of autism – the mice valproic acid (VPA) model – an increased expression of neuro-inflammatory markers in the brain of in utero-exposed male offspring was found. The intestinal tract of VPA mice showed epithelial cell loss and neutrophil infiltration. Interestingly, reduced levels of serotonin were detected in the prefrontal cortex, amygdala, and small intestine. According to the authors [50], enterochromaffin cells and intestinal inflammatory cells (i.e., mast cells and platelets) release serotonin during inflammatory processes. Released serotonin is responsible to increase the secretions, vasodilation, and vascular permeability, resulting in functional dysmotility, stool alterations (diarrhea or constipation), and infiltration of leukocytes in the intestinal wall. Cells that release serotonin utilize much tryptophan, the substrate of the 5-HT synthesis reaction; for this reason, less tryptophan will be available to cross the blood–brain barrier, and brain serotonin levels will be reduced. Decreased levels of brain sero-tonin are responsible of cognitive dysfunctions found in ASD. Furthermore, sero-tonin contributes to both innate and adaptive immune responses [51]. The immune system communicates with the brain via both humoral and neuronal mechanisms, among which serotonin-releasing neurons.

Beyond dietary peptides, other molecules of dietary origins could affect ASD development. The dietary short-chain fatty acid propionic acid (PA) (used as food preservative, but it is also a metabolic end product of gut enteric bacteria) has been reported to induce autism-like behavioral changes and neuro-inflammatory responses in rats. This fatty acid is able to cross the gut–blood and blood–brain barriers and then cell membranes. Once inside the cell, PA provokes intracellular acidification. Decreased pH alters neurotransmitter release, thus influencing the behavior. Intraventricular infusion of PA has been proposed as rodent model of autism [52].

It is noteworthy to consider that dietary fat intake and fat quality are generally deficient in autistic children, as they show low saturated fatty acids and ω-3 poly-unsaturated fatty acids (PUFAs) intakes. Change in the ratio of ω-6/ω-3, espe-cially during early life, may induce developmental changes in brain connectivity, synaptogenesis, cognition, and behavior [53]. Confirmation that abnormal lipid metabolism is implicated in autism arises from a recent study on 121 autistic chil-dren that showed lower percentage of total PUFA (above all omega-6 arachidonic acid and omega-3 docosahexaenoic acid) than 110 non-autistic children [54]. PUFA are essential components of neuronal membrane fluidity and take a role in the structure and function of transmembrane proteins. Among these proteins, the G-coupled protein receptors (GPCRs) activate several downstream signaling pathways and are involved in autism-related cellular and molecular changes [55]. Interestingly, gluten-free/casein-free diet improves the quality of fat intake [56]. ASD children suffering of gastrointestinal perturbations also show altered metab-olomic profiles [57].

4.5   Other Neurological Diseases: Schizophrenia, Parkinson's Disease, etc.

Parkinson's disease (PD) is a neurodegenerative disease with potential involvement of the gastrointestinal tract [58]. Accumulation and aggregation of the alfa-synuclein protein into the substantia nigra (synucleinopathy) leads to PD [59]. Recently, it was proposed that PD pathogenesis could be affected by trans-synaptic cell-to-cell transmission from the enteric nervous system (ENS) to the substantia nigra [11]. Accordingly, the alfa-synuclein accumulation could start in the GI submucosal plexus and then propagate retrogradely to the CNS via vagal preganglionic axons of the dorsal motor nucleus of the vagus nerve (DMVN) finally reaching the substantia nigra. There also is the possibility of a bidirectional, concomitant movement: the disease could start in the ENS and then spread retrogradely toward the CNS (from the gut to the brain) or vice versa (from the brain to the gut) [60]. Interestingly, in PD neurodegenerative processes are accompanied by GI symptoms [10]. Gut dysbiosis, intestinal permeability, and gut microbiota changes participate in the activation of the pro-inflammatory state of neurons and glia cells of the ENS. Prolonged intestinal permeability dysfunction could lead to chronic inflammation and neuronal damage. In support of the hypothesis that PD might start in the gastrointestinal tract, there are evidences relating PD to environmental factors. Pesticides, insecticides, herbicides, and metals are all correlated to high levels of alfa-synuclein and PD development [11]. Generally speaking, all the substances or molecules that trigger a pro-inflammatory state, which in turn is responsible for alfa-synuclein protein aggregation, of the gastrointestinal system could be able to induce PD. It has been proposed that prebiotics, probiotics, and dietary modifications, beneficially impacting intestinal barrier integrity, could be effective in PD treatment [61].

Schizophrenia, the mental disorder characterized by abnormal social behavior and unrecognizing real world, is linked to genetic and environmental factors. Several risk factors with common pathway in the intestinal tract have been associated to schizophrenia [9]: GI barrier dysfunction, food antigen sensitivity, autoimmunity, and inflammation, all of them potentially related to gut microbiota. Indeed, the risk factors for schizophrenia (inflammation, food intolerances, *Toxoplasma gondii* exposure, cellular barrier defects) are part of biological pathways that intersect those of the gut [62]. Prebiotics, probiotics, and therapies to correct GI dysfunction could be useful to improve the symptoms of schizophrenia.

Depression is a complex chronic mood disorder associated with many factors influencing its etiology, including genetics and the environment. It has recently been linked to alterations of the microbiota–gut–brain axis [63]. Correlation between microbiota alterations and depression in humans has been found by the analysis of fecal microbiome of patients diagnosed with depressive disorder compared to non-depressed controls [64]. The study found that *Alistipes*, a genus in the phylum of *Bacteroidetes*, was over-represented in depressed patients. *Alistipes* is associated with inflammation and thus potentially linked to depression through inflammatory pathways.

Immunological factors (T and B cell activity) are associated with the gut microbiota also in autoimmune diseases [65]. Indeed, the gut microbiota is a key factor for the complete development of the immune system. The microbiota interacts with the host providing important immune and physiologic functions [66]. Gut microbiota alterations could influence the disease progression. Targeting the gut microbiome could represent a potential new treatment of autoimmune disease. Among these diseases, systemic lupus erythematosus (SLE) also shows gut microbiota influences [67]. Indeed, recent evidences suggest a strong connection between SLE and the composition of gut commensals, as one of the main environmental factors linked to this disease [68].

References

1. Rhee SH, Pothoulakis C, Mayer EA (2009) Principles and clinical implications of the brain–gut–enteric microbiota axis. Nat Rev Gastroenterol Hepatol 6(5):306–314. doi:10.1038/nrgastro.2009.35306-14
2. Carabotti M, Scirocco A, Maselli MA, Severi C (2015) The gut-brain axis: interactions between enteric microbiota, central and enteric nervous systems. Ann Gastroenterol 28:203–209
3. Burokas A, Moloney RD, Dinan TG, Cryan JF (2015) Microbiota regulation of the mammalian gut-brain axis. Adv Appl Microbiol 91:1–62, chapter 1, Elsevier Inc
4. Mayer EA, Savidge T, Shulman RJ (2014) Brain-gut microbiome interactions and functional bowel disorders. Gastroenterology 146:1500–1512
5. Chen J, Li Y, Tian Y, Huang C, Li D, Zhong Q, Ma X (2015) Interaction between microbes and host intestinal health: modulation by dietary nutrients and gut-brain-endocrine-immune axis. Curr Protein Pept Sci 16:1–12
6. Petra AI, Panagiotidou S, Hatziagelaki E, Stewart JM, Conti P, Theoraides TC (2015) Gut-microbiota-brain axis and its effect on neuropsychiatric disorders with suspected immune dysregulation. Clin Ther 37:984–995
7. Van De Sande MMH, Van Buul VJ, Brouns FJPH (2014) Autism and nutrition: the role of the gut-brain axis. Nutr Res Rev. doi:10.1017/S0954422414000110
8. Mezzelani A, Landini M, Facchiano F, Raggi ME, Villa L, Molteni M, DeSantis B, Brera C, Caroli AM, Milanesi L, Marabotti A (2015) Environment, dysbiosis, immunity and sex-specific susceptibility: a translational hypothesis for regressive autism pathogenesis. Nutr Neurosci 18:145–161
9. Nemani K, Hosseini Ghomi R, McCormick B, Fan X (2015) Schizophrenia and the gut-brain axis. Prog Neuropsychopharmacol Biol Psychiatry 56:155–160
10. Mulak A, Bonaz B (2015) Brain-gut-microbiota axis in Parkinson's disease. World J Gastroenterol 21(37):10609–10620
11. Klingelhoefer L, Reichmann H (2015) Pathogenesis of Parkinson disease-the gut-brain axis and environmental factors. Nat Rev Neurol 11(11):625–636
12. Jackson JR, Eaton WW, Cascella NG, Fasano A, Kelly DL (2012) Neurologic and psychiatric manifestations of celiac disease and gluten sensitivity. Psychiatr Q 83(1):91–102
13. Catassi C, Elli L, Bonaz B, Bouma G, Carroccio A, Castillejo G, Cellier C, Cristofori F, de Magistris L, Dolinsek J, Dieterich W, Francavilla R, Hadjivassiliou M, Holtmeier W, Körner U, Leffler DA, Lundin KE, Mazzarella G, Mulder CJ, Pellegrini N, Rostami K, Sanders D, Skodje GI, Schuppan D, Ullrich R, Volta U, Williams M, Zevallos VF, Zopf Y, Fasano A (2015) Diagnosis of Non-Celiac Gluten Sensitivity (NCGS): the Salerno experts' criteria. Nutrient 7(6):4966–4977
14. Wakefield AJ (2002) The Gut–Brain Axis in childhood developmental disorders. J Pediatr Gastroenterol Nutr 34:S14–S17
15. Butterworth RF (2000) Complications of cirrhosis III hepatic encephalopathy. J Hepatol 32(suppl 1):171–180
16. Fadgyas-Stanculete M, Buga AM, Popa-Wagner A, Dumitrascu DL (2014) The relationship between irritable bowel syndrome and psychiatric disorders: from molecular changes to clinical manifestations. J Mol Psychiatry 2:4–11
17. Gershon MD (1988) The second brain: a groundbreaking new understanding of nervous disorders of the stomach and intestine. Harper & Collins, New York
18. Mayer EA (2000) The neurobiology of stress and gastrointestinal disease. Gut 47:861–869
19. De Magistris L, Picardi A, Sapone A, Cariello R, Siniscalco D, Bravaccio C, Pascotto A (2014) Intestinal barrier in autism. In: Patel VB (ed) Comprehensive guide to autism. Springer, New York, p 123
20. Sekirov I, Russell SL, Antunes LC, Finlay BB (2010) Gut microbiota in health and disease. Physiol Rev 90:859–904

21. Solanas G, Cortina C, Sevillano M, Battle E (2011) Cleavage of E-cadherin by ADAM10 mediates epithelial cell sorting downstream of EphB signalling. Nat Cell Biol 13:1100–1107
22. Ulluwishewa D, Anderson RC, McNabb WC et al (2011) Regulation of tight junction permeability by intestinal bacteria and dietary components. J Nutr 141:769–776
23. Catassi C, Fasano A (2008) Celiac disease. Curr Opin Gastroenterol 24:687–691
24. Vaarala O (2011) The gut as a regulator of early inflammation in type 1 diabetes. Curr Opin Endocrinol Diabetes Obes 18:241–247
25. Bjarnason I, MacPherson A, Hollander D (1995) Intestinal permeability: an overview. Gastroenterology 108:1566–1581
26. Fasano A (2011) Zonulin and its regulation of intestinal barrier function: the biological door to inflammation, autoimmunity and cancer. Physiol Rev 91:151–175
27. D'Eufemia P, Celli M, Finocchiaro R et al (1996) Abnormal intestinal permeability in children with autism. Acta Paediatr 85:1076–1079
28. De Magistris L, Familiari V, Pascotto A et al (2010) Alterations of the intestinal barrier in patients with autism spectrum disorders and in their first-degree relatives. J Pediatr Gastroenterol Nutr 51:418–424
29. De Magistris L, Picardi A, Siniscalco D et al (2013) Antibodies against food antigens in patients with Autistic Spectrum Disorder. Biomed Res Int. doi:10.1155/2013/729349
30. Lerner A, Matthias T (2015) Changes in intestinal tight junction permeability associated with industrial food additives explain the rising incidence of autoimmune disease. Autoimmun Rev 14:479–489
31. Kramer P, Bressan P (2015) Human as superorganisms: how microbes, viruses, imprinted genes, and other selfish entities shape our behaviour. Perspect Psychol Sci 10:464–481
32. Rizzetto L, Weil T, Cavalieri D (2015) Systems level dissection of Candida recognition by Dectins: a matter of fungal morphology and site of infection. Pathogens 4:639–661
33. Crumeyrolle-Arias M, Jaglin M, Bruneau A, Vancassel S, Cardona A, Daugé V, Naudon L, Rabot S (2015) Absence of the gut microbiota enhances anxiety-like behavior and neuroendocrine response to acute stress in rats. Psychoneuroendocrinology 42:207–217
34. Wang Y, Kasper LH (2014) The role of microbiome in central nervous system disorders. Brain Behav Immun 38:1–12
35. Critchfield JW, van Hemert S et al (2011) The potential role of probiotics in the management of childhood autism spectrum disorders. Gastroenterol Res Pract 2011:161358
36. Ghaisas S, Maher J, Kanthasamy A (2015) Gut microbiome in health and disease: linking the microbiome-gut-brain axis and environmental factors in the pathogenesis of systemic and neurodegenerative diseases. Pharmacol Ther 158:52–62, pii: S0163-7258(15)00225-9
37. Sandler RH, Finegold SM, Bolte ER et al (2000) Short-term benefit from oral vancomycin treatment of regressive-onset autism. J Child Neurol 15:429–435
38. Serda Kantarcioglu A, Kiraz N, Aydin A (2015) Microbiota-Gut-Brain axis: yeast species isolated from stool samples of children with suspected or diagnosed autism spectrum disorders and in vitro susceptibility against nystatin and fluconazole. Mycopathologia. doi:10.1007/s11046-015-9949-3
39. Semon BA (2014) Dietary cyclic dipeptides, apoptosis and psychiatric disorders: a hypothesis. Med Hypotheses 82:740–743
40. Zhou L, Foster JA (2015) Psychobiotics and the gut-brain axis: in the pursuit of happiness. Neuropsychiatr Dis Treat 11:715–723
41. Siniscalco D, Antonucci N (2013) Involvement of dietary bioactive proteins and peptides in autism spectrum disorders. Curr Protein Pept Sci 14(8):674–679
42. Reichelt KL, Knivsberg AM (2009) The possibility and probability of a gut-to-brain connection in autism. Ann Clin Psychiatry 21(4):205–211
43. Trivedi MS, Shah JS, Al-Mughairy S, Hodgson NW, Simms B, Trooskens GA, Van Criekinge W, Deth RC (2014) Food-derived opioid peptides inhibit cysteine uptake with redox and epigenetic consequences. J Nutr Biochem 25(10):1011–1018
44. Melnyk S, Fuchs GJ, Schulz E, Lopez M, Kahler SG, Fussell JJ, Bellando J, Pavliv O, Rose S, Seidel L, Gaylor DW, James SJ (2012) Metabolic imbalance associated with methylation dys-

regulation and oxidative damage in children with autism. J Autism Dev Disord 42(3):367–377
45. Lionetti E, Leonardi S, Franzonello C, Mancardi M, Ruggieri M, Catassi C (2015) Gluten psychosis: confirmation of a new clinical entity. Nutrients 7(7):5532–5539
46. Shattock P, Whiteley P (2002) Biochemical aspects in autism spectrum disorders: updating the opioid-excess theory and presenting new opportunities for biomedical intervention. Expert Opin Ther Targets 6(2):175–183
47. Siniscalco D, Sapone A, Giordano C, Cirillo A, de Magistris L, Rossi F, Fasano A, Bradstreet JJ, Maione S, Antonucci N (2013) Cannabinoid receptor type 2, but not type 1, is up-regulated in peripheral blood mononuclear cells of children affected by autistic disorders. J Autism Dev Disord 43(11):2686–2695
48. Siniscalco D, Bradstreet JJ, Cirillo A, Antonucci N (2014) The in vitro GcMAF effects on endocannabinoid system transcriptionomics, receptor formation, and cell activity of autism-derived macrophages. J Neuroinflammation 11:78
49. O'Mahony SM, Clarke G, Borre YE, Dinan TG, Cryan JF (2015) Serotonin, tryptophan metabolism and the brain-gut-microbiome axis. Behav Brain Res 277:32–48
50. de Theije CG, Koelink PJ, Korte-Bouws GA, Lopes da Silva S, Korte SM, Olivier B, Garssen J, Kraneveld AD (2014) Intestinal inflammation in a murine model of autism spectrum disorders. Brain Behav Immun 37:240–247
51. Baganz NL, Blakely RD (2013) A dialogue between the immune system and brain, spoken in the language of serotonin. ACS Chem Neurosci 4(1):48–63
52. MacFabe DF, Cain DP, Rodriguez-Capote K, Franklin AE, Hoffman JE, Boon F, Taylor AR, Kavaliers M, Ossenkopp KP (2007) Neurobiological effects of intraventricular propionic acid in rats: possible role of short chain fatty acids on the pathogenesis and characteristics of autism spectrum disorders. Behav Brain Res 176(1):149–169
53. Van Elst K, Bruining H, Birtoli B, Terreaux C, Buitelaar JK, Kas MJ (2014) Food for thought: dietary changes in essential fatty acid ratios and the increase in autism spectrum disorders. Neurosci Biobehav Rev 45:369–738
54. Brigandi SA, Shao H, Qian SY, Shen Y, Wu BL, Kang JX (2015) Autistic children exhibit decreased levels of essential fatty acids in red blood cells. Int J Mol Sci 16(5):10061–10076
55. Siniscalco D (2014) Adhesion G-protein coupled receptors in autism. Autism Open Access 4, e126. doi:10.4172/2165-7890.1000e126
56. Marí-Bauset S, Llopis-González A, Zazpe I, Marí-Sanchis A, Suárez-Varela MM (2015) Nutritional impact of a gluten-free casein-free diet in children with autism spectrum disorder. J Autism Dev Disord 46:673–684 [Epub ahead of print]
57. Ming X, Stein TP, Barnes V, Rhodes N, Guo L (2012) Metabolic perturbance in autism spectrum disorders: a metabolomics study. J Proteome Res 11:5856–5862
58. Fang X (2015) Potential role of gut microbiota and tissue barriers in Parkinson's disease and amyotrophic lateral sclerosis. Int J Neurosci Oct 16:1–6
59. Dickson DW, Fujishiro H, Orr C, DelleDonne A, Josephs KA, Frigerio R, Burnett M, Parisi JE, Klos KJ, Ahlskog JE (2009) Neuropathology of non-motor features of Parkinson disease. Parkinsonism Relat Disord 15(Suppl 3):S1–S5
60. Natale G, Pasquali L, Paparelli A, Fornai F (2011) Parallel manifestations of neuropathologies in the enteric and central nervous systems. Neurogastroenterol Motil 23:1056–1065
61. Kelly LP, Carvey PM, Keshavarzian A, Shannon KM, Shaikh M, Bakay RA, Kordower JH (2014) Progression of intestinal permeability changes and alpha-synuclein expression in a mouse model of Parkinson's disease. Mov Disord 29(8):999–1009
62. Severance EG, Prandovszky E, Castiglione J, Yolken RH (2015) Gastroenterology issues in schizophrenia: why the gut matters. Curr Psychiatry Rep 17(5):27
63. Dash S, Clarke G, Berk M, Jacka FN (2015) The gut microbiome and diet in psychiatry: focus on depression. Curr Opin Psychiatry 28(1):1–6
64. Naseribafrouei A, Hestad K, Avershina E et al (2014) Correlation between the human fecal microbiota and depression. Neurogastroenterol Motil 26(8):1155–1162

65. Telesford K, Ochoa-Repáraz J, Kasper LH (2014) Gut commensalism, cytokines, and central nervous system demyelination. J Interferon Cytokine Res 34(8):605–614
66. Ochoa-Repáraz J, Kasper LH (2014) Gut microbiome and the risk factors in central nervous system autoimmunity. FEBS Lett 588(22):4214–4222
67. Mu Q, Zhang H, Luo XM (2015) SLE: another autoimmune disorder influenced by microbes and diet? Front Immunol 6:608
68. Sánchez B, Hevia A, González S, Margolles A (2015) Interaction of intestinal microorganisms with the human host in the framework of autoimmune diseases. Front Immunol 6:594

Does Diet Still Retain a Value in Gastrointestinal Pathology?

5

Lucio Lucchin and Marion Schrei

Despite clinical nutrition has strong evidence on a preventive and a therapeutic level, its value is still underestimated by physicians and health-care professionals (HCPs) [1, 2]. Data showing this problem are listed below:

1. Forty percent of Europeans lose weight before hospitalization [3], while 61.9 % lose weight during hospitalization [4–6]. Italians show 30.7 % of "undernutrition" (protein-energy malnutrition or PEM) at admission, whereas 21 % shows "overnutrition" (obesity) [7, 8]. Moreover, in case of acute illness, malnutrition prevalence exceeds 40 % among adults and 70 % among elderly people [9, 10]. PEM is often underdiagnosed because fluid retention is not monitored by bioelectrical impedance analysis (BIA, e.g., 40–80 % of cirrhotic patients) [11, 12].
2. Indicators of nutritional status, especially weight, height, and body mass index (BMI), are poorly measured, despite the evidence of their value in terms of clinical, economic, and quality of life advantages [7–13]. BMI <20 is found in 10–47 % of gastroenterological patients [14].
3. Nutritional screening tools are not enough employed in order to estimate PEM risk (to be confirmed later clinically). Indeed, they are applied in 21–73 % of clinical departments and, on average, in 52 % of highly specialized ones (33 % in Italy). In most gastroenterological studies, the tool employed is the Subjective Global Assessment (SGA, sensitivity 82 % and specificity 72 %). Other validated tests are the Malnutrition Universal Screening Tool (MUST, sensitivity 61 % and specificity 76 %), the Nutritional Risk Screening 2002 (NRS 2002, sensitivity 62 % and specificity 93 %), and, in the elderly (>65 years), the Mini-Nutritional Assessment (MNA, sensitivity 96 % and specificity 98 %) [15]. Caloric intake is

L. Lucchin (✉) • M. Schrei
Division of Clinical Nutrition, Central Hospital Bolzano, Bolzano, Italy
e-mail: lucio.lucchin@nucl.it

© Springer International Publishing Switzerland 2016
E. Grossi, F. Pace (eds.), *Human Nutrition from the Gastroenterologist's Perspective*,
DOI 10.1007/978-3-319-30361-1_5

calculated only in 35 % of risk patients [16]. Finally, the professional that carries out screenings is given just in 13 % of scientific articles, which denotes carelessness on the subject [17].

4. The degree of inappropriateness of natural and/or artificial nutritional interventions is high. In fact, 35–43 % of patients do not assume more than 1500 kcal/day, and 55 % of those with PEM take spontaneously less than 50 % of recommended requirements [18]. Moreover, iatrogenic PEM, which probably interests between 15 and 27 % of hospital patients, keeps to be ignored although 60–66 % of hospitalization days are used by malnourished patients (average lengthening of the stay 54.9 %) [19], who determine about 70 % of the costs. Each day of delay of a malnutrition treatment causes an extra cost of about 55 euro for the treatment itself [20].

5. There is a wrong concern that the improvement in the care for nutritional state will determine an unjustified increase in the workload for health-care professionals.

This situation is partly explained by the following:

- The unacceptable lack of training of physicians in clinical nutrition, even at the level of specialization schools
- The professional inconsistency of many people who realize the strategic role of nutritional intervention, but continue to ignore it because they consider it less noble than other technologically advanced operations (although not necessarily more effective)
- The discomfort in realizing the complexity (the real challenge of future health) of feeding behavior (biological, psychological, and sociocultural components) that requires multidimensional and not super-sectorial knowledge
- The long time (years) required for an effective implementation of scientific evidences [8]

There is an intuitive connection between food and digestive system, as there is an intuitive cause-effect relationship between them from a pathogenetic or preventive point of view. This connection is perceived especially by patients, who often do not receive scientifically acceptable answers by physicians, and also specialists, with the consequent development of prejudices and misconceptions among them. For example, the so-called dieta in bianco (a diet poor in fats and fibers that are easy to digest and stimulate little gastrointestinal motility) is deeply rooted in Italy, while the recourse to food intolerance tests, which don't have any scientific value, is more and more common. The rising desire of people to handle personally the own health, favored by an easy access to information, determines paradoxically an increase in confusion and uncertainty among them as they cannot distinguish between what is right and what is wrong.

Digestive system, and particularly intestine, is strongly connected to the brain that, in turn, deeply influences our feeding behavior. Indeed, there is an indissoluble triangulation among the food, digestive system, and brain. Nerves controlling the central nervous system and digestive system (the number of neurons of the second one is equal or superior to that of the spinal cord) are called, respectively, the first and second brain, and both of them are underestimated. Gastrointestinal symptoms that are often labeled as "functional" correlate precisely with the number of inflammatory cells in the intestinal mucosa [21]. This inflammation increases the permeability of the mucosa allowing bacterial translocation. The prevalence of symptoms (six out of ten Italians suffer from gastrointestinal disturbances at least once every 2 months) [22] and gastrointestinal disorders (digestive diseases affect around 7.5 % of hospital admissions in Italy, approximately 714,000 patients – Federazione Italiana Malattie Apparato Digerente, 2013) justifies the need for a nutritional intervention.

PEM affects an average of 20–48 % patients with gastroenterological pathology (excluding cancer) [23] and in particular:

- Among patients with advanced liver disease, its prevalence is about 39.4 %, while among those with cirrhosis, it varies from 25 to 65 %. Sarcopenia is an independent predictor of survival. Finally, 15–33 % of cirrhotic patients show a REE >120 % compared to the theoretical one (hypermetabolism with loss of lean body mass, partly due to an increased beta-adrenergic activity), whereas 8–31 % of them present a hypometabolism [24].
- Among cancer patients at early stage, PEM prevalence is about 26.8 %; among those with stomach cancer, its prevalence is 19 % [25].
- Among patients with inflammatory bowel diseases, PEM prevalence is 30.6 %, but it can reach 85 % among those hospitalized with acute forms.
- Among patients with pancreatic disease, PEM prevalence is 23 %. In addition, about 50 % of patients with chronic forms are overweight, but their average BMI is lower than that of healthy people. Vitamin deficiencies are often found, and, in particular, vitamins A and E are present, respectively, in 14 and 25 % of cases. On the contrary, 19 % of pancreatopathic patients have a vitamin A excess [26].
- Among patients with gastroesophageal reflux disease, PEM prevalence is about 23 % [27].

It is necessary to realize that nutritional evaluation of gastroenterological patients must be included in the compulsory medical intervention [28].

The following is a summarized evidence of the practical importance of nutrition at the preventive and therapeutic level:

- Gastroesophageal reflux disease occurs more frequently with irregular eating patterns [27]. Moreover, obesity is a clear predisposing and worsening factor for this pathology, and the ability to treat it without trivializing the intervention is vital. Abdominal obesity increases intragastric pressure and gastroesophageal gradient, reduces the pressure of the lower esophageal sphincter (LES), promotes the formation of hiatal hernia, decreases esophageal motility, and thus reduces esophageal clearance. In addition, 88 % of patients with reflux refer exacerbation of symptoms by eating spicy foods [29] even though the trigger dose is not defined. No correlation is found between reflux and fat or coffee (metabolized differently among men and women) intake [30]. Finally, acute and chronic alcohol consumption have opposite effects on the inflammatory response [31]. White wine causes more easily reflux symptoms because of its greater inhibition of the LES, and the average amount of wine that produces symptoms is about 300 cc (1 glass of wine = 12 g of alcohol). Nonetheless, the relationship between alcohol and reflux disease remains controversial [32].

- With pancreatic pathology meals of up to 500 kcal are recommended in order to put aside the organ. Monitoring zinc, selenium, folate, and vitamin B12 levels is also recommended.
- Among patients affected by hepatitis C (European prevalence about 1 %) [33], a low-calorie and low-fat diet is recommended.
- Among people suffering from cirrhosis, nutritional assessment (anthropometric measures, handgrip strength, indirect calorimetry – almost ignored in gastroenterology departments, as well as BIA and DEXA) and sarcopenia investigation, present in about 40 % of cases, are required. In the absence of complications, overweight should be verified, and, if present, caloric restriction should be applied [34]. With ascites, encephalopathy, portal hypertension, and hepatopulmonary syndrome, food intake should be 35–40 kcal/kg of desirable weight/day with 1.2–1.5 g proteins/kg/day (well tolerated by cirrhotic patients and encephalopathy risk-free), of which 0.2–0.3 g/kg/day should be constituted by branched amino acids. A moderate physical activity (at least 5000 steps a day) is also indispensable. With severe encephalopathy a protein intake reduction (0.5–1 g/kg/day) for up to 48 h is possible, and parenteral administration of BCAA (0.25 g/kg) may lead to a faster resolution of neurologic symptoms [35]. Moreover, a fiber intake of 25–45 g/diet, able to modulate positively the microbiota, i.e., reducing Bacteroidetes, Enterobacteriaceae, and Clostridium, can also be useful [36]. On the contrary, diets high in fat or protein increase Firmicutes and reduce Bacteroidetes phylum. Lysozyme and milk oligosaccharides have a positive action on the microbiota of cirrhotic patients [37]. In addition, zinc, magnesium, vitamin B1, and folate supplementation is frequently required [38]. Selenium deficiency correlates with fibrosis and insulin resistance. Iron, manganese, and copper intakes should be pondered carefully, because they may promote fibrogenesis. In the cirrhotic patient, muscle may become an alternative site of ammonia detoxification, and depletion of the protein compartment is detected in 63 % of males and 28 % of females. However, among women the loss of fatty tissue is more intense, maybe because of gender differences in body composition and hormonal status. Furthermore, among cirrhotic patients indirect calorimetry, especially in telemetry, is useful. An evening snack helps in preventing fasting hypersensitivity and muscle loss among these patients. Proteins that have proven to trigger encephalopathy the least are dairy and vegetable ones. In order to prevent a refeeding syndrome, too often ignored and underestimated, it is recommended to start a nutritional intervention with a small caloric provision and to increase it gradually. When malnutrition is present, a protein integration is needed. Finally, in case of dilution caused by renal failure, liquid restriction (1000–1500 ml daily) is controversial.

- Among people affected by Nonalcoholic Fatty Liver Disease, NAFLD (approximately one-third of Americans), the role of the microbiota is increasingly important. For example, *Saccharomyces ellipsoideus* produces alcohol by fermentation. Dysbiosis can also be produced by a high-fat diet (increase of Bacteroidetes and reduction of Firmicutes), which causes microbial overgrowth. As a result there is a greater fermentation of indigestible fibers into oligo- and monosaccharides and into short-chain fatty acids (SCFAs), partly through the inhibition of the adipose factor that induces fasting (FIAF – fasting-induced adipocyte factor) with a consequent increase in the activity of the lipoprotein lipases (LPL). Moreover, the microbiota metabolizes food choline into trimethylamine causing a choline deficiency that impairs the VLDL outflow from the liver, therefore favoring steatosis. Dysbiosis disrupts enterocytes' tight junctions (through chemokine and ligands) resulting in a translocation of microbial and inflammatory metabolites to the liver [39]. In NAFLD advantages are obtained by a moderate caloric (−500–1000 kcal/day) and carbohydrate restriction (40–45 % of total calories, i.e., 25–30 kcal/kg or 1200–1500 kcal/day), by an increase in omega-3 fats and a reduction of saturated fat (SFAs) to less than 10 % of daily calorie intake [40]. However, too restrictive diets result in poor compliance and in a quick mobilization of free fatty acids from adipose tissue that reaches the liver inducing steatosis and gallstone formation. Lastly, a high intake of fiber and carbohydrates with low glycemic index is effective in controlling hyperinsulinemia [41].
- Colic functional disorders are common, and food is the element on which patient attention focuses. The most involved foods are milk and unseasoned dairy products, chocolate, sweeteners (sorbitol, fructose), jam, fruits (pear, peach, plum), and vegetables (cabbage, artichoke, spinach, onion, arugula, cucumber, celery). Some patients report worsening of symptoms with fiber and whole foods, spices, coffee, tea, and caffeinated or carbonated beverages. At least, foods with a high salt content (stock cubes, sausages) may have an indirect effect. The response to exclusion diets varies between 12 and 67 % [42]. In addition, a fiber intake of 15–25 g/day is useful in asymptomatic stages. Infusions or decoctions of peppermint (12 g to steep in 350 cc of water for 10 min) can relieve painful symptoms [43]. Also a limitation in fermentable oligo-, di-, and monosaccharides and polyols (FODMAPs) can help: fructose (apple, pear, banana, peach, fruit juices), lactose (dairy products), fructans and galactans (artichoke, asparagus, cauliflower, broccoli, fennel, garlic, onion, cereals, legumes, watermelon, peach, palm date, khaki), and polyols (apple, apricot, tangerine, pear, peach, plum, watermelon, cauliflower, mushrooms, pea, sorbitol, mannitol, xylitol) [44].
- The etiology of inflammatory bowel diseases results from a complex interaction between genetics (163 identified susceptible alleles), epigenetics, environmental factors, and immune response. Diet can alter the microbiota and this can have a causal role. Dietary fats affect indeed inflammation and regulate mucosal immunity. A high uptake of omega-3 (which inhibits prostaglandins and leukotrienes through arachidonic acid and contrasts vascular adhesion and migration, angiogenesis, and immune response through PPAR-gamma and NF-kB) can be useful in the treatment of ulcerative colitis, while a high intake of trans-fatty acids is

unfavorable in all diseases. Fiber does not seem to affect Crohn's disease, while it may play a slight role in ulcerative colitis. On the contrary, a positive action of fiber has been demonstrated in pouchitis. Furthermore, an exclusive enteral feeding is generally accepted for symptom improvement, but there is limited data about its role in helping the mucosa to heal. Consumption of refined sugars appears to be a risk factor for Crohn's disease but not for ulcerative colitis, which, conversely, correlates with the consumption of fat and red meat [45]. In any case, an excessive intake of sugar promotes obesity and consequently inflammation [46]. A regular intake of vegetables reduces the risk for Crohn's disease [47]. An integration with folate, vitamin B12, iron, magnesium, and zinc is recommended to support postsurgical wound healing and fistulae closure. In addition, calcium and vitamin D are important to prevent osteoporosis [48]. However, in Crohn's disease, the efficacy of nutritional intervention without the coadministration of steroids is inferior than that of steroid treatment [49].

- Polyphenols appear to play a positive role in the treatment of peptic ulcers: cytoprotection, reepithelialization, angiogenesis and neovascularization, upregulation of tissue growth factors and prostaglandins, downregulation of antiangiogenic factors, enhancing nitric oxide synthase-derived NO, inhibition of mucosal oxidative damage, antioxidant strengthening, antacid and antisecretory activity, increase in mucosal defensive factors, block of *Helicobacter pylori* colonization, and anti-inflammatory activity [50], while, the most powerful stimulants of gastric secretion are beer, milk, broth, and pure caffeine. A more bland effect is induced by coffee (even decaf) and cola. In addition, the buffering effect of food is higher in the first 2–4 postprandial hours.

- The spread of dyspeptic symptoms is a difficult challenge when it comes to give nutritional advices. Fatty foods are associated with dyspepsia (evidence type A) because of relaxation of the lower esophageal sphincter, delayed gastric emptying, and increased flatulence. These effects are reduced by the inhibitors of CCK-A and lipase receptors. Besides, the products of lipid hydrolysis, and not the indigestible fats, seem to be responsible for these symptoms. Furthermore, coffee reduces LES pressure and increases gastric secretion by gastrin release. There is an association of symptoms of 70 % with mayonnaise, 60 % with peanuts and fish, and 50 % with chocolate [51]. A lower number of meals are associated with a greater frequency of symptoms, as well as a greater caloric intake. In addition, carbohydrate intake correlates with lower postprandial fullness. Other foods and drinks that evoke symptoms in more than 50 % of patients are sodas (if taken at a temperature below 10 °C, they can bring triplication of the original amount of gas ingested [52]), fried foods, chili, coffee, red meat, and bananas. Frying fatty foods increases gastric emptying time [53]. This is partly explained by a negative feedback of the slower fatty acid absorption. At least, there seems also to be a circadian rhythm of gastric motility which is more active in the morning hours, and temperatures far from 10 °C activate the vagal reflex of pylorus closure.

- In malabsorption, for a rapid reintegration of vitamins, iron, calcium, magnesium, and other trace elements, supplementation should correspond to a requirement five to ten times higher than the normal average.

- Foods like bananas and shared apple pulp have a mild astringent effect [54].
- Eight foods cause 90 % of allergies: milk, nut, peanut, wheat, soy, egg, fish, and shellfish [55]. Moreover, foods causing symptoms similar to IgE-mediated allergy are milk and dairy products, yeast, wheat, vegetable oil, and olive oil. Foods high in sugar seem to be those most prone to provoke intolerances (fruit juices, legumes, sweeteners). Finally, foods such as chocolate, strawberry, exotic fruits, shellfish, and fermented cheese can cause histamine release with urticaria, while there are foods that naturally contain this amine like sardines, herring, mackerel, blue cheese, salami, wine, and beer.
- The relationship between diet and digestive tract tumors is controversial. A diet rich in vegetables and low in starch and salt has a protective effect against gastric cancer (risk reduction of 25 %) [56], while an adequate intake of plant foods seems to have a protective effect against gallbladder cancer [57]. An increased intake of carbohydrates with high glycemic index does not seem to be associated with an increased risk of cancer of the liver and biliary tract. A protective effect, however, was demonstrated for a diet rich in fiber [58]. Furthermore, in pancreatic cancer nutritional and hydrating perioperative intervention is essential [59]. An anti-inflammatory diet is helpful. Finally, vegetarians, fish eaters, and people eating meat one time/week do not show a significant risk reduction for colon cancer compared to those who eat meat six to seven times a week. Conversely, a protective effect is clear for vegetable intake [60]. Red meat (muscular parts of beef, veal, pork, lamb, mutton, horse, and goat) intake determines a variable risk for colorectal cancer. When not processed, red meat has been cataloged in group 2A (limited evidence) and, when processed, in group 1 (definitely carcinogenic) of carcinogenic substance classification. The risk would be 18 % every 50 g of processed meat consumed on a daily basis and 17 % every 100 g of red meat [61]. Cooking meat at high temperatures generates carcinogenic chemical compounds.

Conclusions

Data presented are so indicative that keeping to neglect the nutritional aspects of gastrointestinal disease is no longer ethically acceptable. In a very technological and interventional moment of medical history, the attractiveness for the physician from areas other than nutrition is strong. The reductionist attitude is still predominant in comparison to the holistic one, even though it does not satisfy expectations. What is emerging is a complexity (that does not mean complication), which is more and more confusing and for which we do not have yet adequate dealing skills. However, this is the challenge for the future, as it is moving toward a "positive medicine" instead of a "negative one" (how to solve the problem when it has already arisen). Some factors slow the changing process like the strong hyper-specialistic tendency, the experience/age of the operator, the guidelines, the patients' expectations, and the ambivalence between professional honesty and simplification need. Other factors that complicate the picture are the big funding cuts forecasted in future years (that are not going to ease interaction among professionals), the rise of defensive medicine, the need to improve service quality and public satisfaction, and the increase of request of assistance because of population aging and chronic pathology boost. Lifestyles are the main positive and negative determinant in the development of chronic pathologies, and nutrition plays a main role. Today, the specialist experiences a situation of increasing uncertainty. On one hand, the attitude to stop at sectorial professional competence, believed to be ethic, is more and more rooted, even when there is not the possibility of a multi-professional consultation. On the other hand, there is the attitude to simplify in order to manage complexity. Simplification is actually the only way to improve knowledge, but trivializing is more dangerous. It seems that there is not any other way-out from this situation than looking for the right balance between reductionism and holism, and single- and multi-professional treatment. Consequently, it comes that multidimensionality, i.e., obtaining deeper knowledge of contiguous and complementary fields, as the nutritional one, by the same professional, is a possible solution. Keeping to ignore the role of clinical nutrition is a hypocrisy that medicine and gastroenterology, primarily, cannot indulge.

References

1. Godlee F (2014) Nutrition matters. BMJ 349:g7255
2. Lucchin L (2015) La Nutrizione Clinica conta? Perché è così ignorata negli ospedali italiani? Recenti Prog Med 106:74–77
3. Schindler K, Pernicka E, Laviano A, Howard P, Schütz T, Bauer P et al (2010) How nutritional risk is assessed and managed in European hospitals: a survey of 21.007 patients findings from the 2007–2008 cross-sectional Nutrition Day survey. Clin Nutr 29(5):552–559
4. Kob K, Lucchin L, Wegher L (2001) Stato dell'arte sull'epidemiologia e la prevenzione della malnutrizione ospedaliera. L'Ospedale Periodico ANMDO Edicom 1:8–12
5. Dzieniszewski J, Jarosz M, Szezygiel B et al (2005) Nutritional status of patients hospitalised in Poland. Eur J Clin Nutr 59(4):552–560
6. Kyle U, Kossovsky MP, Karsegard L, Pichard C (2005) Comparison of tools for nutritional assessment and screening at hospital admission: a population study. Cl Nutr 25(3):409–417
7. Lucchin L, D'Amicis A, Gentile MG, Battistini NC, Fusco MA, Palmo A et al (2009) A nationally representative survey of hospital malnutrition: the Italian PIMAI (Project: Iatrogenic Malnutrition in Italy) study. Mediterr J Nutr Metab 2:171–179
8. Sandlers L (2009) Every patient tells a story: medical mysteries and the art of diagnosis. Broadway Books, New York
9. Kubrak C, Jensen L (2007) Malnutrition in acute care patients: a narrative review. Int J Nurs Stud 44:1036–1054
10. Correia MITD, Waitzberg DL (2003) The impact of malnutrition on morbidity, mortality, length of hospital stay and costs evaluated through a multivariate model analysis. Clin Nutr 22:235–239
11. Talluri A, Maggia G (1995) Bioimpedance analysis (BIA) in hemodialysis: technical aspects. Int J Artif Organs 18(11):687–692
12. Peng S, Plank LD, McCall JL, Gillanders LK, Mcllroy K, Gane EJ (2007) Body composition, muscle function, and energy expenditure in patients with liver cirrhosis: a comprehensive study. Am J Clin Nutr 85:1257–1266
13. Lennard-Jones JE, Arrowsmith H, Davison C, Denham AF, Micklewright A (1995) Screening by nurses and junior doctors to detect malnutrition when patients are first assessed in hospital. Clin Nutr 14(6):336–340

14. Gheorghe C, Pascu O, Iacob R, Vadan R, Iacob S, Goldis A, Tantau M, Dumitru E, Dobru D, Miutescu E, Saftoiu A, fraticiu A, Tomescu D, Gheorghe L (2013) Nutritional risk screening and prevalence of malnutrition on admission to gastroenterology departments: a multicentric study. Chirurgia 108:535–541
15. da Silva FJ, de Mello PD, de Mello ED (2015) Subjective global assessment of nutritional status. A systematic review of the literature. Clin Nutr 34:785–792
16. Sorensen J, Kondrup J, Prokopowicz J, Schiesser M, Kraehenbuehl L, Liberda M, EurOOPS study group (2008) EuroOOPS: an international, multicentre study to implement nutritional risk screening and evaluate clinical outcome. Clin Nutr 27(3):340–349
17. Steenson J, Vivanti A, Isenring E (2013) Inter-rater reliability of the subjective global assessment: a systematic literature review. Nutrition 29:350–352
18. Agarwal E, Ferguson M, Banks M, Batterham M, Bauer J, Capra S et al (2013) Malnutrition and poor food intake are associated with prolonged hospital stay, frequent readmissions, and greater in-hospital mortality: results from the Nutrition Care Day survey 2010. Clin Nutr 32(5):737–745
19. Lucchin L, D'Amicis A, Gentile MG, Fusco MA, Battistini N, Palmo A, Muscaritoli M, e il gruppo di collaborazione PIMAI (2006) Project Iatrogenic Malnutrition in Italy(PIMAI) parte prima. Da: Gentile MG. Aggiornamenti in Nutrizione Clinica 14.Il Pensiero Scientifico Editore Roma. 25–4
20. Kruizenga HM, van Tulder MW, Seidell JC et al (2005) Effectiveness and cost-effectiveness of early screening and treatment of malnourished patients. Am J Clin Nutr 82:1082–1089
21. Barbara G, Stanghellini V, De Giorgio R et al (2004) Activated mast cells in proximity to colonic nerves correlate with abdominal pain in irritable bowel syndrome. Gastroenterology 126:693–702
22. Anifa 28 novembre 2012. Indagine Associazione Nazionale Industria Farmaceutica dell'Automedicazione. Campione di 1000 individui di 15–64 anni
23. Norman K, Kirchner H, Lochs H, Pirlich M (2006) Malnutrition affects quality of life in gastroenterology patients. World J Gastroenterol 7(12):3380–3385
24. Cheung K, Lee SS, Raman M (2012) Prevalence and mechanisms of malnutrition in patients with advanced liver diseases and nutrition management strategies. Clin Gastroenterol Hepatol 10:117–125
25. Fukuda Y, Yamamoto K, Hirao M, Nishikawa K et al (2015) Prevalence of malnutrition among gastric cancer patients undergoing gastrectomy and optimal preoperative nutritional support for preventing surgical site infections. Ann Surg Oncol 19:332
26. Duggan SN, Smyth ND, O'Sullivan M, Feehan S, Ridgway PF, Conlon KC (2014) The prevalence of malnutrition and fat-soluble vitamin deficiencies in chronic pancreatitis. Nutr Clin Pract 29(3):348–354
27. Esmaillzadeh A, Keshteli AH, Feizi A, Zaribaf F, Feinle-Bisset C, Adibi P (2013) Patterns of diet-related practices and prevalence of gastro-esophageal reflux disease. Neurogastroenterol Motil 25(10):831–e638
28. Lucchin L, Chilovi F (2009) Nutrizione e patologia gastrointestinale. Il Pensiero Scientifico, Roma
29. Nebel OT, Fornes MF, Castell DO (1976) Symptomatic gastroesophageal reflux: incidence and participating factors. Am J Dig Dis 21:953–956
30. Graham TE, McLean C (1999) Gender differences in the metabolic response to caffeine. In: Tarnopolsky M (ed) Gender differences in metabolism. CRC Press LLC, Boca Raton, p 307
31. Szabo G (2007) Moderate drinking inflammation and liver disease. Ann Epidemiol 17(5):S49–S54
32. Nilsson M, Johnse R, Ye W, Hveem K, Lagergren J (2004) Lifestyle related risk factors in the aetiology of gastro-oesophageal reflux. Gut 53:1730–1735
33. Rasu E, Jinga M, Enache G, Rusu F, Dragomir AD et al (2013) Effects of lifestyle changes including specific dietary intervention and physical activity in the management of patients with chronic hepatitis C-a randomized trial. Nutr J 12:119

34. Toshikuni N, Arisawa T, Tsutsumi M (2014) Nutrition and exercise in the management of liver cirrhosis. World J Gastroenterol 20(23):7286–7297
35. Heyman JK, Whitfield CJ, Brock KE, Mc Caughan GW, Donaghy AJ (2006) Dietary protein intakes in patients with hepatic encephalopathy and cirrhosis: current practice in NSW and ACT. Med J Aust 185:542–543
36. Bèmeur C, Butterworth RF (2014) Nutrition in the management of cirrhosis and its neurological complications. J Clin Exp Hepatol 482:141–150
37. Merli M, Iebba V, Giusto M (2015) What is new about diet in hepatic encephalopathy. Met Brain Dis. 2015 online 29 Sep
38. O'Brien A, Williams R (2008) Nutrition in end stage disease: principles and practice. Gastroenterology 134:1729–1740
39. Abdul-Hai A, Abdallah A, Malnick SDH (2015) Influence of gut bacteria on development and progression of non alcoholic fatty liver disease. World J Gastroenterol 7(12):1679–1684
40. Rusu E, Enache G, Jinga M, dragut R, Nan R et al (2015) Medical nutrition therapy in non alcoholic fatty liver disease-a review of literature. J Med Life 8(3):258–262
41. Riccardi G, Giacco R, Rivellese A (2004) Dietary fat, insulin sensitivity and the metabolic syndrome. Clin Nutr 23:447–456
42. Petitpierre M, Gumowsky P, Girard JP (1985) Irritable bowel syndrome and hypersensitivity to food. Ann Allergy 54:538–540
43. Hills JM, Aaronson PI (1991) The mechanism of action of peppermint oil in gastrointestinal smooth muscle. Gastroenterology 101:55–65
44. Gibson PR, Shepard SJ (2010) Evidence-based dietary management of functional gastrointestinal symptoms. The FODMAP approach. J Gastroenterol Hepatol 25:252–258
45. Ananthakrishnan AN, Khalili H, Konijeti GG, Higuchi LM et al (2014) Long term intake of dietary fat and risk of ulcerative colitis and Crohn's disease. Gut 63(5):776–784
46. Chan SSM, Chir MBB, Luben R, Van Schaik F et al (2014) Carbohydrate intake in the etiology of Crohn's disease and ulcerative colitis. Inflamm Owel Dis 20:2013–2021
47. Danese S, Sans M, Fiocchi C (2004) Inflammatory bowel disease: the role of environmental factors. Autoimmun Rev 3(5):394–400
48. Bernstein CN, Blanchard JF, leslie W, Wajda A, Yu BN (2000) The incidence of fracture among patients with inflammatory bowel disease. A population based cohort study. Ann Intern Med 133(10):795–799
49. Messori A, Trallori G, D'Albasio G, Milla M, Vannozzi G, Pacini F (1996) Defined formula diets versus steroids in the treatment of active Crohn's disease: a meta analysis. Scand J Gastroenterol 31(3):267–272
50. Farzaei MH, Abdollahi M, rahimi R (2015) Role of dietary polyphenols in the management of peptic ulcer. World J Gastroenterol 21(21):6499–6517
51. Feinle-Bisset C, Vozzo R, Horowitz M, Talley NJ (2004) Diet, food intake, and disturbed physiology in the pathogenesis of symptoms in functional dyspepsia. Am J Gastroenterol 99:170
52. Dobrilla G (2002) La digestione difficile. Il Pensiero Scientifico Editore, Roma
53. Benini L, Brighenti F, Castellani G, Brentegani MT et al (1994) Gastric emptying of solids is markedly delayed when meals are fried. Dig Dis Sci 39(11):2288–2294
54. Dinella C, Recchia A, Tuorila H, Monteleone E (2011) Individual astringency responsiveness affects the acceptance of phenol-rich foods. Appetite 56(3):633–642
55. Hefle SL (1996) The chemistry and biology of food allergens. Food Technol 50:86–92
56. Bertuccio P, Rosato V, Andreano A, ferraroni M, decarli A, Edefonti V, la Vecchia C (2013) Dietary patterns and gastric cancer risk. A systematic review and meta-analysis. Ann Oncol 24:1450–1458
57. Vieira AR, Vingeliene S, Chan DSM, Aune D et al (2015) Fruits, vegetables and bladder cancer risk: a systematic review and meta-analysis. Cancer Med 4(1):136–146

58. Fedirko V, Lukanova A, Bamia C, Trichopolou A et al (2012) Glycemic index, glycemic load, dietary carbohydrate, and dietary fiber intake and risk of liver and biliary tract cancers in Western Europeans. Ann Oncol 24:543–553
59. Afaneh C, Gerszberg D, Slattery E et al (2015) Pancreatic cancer surgery and nutrition management: a review of the current literature. Hepato Biliary Surg Nutr 4(1):59–71
60. Gilsing AMJ, Schouten LJ, Goldbohm RA, Dagnelie PC, van den Brandt PA, Weijenberg MP (2015) Vegetarianism, low meat consumption and the risk of colorectal cancer in a population based cohort study. Sci Rep 5:13484. doi:10.1038/srep13484
61. Bouvard V, Loomis D, Guyton KZ, Grosse Y et al (2015) Carcinogenicity of consumption of red and processed meat. Lancet Oncol 16:1599–1600, online 26 october

Diet as Therapy for IBD?

6

Aronne Romano and Valeriano Castagna

In a clinical context, the question of what to eat is one of the most commonly asked by patients and also, at least as inflammatory bowel disease (IBD) is concerned, among the most difficult to answer by physicians. In published guidelines for management of IBD, dietary advice plays only a minor part, while public guidance, as provided by professional bodies, varies and is often based on consensus rather than on evidence [1]. In the last few years, excellent reviews of the epidemiological, clinical, and experimental works addressing the role of nutrition in IBD have been published [2–8]. The aim of this chapter is to revise the emerging knowledge, introduce some ideas and new data from recent research, and explain the authors' point of view.

Crohn's disease (CD) and ulcerative colitis (UC) are parts of the spectrum of IBD. They are characterized by a condition of chronic intestinal inflammation of relapsing and remitting nature. In UC this is confined to the large-bowel mucosa, while in CD it can virtually affect any segment in the digestive tract, and it is typically transmural, resulting in stricture and fistula formation. Clinical features include diarrhea, abdominal pain, weight loss, malaise, anorexia, fever, rectal bleeding and urgency, as well as extra-intestinal manifestations (e.g., spondylitis, uveitis, erythema nodosum) [2].

The last half century has witnessed a dramatic increase in the rates of CD and UC, along with other so-called diseases of affluence: in 40 years there has been approximately a fourfold rise in IBD incidence in Western Europe and a fourfold increase in Japan in 15 years [1]. In North America, the prevalence of UC has

A. Romano
Associazione Etica Nutrizionale Gerona 2005, Vicolo Filatoio 19, Rezzato, BS, Italy
e-mail: arosatu@libero.it

V. Castagna (✉)
UOC di Gastroenterologia ed Endoscopia Digestiva, ASST Bergamo Est, Seriate, BG, Italy
e-mail: valcasta@libero.it

© Springer International Publishing Switzerland 2016
E. Grossi, F. Pace (eds.), *Human Nutrition from the Gastroenterologist's Perspective*,
DOI 10.1007/978-3-319-30361-1_6

reached 249 per 100,000 persons, and 319 per 100,000 people have CD [2, 9]. Possible explanations include increased hygiene during infancy, or greater exposure to antibiotics, but circumstantial evidence seems to implicate changes in dietary habits both in countries shifting to a Western diet (e.g., Japan, India) and in ethnic groups adopting a Western diet after migrating to a Western nation [2].

The etiology of IBD is still not completely understood. There is general agreement on the concurrence of genetic predisposition and immune dysfunction, together with the enteric microbiota and environmental factors [2], although it is far from clear whether these components are equally necessary and sufficient, and exactly how they interact [10]. Modern research has delved deeply into the underlying fine genetic, epigenetic, and immunological mechanisms, and increasing effort is conveyed to uncover the complex role of microbiota and its relation with the host. So far, assessment of environmental effect has been limited by the extent to which we are able to measure the environment [1].

Along with changes in lifestyle such as improved hygiene, alcohol consumption, smoking, and altered sleep habits, environmental triggers linked to IBD must include dietary intake, as diet, together with the microbiota, provides most of the luminal antigens [11]. Food may influence intestinal inflammation via direct antigenic effect, alteration of gene expression, modulation of inflammatory mediators (e.g., eicosanoids), change of mucosal permeability, and impact on the composition of enteric flora [12].

6.1   What Have We Acknowledged So Far About Diet and IBD?

Diet is the primary behavioral factor manipulated by patients with IBD, through a frustrating trial-and-error process of identification of foods that trigger symptoms. Information is often sought by patients wherever available, such as traditional or alternative health practitioners, published literature, and the Internet. Food avoidance is far more common than in the general population, but sugar consumption from sweetened beverages is far greater in those with active IBD [3], potentially giving rise to undernutrition or overnutrition. In fact, overall adherence to national dietary guidelines is poor, and food avoidance strategies may lead to nutritional inadequacy [3]. In an Internet query of dietary advice in IBD [6], examining 28 food categories, patient-targeted recommendations were similar for CD and UC and appeared to be highly restrictive and frequently conflicting, fostering confusion and possibly nutritional deficiencies, which patients are already prone to experience.

It appears that a large gap exists in translating research-based dietary knowledge to clinical practice for the IBD population [13]. Creating evidence-based dietary recommendations for people with IBD is an unaddressed need.

6.2   Insight from Epidemiology: Can Diet Prevent the Onset of IBD?

Several approaches have been taken to identify candidate dietary patterns that contribute to the risk of IBD, after hypotheses supported by preliminary observations. A due premise is that methodology flaws can be recognized in many publications. Recall bias in retrospective studies represent a major limiting factor, as dietary changes may have occurred soon after the development of symptoms, perhaps years before diagnosis. Other sources of bias are found in the process of recruitment and selection, in dietary assessment methods, and in the multiple comparisons carried out, often seen in case-control and cohort studies [2]. Anyway, prospective surveys together with intervention studies seem the most powerful and accurate way of identifying causal relationships with susceptibility to IBD [3].

Despite the fact that large studies on the identification of dietary risk factors have been published, there are major limitations to reported data. First, these studies have largely examined diet of adults to determine predictors of the onset of new IBD in mature persons (fifth decade), in an age range not comprising peak incidence (15–30 years of age) [3]. Whether associations observed in late-onset IBD apply to the whole temporal spectrum of disease is uncertain. For instance, in the large US Nurses' Health Study (NH, $n=72,719$), no association was recognized between breastfeeding and the risk of CD, while a preceding high-quality retrospective population-based study reported long-term breastfeeding (>3 months) to be protective [3]. It is likely that the effect wanes with age, as in another systematic review breastfeeding seems to preserve children from developing IBD (OR 0.69; 95 % CI 0.51–0.94) [3]. A second limitation is that food intake data are based on rather old food-frequency questionnaires providing limited details on food composition and entailing considerable variability in their interpretation.

An epidemiological study from Japan showed correlation between dietary changes and the incidence of CD from 1966 to 1985 [1]. By univariate analysis, the increased incidence of CD was strongly correlated ($P<0.001$) with increased intake of total fat ($r=0.919$), animal fat ($r=0.880$), n-6 polyunsaturated fatty acids (PUFAs; $r=0.883$), animal protein ($r=0.908$), milk protein ($r=0.924$), and the ratio of n-6 to n-3 FAs intake ($r=0.792$). There was a weaker correlation with intake of total protein ($r=0.482$, $P<0.05$). There was no correlation with intake of fish protein ($r=0.055$, $P>0.1$) and an inverse correlation with intake of vegetable protein ($r=0.941$, $P<0.001$). Multivariate analysis showed that increased intake of animal protein was the strongest independent factor.

A separate study from Japan identified consumption of margarine as a significant risk factor (P for trend = 0.005) for the development of UC [1]. Also an Italian study showed high consumption of margarine to be strongly associated with the risk for UC [OR, 21.37; CI, 2.32–196.6], but not CD [1].

A systematic review that included 19 studies reporting pre-illness diet in IBD found a positive association between the risk for CD and a high intake of saturated fats, monounsaturated fatty acids, total PUFAs, total n-3 FAs, n-6 FAs, mono- and disaccharides, meat, and low intake of dietary fiber and fruits [1]. Increased risk for UC was associated with high intakes of total fats, total PUFAs, n-6 PUFAs, and a low vegetable intake.

Intriguing data have come from the European Prospective Investigation into Cancer and Nutrition (EPIC) study, designed to investigate the relationships between diet, nutritional status, lifestyle, and environmental factors and the incidence of cancer and other chronic diseases, involving 203,193 people in ten European countries. A nested case-control study within the EPIC cohort included 126 cases with subsequent UC matched with 504 healthy controls. Multivariate analysis showed that the highest quartile of intake of linoleic acid (LA, an n-6 PUFA found in red meat, corn, and sunflower oils and margarine) was associated with an increased risk of UC (OR = 2.49; 95 % CI, 1.23–5.07; $P=0.01$) when adjusted for age at recruitment, gender, center, energy intake, and cigarette smoking [5]. In contrast, people who consumed higher levels of n-3 PUFA docosahexaenoic acid (DHA) were less likely to be diagnosed with UC.

Another very large prospective cohort study involving 67,581 women aged 40–65 in France (E3N Study) showed a similar association between high animal protein intake (meat or fish but not eggs or dairy products) and IBD, particularly UC (HR = 3.29 for top tertile vs. bottom tertile, CI, 1.34–8.04; $P=0.005$) [5]. An association of risk of IBD and elevated protein intake was confirmed in another study from Japan [3]. Moreover, a study of environmental factors on IBD in twins demonstrated that a high intake of processed meat conveyed a high risk for both CD (OR = 7.9 in monozygous twins, CI, 2.15–38.12, and OR = 10.75 in dizygous twins, CI, 4.82–25.55) and UC (OR = 5.69 in monozygous twins, CI, 1.89–19.48, and OR = 18.11 in dizygous twins, CI, 7.34–50.85) [1].

Epidemiological studies have yielded conflicting data regarding the role of carbohydrate exposure as risk factor for IBD [8]. Nevertheless, the same systematic review already mentioned showed a very consistent reporting of high pre-illness intake of refined sugar among patients with CD [5], while in the EPIC study, no association was found between carbohydrate intake and onset of UC during the follow-up [8]. However, a more recent article concludes that a diet imbalance with high consumption of sugar and soft drinks and low consumption of vegetables is associated with higher UC risk [14].

The NH study has examined the association between fiber intake and incidence of IBD: nurses consuming large amounts of fiber, particularly fruits, were approximately 40 % less likely to be diagnosed with CD, although no association was observed for UC [3].

6.3   Dietary Interventions in Active Inflammatory Bowel Disease: Can Diet Cure Active Disease?

In the 1970s, total bowel rest and intravenous glucose were deemed appropriate for active disease, but patients soon developed protein-energy malnutrition. Total parenteral nutrition (TPN) overcame this issue [2], but because of its invasiveness, risks of serious complications, and gut atrophy, more recently enteral nutrition (EN) has been considered more suitable when viable.

Exclusive enteral nutrition (EEN) is a well-established method for inducing remission in children with recent-onset Crohn's disease [8]. It also improves nutritional status, growth, and development, and, according to a prospective Australian study, 8-week long EEN is accompanied by mucosal healing, either complete (42 %) or nearly complete (58 %) [8]. The majority of children relapse during the first year, but 66 % respond with remission to a second course of EEN [8]. Early EN was based on an elemental formula, but later equally efficacious, more palatable peptide and whole-protein formulas have been introduced [2]. Partial enteral nutrition (PEN) associated to a free diet seems to be ineffective for the induction of remission [8]. In adults with CD, the evidence is not so strong and EN is less effective than corticosteroids [2]. It can be useful as an adjunctive treatment to other therapeutic measurements and when the benefits of nutritional support are warranted [2].

EN does not provide a primary therapeutic option in UC, but can be used for nutritional support [2].

Postulated mechanisms of response have included the effect of EEN on the gut microbiome (improvement in diversity, in protective species, in butyrate production) [8]. However, in a Scottish study on 15 children with CD in successful remission with EEN, compared to 21 controls, contrary to the expectations, EEN was associated with a further decrease in diversity, decrease in specific "protective species," and a reduction in butyrate in fecal samples.

Investigators from Israel have hypothesized that the major mechanism lies in the exclusion of dietary components thought to affect the microbiome or intestinal permeability [8]. They treated for 6 weeks 47 patients with active CD with PEN (up to 50 % of dietary calories) and an exclusion diet that allowed access to specific foods (lean chicken breast, fish, eggs, vegetables, and rice) and restricted exposure to all other foods. The use of this diet led to clinical remission in 70 % of patients by week 6, accompanied by a significant drop in C-reactive protein (CRP) and erythrocyte sedimentation rate (ESR) through week 12, normalization of CRP in 70 % of patients in remission, and mucosal healing in a subset of responders (11 of 15). If confirmed, the results suggest that specific dietary products do play a role in gut inflammation.

Success of EN for active CD has led to the evaluation of the same approach to other gut inflammatory conditions. Investigators from London evaluated the use of an elemental diet for chronic pouchitis [8]. Seven patients with pouchitis were treated with an EEN for 28 days. The use of EEN led to a significant decrease in stool frequency and in the Pouch Disease Activity Index (PDAI), but there was no improvement in the endoscopic or histology scores.

In active UC, the use of TPN provided no advantage in one small RCT [3], and most other dietary interventional studies have been mainly applied to preventing relapse. However, Kyaw et al. [8] treated 61 UC adult patients over 4–6 weeks during a disease flare. Their dietary intervention was based on reduced exposure to fat, simple carbohydrates, red meat, and processed food. By week 24, there was a modest but significant improvement in the activity score, suggesting that this may improve disease activity, although it could not induce remission.

Interventions with increased fiber intake have all involved using supplemental fiber (including non-starch polysaccharides, oligosaccharides, and germinated barley), not taking account of habitual intake [3]. A recent systemic review, involving 23 clinical trials (1,296 patients) on the effects of fiber on clinical end points (primarily disease activity, for treatment or maintenance) or physiological outcomes, found no effect for the supplementation of dietary fiber in CD, a possible weak effect in UC, and a possible effect in pouchitis [3]. Despite this, a few of the studies reported favorable intragroup effects on physiological outcomes, including fecal butyrate, fecal calprotectin, inflammatory cytokines, microbiota, and gastrointestinal symptom indices. Most important, contrary to common belief, there was no evidence that fiber intake should be restricted in patients with IBD (cfr. also next paragraph).

Interventions aimed at changing fat intake in IBD have been restricted to the use of n-3 PUFA supplements, whereby efficacy has not been established for either active disease or in prevention of relapse [3]. Elimination of cow's milk protein in UC has obtained inconsistent evidence [8].

6.4 Dietary Interventions After Induction of Remission: Can Diet Help Maintain Remission?

Multiple small studies have shown that PEN may be effective as a maintenance therapy to prevent clinical recurrence of CD [8]. Postoperative PEN with nightly tube feeding and a daily low-fat diet prevented endoscopic recurrence at 1 year; at 5 years, significantly more patients in the control group required biological therapy. As to UC, there is no evidence to support EN in the maintenance of disease remission.

Maintenance of clinical remission of CD induced by a variety of techniques can be improved to a small extent by an individualized food exclusion diet [3]. One of the most successful is the low-fat fiber-limited exclusion (LOFFLEX) diet: it not only helps maintain disease remission [2], but it helps to identify potentially problematic foods that are poorly tolerated. In 2–4 weeks, LOFFLEX foods are introduced to quickly provide a nutritionally complete, whereas the EN is reduced and usually discontinued. A slow reintroduction of a new food every 2–4 days allows patients to determine tolerance.

In another small study ($n=22$) from Japan, Chiba et al. [6] demonstrated superiority of a semi-vegetarian diet (SVD) to maintain clinical remission (absence of symptoms). The study included patients with medically ($n=17$) or surgically ($n=5$) induced remission who had already received an in-hospital lacto-ova-vegetarian diet. After discharge, patients could choose to continue the diet or revert to a traditional one (undefined, considered "omnivorous"). The diet comprised brown rice, miso (fermented bean paste) soup, vegetables, fruits, legumes, potatoes, pickled vegetables, and plain yogurt daily. Fish was allowed once a week and meat once every 2 weeks, no limitation was imposed for eggs and milk. Beverages only included green tea and water. The SVD was continued by 73 % of patients ($n=16$).

Remission over 2 years was maintained in 94 % (SVD) vs. 33 % of patients in the control group. There was no untoward effect of SVD.

Conversely, both low-residue and an unrefined carbohydrate or fiber-rich diets showed no apparent effects on clinical outcomes after steroid-induced remission over at least 2 years [3].

In a study conducted in Australia, 25 patients with UC in remission and 12 healthy controls were randomized to receive either a low-resistant starch, low-wheat bran exposure diet, or a high-resistant starch with high-wheat bran diet over 2 weeks; then each group crossed over to the second diet after a washout period. Surprisingly, increased exposure to starch and fiber in the UC group did not increase short-chain fatty acid production and did not lead to a change in the composition of the microbiome. The authors concluded that individuals with UC have decreased ability to ferment non-starch polysaccharides and starch [8].

6.5   Dietary Interventions for Symptomatic Relief: Can Diet Afford Control of Symptoms?

In everyday practice, it is usual for gastroenterologists to prescribe a low-fiber diet during a flare-up, and a low-residue diet in patients with known stricturing CD. Also frequently prescribed is the decrease in the consumption of greasy foods, caffeine, alcohol, and dairy products, depending on individual tolerance. However, while agreed on by common sense, these measures do not seem to stem from sound evidence. Few trials have examined dietary manipulation to treat symptoms of IBD, perhaps because of the difficulty to design a randomized control trial with all dietary variables under control (unless all meals are provided by the researchers), or for the poor funding of research in this area [7]. An issue with all studies investigating the effects of diet on IBD symptoms is the low-sample size that limits the generalizability one can draw from any of these interventions.

Low-residue or low-fiber diet trials have shown no significant difference in symptom control between treatment and control groups [7].

On the other hand, in exclusion diets studies, significant improvements in symptoms post diet intervention have been reported for CD as well as for UC patients [7]. These diets imply gradual introduction of foods, after induction of remission, and elimination of those that cause symptoms. In general, a single new item is introduced each day, and any food provoking symptoms is discarded. Once the testing stage is completed, suspect foods are retested, to confirm negative effects on symptoms, and eventually definitely excluded. Dietary assessment is provided, to ensure nutritional adequacy.

An interesting extension of these diets is based on IgG-guided elimination of foods. A pilot trial evaluated CD patients with active disease, whose serum was tested for IgG4 antibodies to 14 specific food antigens; each patient's four most reactive foods were then removed from their meals for 4 weeks [7]. Eggs and beef were the items most commonly associated with high IgG4 antibody levels and were therefore excluded by the greatest number of patients. Significant symptomatic improvement was reported, mostly in number of bowel movements per day (mean reduction from 4 to 2, $P=0.0001$), followed by mean pain-rating reduction (from 0.71 to 0.43, $P=0.030$), and general well-being improvement (from 0.88 to 0.63, $P=0.045$).

A second randomized, double-blind, cross-over intervention trial [7] further examined an IgG-guided exclusion diet in active CD ($n=23$). The first step involved measuring the reactivity of T cells, CD4, and CD25 to patient-specific food antigens in vitro. Patients receiving a specific elimination diet for 6 weeks, based on these IgG results, then crossed over to the sham diet. The control group received a sham diet during the same time, but patients eliminated certain foods that differed from those specified by IgG results, and then crossed over to the exclusion diet. Stool frequency was significantly lower during the IgG-selected diet. There was a nonsignificant improvement in the combined score to rate general well-being and abdominal pain for the IgG diet group.

Defined diets are dietary regimens based on an underlying "theory" of food-body interactions. To date they still await rigorous scientific assessment [6].

The *Specific Carbohydrate Diet* (SCD) was first described by Dr. Sidney Haas in 1924, as a means to treat celiac disease, and later popularized by biochemist Elaine Gottschall [6]. The underlying theory of the SCD is that disaccharide and polysaccharide carbohydrates are poorly absorbed in the intestinal tract, resulting in bacterial and yeast overgrowth and subsequent overproduction of mucus. Resulting small bowel injury is hypothesized that further worsens carbohydrate malabsorption and subsequent intestinal injury [6]. The diet excludes all but simple carbohydrates (glucose, fructose, and galactose). All fresh fruits and vegetables are acceptable with the exception of potatoes and yams. Only certain legumes are permitted, and no grains are allowed. Patients can use saccharin and honey, in addition to moderate sorbitol and xylitol. Unprocessed meats can be eaten without limitation, while processed, canned, and most smoked meats are restricted (for possible sugars and starches as additives). Milk is forbidden because of lactose content, but certain lactose-free cheeses are allowed, as is homemade lactose-free yogurt.

Derived from the SCD, the *IBD anti-inflammatory diet* (IBD-AID) has been proposed recently by Olendzki [15] to demonstrate the potential of an adjunct dietary therapy for the treatment of IBD. This diet consists of lean meats, poultry, fish, omega-3 eggs, particular sources of carbohydrate (avoiding lactose and refined or processed complex carbohydrates), select fruits and vegetables, nut and legume flours, limited aged cheeses (made with active cultures and enzymes), fresh cultured yogurt, kefir, miso and other cultured products (rich with certain probiotics), and honey. It specifically decreases the total and saturated fats, eliminates hydrogenated oils, and encourages the increased intake of foods with n-3 fatty acids. Oats are permitted, since oats appear to be well tolerated and are useful in regulation of bowel frequency and consistency [15]. Prebiotics, in the form of soluble fiber (containing beta-glucans and inulin, such as bananas, oats, blended chicory root, and flax meal), are suggested. In addition, the patient is advised to begin at a texture phase of the diet matching with symptomatology, starting with phase I (i.e., softer, blended foods) if in an active flare. Many patients require foods to be mechanically softened and devoid of seeds when starting the diet, as intact fiber can be problematic (strictures, highly active mucosal inflammation); some may require lifelong avoidance of intact fiber. Food irritants may also include certain foods, processing agents, and flavorings to which IBD patients may be reactive. The dietary pattern of the IBD-AID is said to be carefully oriented to decrease inflammation, as application of the formerly developed Dietary Inflammatory Index [16, 17], designed to assess the inflammatory potential of diet.

In a retrospective case series report, patient started the diet while in a flare. As symptoms improved, they were advanced to more whole foods, but within the guidelines of the IBD-AID. Twenty-seven patients (out of 40 originally included) attended a follow-up visit: 24 reported a good or very good response to the diet, as measured by self-report of symptoms and compliance with the diet through food records. The investigators had complete medical records of 11 patients (8 CD, 3 UC; age range, 19–70), 7 had experienced one or more treatment failures; diet was followed for at least 4 weeks. After the IBD-AID, the only additional intervention added, all of the patients succeeded in downscaling their medication regimen, and their IBD symptoms were reduced.

The acronym "FODMAPs" (Fermentable Oligo-, Di-, and Monosaccharides and Polyols) describes a group of short-chain carbohydrates and sugar alcohols (polyols). FODMAPs are widespread in the diet, and their ingestion increases delivery of readily fermentable substrate and water to the distal small intestine and proximal colon, which are likely to induce luminal distension and induction of functional gut symptoms. Poorly absorbed carbohydrates result in bacterial overgrowth [6]. The FODMAP diet has been studied primarily for irritable bowel syndrome and functional gastrointestinal disorders. The underlying mechanistic theory overlaps with the SCD. However, although they are similar in the restrictions of cereal grains and unrestricted meat, the FODMAP diet is highly restrictive on certain fruit and vegetable intake, whereas the SCD has unrestricted fruit and vegetable, except potatoes and yams.

There have been two small retrospective studies evaluating the FODMAP diet in IBD [6], supportive of dietary interventions to improve IBD symptoms. However, they lack objective data regarding inflammatory changes associated with dietary intervention. Symptomatic response may also suggest that in some IBD patients with remitting disease, persistence of symptoms may be due to an overlap with functional disorders.

Few studies have addressed the issue of foreign chemical molecules that may be inadvertently ingested by patients. A 2×2 factorial design study assessed a diet low or normal in microparticles (titanium dioxide and particulate silicates) and/or calcium for 16 weeks on patients with active CD [7]. There was no benefit from reducing dietary microparticles or manipulating dietary calcium.

Bartel et al. [7] assessed a diet low in ingested matter from environmental factors (i.e., fertilizers, pesticides, preservatives, food additives). Patients with active stricturing CD followed a restricted diet for 6 weeks, composed of red meat, sourdough bread, rape oil, and fresh butter from intensively monitored organic farming. The control group was instructed to eat a well-balanced, low-fat, high-carbohydrate diet while avoiding fruits and vegetables and red meat. This study showed a significant improvement based on MRI, endoscopic, and ultrasound evaluation but no statistically significant changes on clinical or laboratory parameters.

Finally, Grimstad et al. [7] treated patients with active UC with a salmon-rich (600 g per week) diet for 8 weeks. Levels of n-3 PUFA in plasma and rectal biopsies were significantly augmented, resulting in an increased n-3/n-6 PUFA ratio. There were significant improvements in Simple Clinical Colitis Activity Index (SCCAI) score from visit one (median, 3; range, 0–7) to visit two (1.5, 0–6, $p=0.007$), as well as nonsignificant reductions in CRP ($P=0.066$) and homocysteine levels.

6.6   Which Are the Pathophysiological Mechanisms Involved?

It would be virtually impossible to report all the mechanisms that are thought to link food components to IBD. At least two, though, appear to be particularly important, dysbiosis and increased intestinal permeability.

Martinez-Medina et al. [8] demonstrated that a high-fat, high-sugar diet led to dysbiosis and colonization with adherent-invasive *E. coli* (AIEC), depletion of the mucous layer, and increased intestinal permeability in an IL-10$^{-/-}$ knockout mouse.

The effect of a high-fat diet (HFD) was reproduced in the TNF$^{\Delta Are/wt}$ mouse model of ileitis too. This study demonstrated that HFD can markedly reduce expression of occlusion in tight junctions independent of inflammation and increase translocation of endotoxin. It can also enhance expression of inflammation markers by epithelial cells, along with luminal factors-driven recruitment of dendritic cells and Th17-biased lymphocyte infiltration into the lamina propria [8].

In older mice, a diet rich in n-6 PUFAs led to intestinal inflammation and was associated with dysbiosis, with depletion of Bacteroidetes and Firmicutes [18]. Moreover, a 3-week diet of saturated milk-derived FAs, compared to PUFAs or low-fat diet, increased the formation of taurine-conjugated bile acids in IL-10$^{-/-}$ knockout mouse [4], increasing the availability of organic sulfur in the intestinal lumen and leading to the expansion of the low-abundant, sulfite-reducing *B. wadsworthia*, a pathobiont. Susceptibility to colitis and severity were augmented in IL-10$^{-/-}$ knockout mouse, but not in the wild type.

Even gluten might play a deleterious role in ileitis as well. Gluten can induce zonulin, which increases small intestinal permeability [8]. Wagner et al. [8] compared the development of ileitis in mice fed with standard, gluten-free, or gluten-added diet. Exposure to gluten exacerbated ileitis, most likely by increasing the intestinal permeability.

Two clues may connect diet and AIEC, a possible pathobiont in Crohn's disease. These bacteria can translocate across ileal epithelium, survive in macrophages, and generate TNF-α, leading to granulomas. Strains of AIEC have been isolated from the ileum and the colon of CD patients [8].

Maltodextrin, a thickening and binding agent found in breakfast cereals and artificial sweeteners, was found to promote AIEC biofilms and increase adhesion of AIEC strains to intestinal epithelial cells and macrophages via upregulation of type 1 pili expression [8]. This mechanism is independent from interaction with the usual ligand (CEACAM6), suggesting that exposure to maltodextrin may allow AIEC to attach when it otherwise could not adhere to cells.

Iron and heme may be critical for AIEC penetration and survival in macrophages. The growth of AIEC required iron, and the enrichment of these strains with heme acquisition genes correlated with persistence in macrophages [8].

Red meat was shown to promote inflammation in a dextran sulfate sodium (DSS) colitis model. Interestingly, the effect was amended by resistant starch, one of the sources for butyrate production [8].

n-Butyrate, a product of bacterial fermentation of fibers and starches, was found to reduce the secretion of interleukin 6 (IL-6), IL-12, and nitric oxide synthase directly inhibiting deacetylation of histones [8]. It was also found to induce differentiation of regulatory T cells [8]. However, it was ineffective in ameliorating colitis in a DSS model of colitis [8].

6.7 Some Considerations

With the exception of enteral nutrition in active Crohn's disease, evidence from observational and intervention studies appear still fragmentary and somewhat contradictory. For instance, it is puzzling that different and opposed approaches, like exclusion diets and PEN versus some fiber-rich diets [6, 15], seem to obtain equally good response in CD patients in remission, at least as far as symptoms are concerned. Likewise, we still lack an explanation for the seemingly ambiguous role of carbohydrates and to a lesser extent of polyunsaturated n-6 fatty acids or the inconspicuous role of n-3 PUFA supplements in IBD, which apparently contradicts the anti-inflammatory effects shown by experiments in animal models of IBD, as well as our understanding of their role in the resolution of inflammation.

Some light has been shed by the introduction of the Dietary Inflammatory Index (DII) [17], which has been tested in different contexts, ranging from asthma and other respiratory conditions to lung, breast, prostate, pancreatic, and colorectal cancer, as well as cardiovascular and metabolic diseases. This index has been constructed after reviewing all research articles published from 1950 up to 2010 (some 6,500 papers), which assessed the role of 45 different dietary constituents on specific inflammatory markers (IL-1b, IL-4, IL-6, IL-10, TNF-α, and C-reactive protein). Collected results were used to set the *overall inflammatory effect score* for each dietary item, a positive score meaning pro-inflammatory effect, a negative one the opposite. Based on 11 extensive food consumption data sets from around the world, *global daily mean intakes* were calculated, as well as standard deviations. To assess the actual DII of an individual's diet, the percentile score of each diet component is determined through intermediate steps and multiplied by the corresponding *overall inflammatory effect score*. Finally, all results are added. The computed DII ranges from a theoretical value of 7.98 (pro-inflammatory maximum) and −8.87 (anti-inflammatory maximum). Its application to the analysis of real individual diets acknowledges their inflammatory potential, and several studies have been published, which confirm the value of this approach in appreciating observed dietary patterns and their effects. As an example, it has been recognized that FAs are heterogeneous in their association with postmenopausal breast cancer risk [19], that FAs from marine food are associated with reduced risk of additional breast cancer events and all-cause mortality [20], or that a pro-inflammatory diet, as indicated by higher DII scores, was associated with higher risk of all-cause, CVD, and cancer mortality [21].

Looking through the list of analyzed food parameters, it is noteworthy that the *overall inflammatory effect score* for carbohydrates is positive yet quite small (0.097), while higher values are shown by the total fat (0.298), saturated fat (0.373), and trans fat (0.229). On the other hand, for n-3 PUFAs and n-6 PUFAs, negative values, that is, anti-inflammatory effect, have been registered (−0.436 and −0.159, respectively), so as for monounsaturated FA (MUFA) (0.009). The highest anti-inflammatory effect is shown by turmeric (−0.785), followed by fiber (−0.663), flavones (−0.616), isoflavones (−0.593), beta-carotene (−0.584), and green/black tea (−0.536). The net effect of each component of the diet depends of course on the total amount present; so a diet could be theoretically devised, taking into account individual preferences and needs while addressing maximum anti-inflammatory result. Alternatively, existing dietary patterns could be evaluated and confronted for pro- or anti-inflammatory potential, and some publications have already addressed the issue.

The Dietary Inflammatory Index undoubtedly represents a skilled application of actual knowledge in an extremely compact form; nonetheless, this promising tool is unlikely to clear the problems in nutrition research. The performance of clinical trials in dietary and nutrition studies generally uses principles of good practice that derive from pharmacological trials. However, there are multiple differences between the structure and design of pharmacological and dietary studies. In the latter, issues that are difficult to attain, such as a true placebo diet or unequivocal blinding, have often hindered credibility. Also epidemiological observations have been disappointing in their contribution to the field, despite multiple studies with huge patient populations [3]. The result is the limited high-quality evidence available, which poses serious issues when prompting dietary recommendations to patients with IBD [22].

The theoretical grounds of nutrition research have been questioned lately. The bottom-up reductionist approach has been so far predominant and has unraveled some of the fundamental mechanisms at the basis of food nutrients. Yet, interactions between food compounds and physiological effect cannot be modeled based on a linear cause-effect relation, but rather from multicausal nonlinear relations. Foods composing the diet and the human organism are complex systems that interact before, during, and after food consumption. This is a formidable challenge, one to be addressed under a more holistic perspective, which considers the ecosystem within the context of relations, without dissociating human beings from the society and the natural environment. Some steps along the trail have been taken when dietary patterns rather than isolated food compounds are considered, as foods are perceived not only as the sum of their compounds, but also as complex structures or matrices. The increased use of high-throughput approaches such as metabolomics and transcriptomics to measure the effect of a diet on the overall metabolism or gene expression is another example [23]. Obviously, coupling metabolomics with genomics, transcriptomics, and proteomics will facilitate the development of a more holistic picture, but necessitates the development of dedicated mathematical applications [10].

A top-down approach becomes necessary to investigate complex issues through a holistic view, starting without a priori assumptions with the use of observational tools and unraveling cause-effect relation later, through a specific reductionist approach that explains a particular point when necessary. Thus, both approaches are needed and mutually reinforcing. The holistic approach appears to be empowered to discover hidden associations or new research hypotheses, with techniques that go beyond classic statistical tools to help address them [23].

A different and yet intriguing perspective on nutrition is given by Darwinian/evolutionary medicine. This approach examines how diet helped us evolve among primates and to adapt (or fail to adapt) our metabolome to specific environmental conditions [24].

In 1985, Eaton and Konner published a seminal article in the *New England Journal of Medicine* about Paleolithic nutrition, in which they postulated the evolutionary discordance or "mismatch" model [25]. According to their view, human bodies, reflecting adaptations established in the Paleolithic era (2.6 million to 12,000 years ago), are ill suited to modern industrialized diets and develop rapidly increasing rates of chronic metabolic disease. They suggested that the Paleolithic diet, an ancestral diet characterized by higher protein, less total fat, more essential fatty acids, lower sodium, and higher fiber, should serve as a reference standard for modern human nutrition. Multidisciplinary papers trying to define the nutritional patterns of our ancestors from the Paleolithic era have revealed considerable variety. Cordain et al. [26] estimated macronutrient energy and plant to animal ratio on the data from Murdock's Ethnographic Atlas and found that 73 % of the worldwide hunter-gatherer (HG) societies derived more than 50 % of total daily energy from animal foods and only 14 % used more gathered plant foods. However, the meals of our preagricultural ancestors were virtually devoid of cereals, newborns were fed with breast milk, but children and adults never touched milk products, and heating was probably the only significant food-processing procedure. Konner and Eaton [27] estimated that total fiber intake (TFI) would have averaged 150 g/day and was not likely lower than 70 g/day. They also stated that the low amount of phytic acid, together with the high-calcium intake and the net negative acid load, made HG diet protective for low bone mineral density and fractures.

In the wake of these papers, many others have been issued, most of which have investigated the effects of this diet on metabolic diseases. A recent systematic review and meta-analysis by Manheimer et al. [28] addressed Paleolithic nutrition for metabolic syndrome. Primary outcome measures were changes from the baseline of waist circumference, triglycerides, HDL cholesterol, blood pressure (systolic and diastolic), and fasting blood sugar. Four RCTs with a total of 159 randomly assigned participants met the inclusion criteria. Paleolithic nutrition resulted in greater short-term pooled improvements on each of the five components of the metabolic syndrome than did currently recommended guideline-based control diets. However, the greater pooled improvements did not reach significance for two of the five components (i.e., HDL cholesterol, and fasting blood sugar).

The original article by Eaton has been followed by a lively debate, and controversies about the assumptions that genetic traits evolved largely during the Paleolithic period have been outpaced by cultural change, resulting in a gene-culture mismatch and the epidemic "diseases of civilization" [29]. While critics do not label the hypothesis as incorrect, they contest that it is incomplete in relying primarily on genetic understanding of the human diet. According to current research, human eating habits would have been learned primarily through behavioral, social, and physiological mechanisms that start in utero and extend throughout the life course. Adaptations that appear to be strongly genetic would likely reflect Neolithic, rather than Paleolithic, adaptations and would be significantly influenced by human niche-constructing behavior [30].

An extremely important factor in IBD pathogenesis, gut microbiota, might explain at least some of the characteristics that have been highlighted by nutrition studies as far as fatty acids are concerned in the light of coevolution with our species. It has been proposed that the immune system has evolved a capacity to modify expenditure on inflammation to compensate for the effects of dietary FA on gut microorganisms [31]. The body would upregulate inflammation in response to saturated FAs (SFAs) that promote harmful microbes. In contrast, it would reduce inflammation in response to the many PUFAs with antimicrobial properties. This model is supported by observed contrasts involving shorter-chain FAs (SCFAs) and n-3 PUFAs, with less consistent evidence for trans fatty acids (TFAs), which are a recent addition to the human diet. Modern farmed meat provides a much higher concentration of SFAs than wild game. In addition, the n-3 PUFAs content is higher in wild fish and game than in farmed meat. It has been suggested that the decreased ratio of n-3 to n-6 FAs in the diet is a source of increased pro-inflammatory eicosanoid synthesis [32]. The nutrient signaling model not only helps explain the inflammatory effects of dietary fat, but it also might account for the production and modification of lipids by intestinal bacteria. Predictions could apply to other nutrient classes encountered during human evolution that reliably influence the gut microbiota. Carbohydrates are good candidates, so as many secondary plant compounds (e.g., polyphenols). Simple sugars are known to increase the survival of pathogens in an acidic environment such as that represented by the gut [33]. On the other hand, oligosaccharides are the precursors of SCFAs production in the human colon by bacterial fermentation. These fermentation products lower intestinal pH, inhibiting the growth of pathogenic species [34].

Konner and Eaton published a review article in 2010 [27], some 25 years after their original work, vindicating the validity of the model despite some changes in the original macronutrient estimates. In their opinion evidence from the epidemiological and clinical studies have shown that, at least in some high-risk populations, the Paleolithic diet is superior to those commonly advised.

Since 1997, one of the authors has been using the "Zone diet," introduced by the biochemist Barry Sears, with IBD patients. The intent of Dr. Sears had been to develop a diet able to reduce cellular inflammation, thanks to the hormonal control exerted by food [35]. In 2003 Dr. Aronne Romano thought to apply to the Zone diet the concepts emerging from evolutionary nutrition, as proposed by Boyd Eaton and Loren Cordain. He devised his *PaleoZone* diet [36], which he has been proposing to his IBD patients ever since.

In the *PaleoZone* diet, the ideal protein to carbohydrate ratio is 0.75, with an acceptable tolerance ranging from 0.5 to 1. This means 4 g of carbohydrates every 3 g of protein, the ratio yielding a 40 % carbohydrate, 30 % protein, and 30 % lipid energy distribution, close to the estimation of intakes from an East African Paleolithic diet dating from about 200,000 years ago [37].

When adopting this diet, a pivotal role in defining the patient's nutritional needs is played by the amount of proteins deemed necessary to maintain lean mass and to avoid disorders related to an inadequate protein supply (e.g., immune system deficiencies). Such amount is dependent on the patient's lean body mass and daily physical activities. The quantity of carbohydrates follows directly, defined by the abovementioned protein to carbohydrate ratio. This way insulin secretion is not excessively stimulated by the carbohydrate load in the meal, while glucagon secretion is guaranteed by its protein share, warranting the best hormonal control [35, 36].

Low glycemic load carbohydrate sources are selected, such as non-starchy vegetables and fruit, a good choice for their high content of micronutrients like vitamins, mineral salts, and fiber and for their documented anti-inflammatory effect, eventually due to polyphenols. It has been proven that polyphenols can confer substantial benefits to gut health by increasing eubiotic flora [38]. The best sources of polyphenols are red and green chicories, red and yellow onions, and spinach; among the fruits are prune, plum, apple, black grape, pomegranate, and especially wild berries (blueberry, black currant, blackberry, strawberry, red raspberry, black chokeberry, black elderberry). Herbs like oregano, basil, sage, turmeric, rosemary, spearmint, thyme, and spices represent other good sources of polyphenols, and to complete the list, the *PaleoZone* diet includes cocoa, dark bitter chocolate, green tea, capers, and ginger.

Besides banning junk foods, soft drinks, sweets, and candies, not granted carbohydrate-rich foods in the diet are starchy vegetables, grains, and legumes, in the first place not to allow excessive insulin stimulation, with the resulting proinflammatory hormonal imbalance. Another and most important reason is that cereal grains and legumes, together with pseudocereals (like amaranth, quinoa, chia seeds, and buckwheat), and nightshades (Solanaceae) contain substances able to increase intestinal permeability, either directly damaging enterocytes and/or opening tight junctions or indirectly promoting bacterial and yeast overgrowth in the small bowel. These noxious substances include inhibitors of digestive enzymes, lectins (prolamins and agglutinins), and saponins.

Among enzyme inhibitors, protease inhibitors (like trypsin inhibitors) are well represented in cereal grains, beans, and other legumes [39]. Phytates and phytic acid are present in cereals, pseudocereals, and legumes. They are known to interfere with mineral absorption and can limit activity of proteases like pepsin and trypsin, of amylase, and of glucosidases.

Lectins are present in a variety of plants, especially in seeds, where they serve as defense mechanisms against other plants and fungi. Because of their ability to bind to virtually all cell types and cause damage to several organs, lectins are widely recognized as anti-nutrients within food [40]. Most lectins are resistant to heat and the effects of digestive enzymes.

Prolamins and agglutinins constitute the two main lectin classes. Prolamins abound in cereal grains (wheat, barley, oats), quinoa, rice, peanuts, and soy: among them gluten is the best known. Gluten is the main structural protein complex of wheat consisting of glutenins and gliadins and constituting about 80 % of the total protein of the seed. Gliadin has been shown to increase intestinal permeability [41]: gliadin peptides cross the epithelial layer by transcytosis or paracellular transport, which occurs when intestinal permeability is increased, a feature that is characteristic for CD [42]. Gliadin has been demonstrated to increase permeability in human Caco-2 intestinal epithelial cells by reorganizing actin filaments and altering expression of junctional complex proteins [43]. Several studies show that the binding of gliadin to the chemokine receptor CXCR3 on epithelial IEC-6 and Caco2 cells releases zonulin, a protein that directly compromises the integrity of the junctional complex [44, 45].

Lectin activity has been demonstrated in wheat, rye, barley, oats, corn, and rice; however, the best studied of the cereal grain lectins is wheat germ agglutinin [46]. WGA binds to cell surface glycoconjugates (via N-glycolylneuraminic acid), which allows for cell entry, and can disturb immune tolerance, inducing inflammatory responses by immune cells. Exposure to micromolar concentrations of WGA impairs the integrity of the intestinal epithelial layer, allowing passage of small molecules. At the basolateral side of the epithelium, nanomolar concentrations of WGA induce the secretion of pro-inflammatory cytokines by immune cells [47]. This may further affect the integrity of the epithelial layer, heightening the potential for a positive feedback loop, suggesting that, together with gliadin, WGA can increase intestinal permeability.

Soybean agglutinin and peanut agglutinin seem to cause analogous problems.

Saponins are steroid or triterpenoid glycosides, common in a large number of plants, in which they can be so abundant to reach 30 % of the dry weight of a plant [48]. Their physiological role is not yet fully understood, but saponins may be considered a part of the plants' defense systems. In cultivated crops, the triterpenoid saponins are generally predominant and have been detected in many legumes such as soybeans, beans, and peas. Steroid saponins are found in oats, capsicum peppers, aubergine, tomato seed, alliums, asparagus, yam, fenugreek, yucca, and ginseng. A large number of the biological effects of saponins have been ascribed to their action on membranes, where they express the specific ability to form pores [49]. Johnson et al. [50] found that some saponins increased the permeability of intestinal mucosal cells in vitro, inhibited active mucosal transport, and facilitated uptake of substances that are normally not absorbed. This may have important implications for the uptake of macromolecules, such as allergens, whose passage through the epithelium is normally somewhat restricted [51]. Histological investigation of the mucosal epithelium exposed to saponin revealed damage, especially of the villi, but the mechanism of action on the intestinal membranes in vivo is not yet clearly understood. Absorption of saponin metabolites produced in the intestine by microorganisms into the body of human subjects has been however demonstrated [52]. Furthermore, saponins reduce protein digestibility probably by the formation of sparingly digestible saponin-protein complexes. Cooking does not destroy saponins, and fermentation only partially reduces their concentration.

Even nightshades (Solanaceae) contain saponins called solanines. The content of α-solanine and α-chaconine is rather high in the green peel and in the sprouts of potatoes. They are the main toxic molecules synthetized by the plant, and tubers damaged during harvesting and/or transport produce increased levels of these glycoalkaloids (GAs) that cause sporadic outbreaks of poisoning in humans, as well as many livestock deaths [53]. The accepted concentration of GAs in potatoes intended for human consumption is 200 mg/kg, as we assume that levels below 200 mg/kg are safe, but according to Parnell [53], the 200 mg/kg threshold only relates to acute and/or subacute effects and not to possible chronic effects, raising safety issues.

Therefore, potatoes, with tomatoes, peppers, and chili peppers, are not recommended for patients following the *PaleoZone*.

Protein sources are represented by fish, mollusks and shellfish, white meat, game, or lean cuts of red meat from grazing animals. Meat from grass-fed animals, as compared to animals raised in feedlots, is leaner and with better n-6 to n-3 PUFA ratio; they are also richer in vitamins (beta-carotene, thiamine, riboflavin, vitamin E) and mineral salts such as calcium, magnesium, and potassium.

Milk and dairy products are not allowed (for their content in protease inhibitors); milk exhibits a high insulin index, a factor that can contribute to inflammation and insulin resistance.

Olives, extra-virgin olive oil, avocados, and nuts like walnuts, almonds, and hazelnuts provide a fair amount of monounsaturated fatty acids (MUFA). The use of saturated fats (SF) and arachidonic acid (AA), the precursor of pro-inflammatory eicosanoids (to be found mainly in egg yolk, animal fat, and offal), should be limited. Hydrogenated, partially hydrogenated, fractionated, and refined vegetable oils or oils produced from legumes or cereals (canola oil, corn oil, cotton oil, margarine, palm oil, peanut oil, sunflower oil, soy oil, safflower oil) are excluded. Seeds too must be avoided (i.e., pumpkin seeds, sunflower seeds, etc.), being rich both in n-6 PUFA and phytates.

Hormonal control is provided also from the adequate distribution of food during the day, partitioning the balanced diet in various meals and snacks so that intervals greater than 5 h in between meals can be avoided; this allows to stabilize blood glucose adequately and prevents compensatory secretion of cortisol by (relative) hypoglycemia [54].

Several hundred IBD patients have now adopted the *PaleoZone* at home. One hundred of them, who have consecutively attended courses held in doctor Romano's office especially devised to explain the diet principles and have been following the nutritional instructions for at least 3 months, were subjected to a questionnaire during checkup. Ninety-two (32 CD, 68 UC) patients judged the nutritional approach with *PaleoZone* better than all treatments carried out so far, while eight of them found it to be equivalent.

To the authors' knowledge, no controlled trials have been published so far addressing Paleolithic nutrition and IBD. Nonetheless, the choice of foods allowed by the *PaleoZone* diet almost completely overlaps with the foods enlisted by Olendzki in the IBD-AID, differences apparently limited to oats (not contemplated in the *PaleoZone* diet) and fermented foods (some of which could be considered also in the *PaleoZone* diet). While the Dietary Inflammatory Index has not been computed for the *PaleoZone* diet yet, one would not be surprised to obtain a consistent anti-inflammatory index value, should its application be considered.

By and large, the evidence supports that a Western diet is associated with IBD, although no specific component can account for the disease. The authors' view is that a diet with adequate good-quality protein, correct ratio of polyunsaturated fatty acids, high levels of fiber via increased intake of fruit and vegetables should be considered in IBD patients, with limited access to processed foods, if any. Adequate assessment of the patient's needs is essential and should be provided by an expert physician. Since counseling is of paramount importance, adequate steps should be taken to secure proper dietary instruction and support.

References

1. Richman E, Rhodes JM (2013) Review article: evidence-based dietary advice for patients with inflammatory bowel disease. Aliment Pharmacol Ther 38:1156–1171
2. Lomer MCE (2011) Dietary and nutritional considerations for inflammatory bowel disease. Proc Nutr Soc 70:329–335
3. Halmos EP, Gibson PR (2015) Dietary management of IBD—insights and advice. Nat Rev Gastroenterol Hepatol 12:133–146
4. Lee D, Albenberg L, Compher C, Baldassano R, Piccoli D, Lewis JD, Wu GD (2015) Diet in the pathogenesis and treatment of inflammatory bowel diseases. Gastroenterology 148(6):1087–1106
5. Hou JK, Abraham B, El-Serag H (2011) Dietary intake and risk of developing inflammatory bowel disease: a systematic review of the literature. Am J Gastroenterol 10(4):563–573
6. Hou JK, Lee D, Lewis J (2014) Diet and inflammatory bowel disease: review of patient-targeted recommendations. Clin Gastroenterol Hepatol 12(10):1592–1600
7. Charlebois A, Rosenfeld G, Bressler B (2015) The impact of dietary interventions on the symptoms of inflammatory bowel disease: a systematic review. Crit Rev Food Sci Nutr Jan 8:0. [Epub ahead of print] DOI: 10.1080/10408398.2012.760515
8. Sarbagili-Shabat C, Sigall-Boneh R, Levine A (2015) Nutritional therapy in inflammatory bowel disease. Curr Opin Gastroenterol 31(4):303–308
9. Molodecky NA, Soon IS, Rabi DM et al (2012) Increasing incidence and prevalence of the inflammatory bowel diseases with time, based on systematic review. Gastroenterology 142(1):46–54
10. Fiocchi C (2012) Genes and 'in-vironment': how will our concepts on the pathophysiology of inflammatory bowel disease develop in the future? Dig Dis 30(Suppl 3):2–11

11. Montgomery SM, Ekbom A (2002) Epidemiology of inflammatory bowel disease. Curr Opin Gastroenterol 18:416–420
12. Cabré E, Domènech E (2012) Impact of environmental and dietary factors on the course of inflammatory bowel disease. World J Gastroenterol 18(29):3814–3822
13. Brown AC, Roy M (2010) Does evidence exist to include dietary therapy in the treatment of Crohn's disease? Expert Rev Gastroenterol Hepatol 4(2):191–215
14. Racine A, Carbonnel F, Chan SS (2016) Dietary patterns and risk of inflammatory bowel disease in Europe: results from the EPIC Study. Inflamm Bowel Dis 22(2):345–354
15. Olendzki BC, Silverstein TD, Persuitte GM et al (2014) An anti-inflammatory diet as treatment for inflammatory bowel disease: a case series report. Nutr J 13:5
16. Cavicchia PP, Steck SE, Hurley TG et al (2009) A new dietary inflammatory index predicts interval changes in serum high-sensitivity C-reactive protein. J Nutr 139:2365–2372
17. Shivappa N, Steck SE, Hurley TG et al (2013) Designing and developing a literature-derived, population-based dietary inflammatory index. Public Health Nutr 14:1–8
18. Tilg H, Moschen AR (2015) Food, immunity, and the microbiome. Gastroenterology 148(6):1107–1119
19. Sczaniecka AK, Brasky TM, Lampe JW (2012) Dietary intake of specific fatty acids and breast cancer risk among postmenopausal women in the VITAL cohort. Nutr Cancer 64(8):1131–1142
20. Patterson RE, Flatt SW, Newman VA (2011) Marine fatty acid intake is associated with breast cancer prognosis. Nutrition 141(2):201–206
21. Shivappa N, Steck SE, Hussey JR et al (2015) Inflammatory potential of diet and all-cause, cardiovascular, and cancer mortality in National Health and Nutrition Examination Survey III Study. Eur J Nutr Dec 7. [Epub ahead of print] DOI: 10.1007/s00394-015-1112-x
22. Ioannidis JP (2005) Why most published research findings are false. PLoS Med 2(8):e124
23. Fardet A, Rock E (2014) Toward a new philosophy of preventive nutrition: from a reductionist to a holistic paradigm to improve nutritional recommendations. Adv Nutr 5(4):430–446
24. Lucock MD, Martin CE, Yates ZR, Veysey M (2014) Diet and our genetic legacy in the recent anthropocene: a Darwinian perspective to nutritional health. Evid Based Complement Alternat Med 19(1):68–83
25. Eaton SB, Konner M (1985) Paleolithic nutrition. A consideration of its nature and current implications. N Engl J Med 312(5):283–289
26. Cordain L, Miller JB, Eaton SB, Mann N (2000) Macronutrient estimations in hunter-gatherer diets. Am J Clin Nutr 72:1589–1592
27. Konner M, Eaton SB (2010) Paleolithic nutrition: twenty-five years later. Nutr Clin Pract 25:594–602
28. Manheimer EW, van Zuuren EJ, Fedorowicz Z, Pijl H (2015) Paleolithic nutrition for metabolic syndrome: systematic review and meta-analysis. Am J Clin Nutr 102(4):922–932
29. Eaton SB, Konner MJ, Shostak M (1988) Stone agers in the fast lane: chronic degenerative diseases in evolutionary perspective. Am J Med 84:739–749
30. Turner BL, Thompson AL (2013) Beyond the Paleolithic prescription: incorporating diversity and flexibility in the study of human diet evolution. Nutr Rev 71(8):501–510
31. Alcock J, Franklin ML, Kuzawa CW (2012) Nutrient signaling: evolutionary origins of the immune-modulating effects of dietary fat. Q Rev Biol 87(3):187–223
32. Teitelbaum JE, Allan Walker W (2001) Review: the role of omega 3 fatty acids in intestinal inflammation. J Nutr Biochem 12(1):21–32
33. Goepfert JM, Hicks R (1969) Effect of volatile fatty acids on Salmonella typhimurium. J Bacteriol 97(2):956–958
34. Newburg DS, Ruiz-Palacios GM, Morrow AL (2005) Human milk glycans protect infants against enteric pathogens. Annu Rev Nutr 25:37–58
35. Ludwig DS, Majzoub JA, Al-Zahrani A et al (1999) High glycemic index foods, overeating, and obesity. Pediatrics 103(3):E26
36. Romano A (2013) La PaleoZona. RCS Libri S.p.A, Milano

37. Kuipers RS, Luxwolda MF, Dijck-Brouwer DA et al (2010) Estimated macronutrient and fatty acid intakes from an East African Paleolithic diet. Br J Nutr 104(11):1666–1687
38. Parker SG, Stevenson DE, Skinner MA (2008) The potential influence of fruit polyphenols on colonic microflora and human gut health. Intl J Fd Microbiol 124:295–298
39. Zahnley JC (1984) Stability of enzyme inhibitors and lectins in foods and the influence of specific binding interactions. Adv Exp Med Biol 177:333–365
40. Pusztai A, Ewen SW, Grant G et al (1993) Antinutritive effects of wheat-germ agglutinin and other N-acetylglucosamine-specific lectins. Br J Nutr 70:313–321
41. Hollon J, Puppa EL, Greenwald B et al (2015) Effect of gliadin on permeability of intestinal biopsy explants from celiac disease patients and patients with non-celiac gluten sensitivity. Nutrient 7(3):1565–1576
42. Catassi C, Pierani P, Natalini G et al (1991) Clinical application of a simple HPLC method for the sugar intestinal permeability test. J Pediatr Gastroenterol Nutr 12:209–212
43. Sander GR, Cummins AG, Henshall T et al (2005) Rapid disruption of intestinal barrier function by gliadin involves altered expression of apical junctional proteins. FEBS Lett 579:4851–4855
44. Drago S, El Asmar R, Di Pierro M et al (2006) Gliadin, zonulin and gut permeability: effects on celiac and non-celiac intestinal mucosa and intestinal cell lines. Scand J Gastroenterol 41:408–419
45. Lammers KM, Lu R, Brownley J et al (2008) Gliadin induces an increase in intestinal permeability and zonulin release by binding to the chemokine receptor CXCR3. Gastroenterology 135:194–204
46. Cordain L (1999) Cereal grains: humanity's double-edged sword. World Rev Nutr Diet 84:19–73
47. Dalla Pellegrina C, Perbellini O, Scupoli MT et al (2009) Effects of wheat germ agglutinin on human gastrointestinal epithelium: insights from an experimental model of immune/epithelial cell interaction. Toxicol Appl Pharmacol 237:146–153
48. Moses T, Papadopoulou KK, Osbourn A (2014) Metabolic and functional diversity of saponins, biosynthetic intermediates and semi-synthetic derivatives. Crit Rev Biochem Mol Biol 49(6):439–462
49. Keukens EA, de Vrije T, van den Boom C (1995) Molecular basis of glycoalkaloid induced membrane disruption. Biochim Biophys Acta 1240(2):216–228
50. Johnson IT, Gee JM, Price K et al (1986) Influence of saponins on gut permeability and active nutrient transport in vitro. J Nutr 116(11):2270–2277
51. Gee JM, Wortley GM, Johnson IT et al (1996) Effects of saponins and glycoalkaloids on the permeability and viability of mammalian intestinal cells and on the integrity of tissue preparations in vitro. Toxicol in Vitro 10(2):117–128
52. Wakabayashi C, Hasegawa H, Murata J, Saiki I (1997) In vivo antimetastatic action of ginseng protopanaxadiol saponins is based on their intestinal bacterial metabolites after oral administration. Oncol Res 9(8):411–417
53. Korpan YI, Nazarenko EA, Skryshevskaya IV et al (2004) Potato glycoalkaloids: true safety or false sense of security? Trends Biotechnol 22(3):147–151
54. Sears B (1995) The zone. Regan Books (Harper Collins), New York

Diverticular Diseases and Western Diet: Another Metropolitan Legend?

7

Paolo Andreozzi and Gianpiero Manes

7.1   Introduction

The prevalence of colonic diverticula in the general population is estimated to range from 20 to 60 % [1]. The prevalence of diverticulosis and diverticular disease increases with age, since diverticula were found in ~70 % of screening colonoscopies in individuals over the age of 80 [2].

Diverticula of the large bowel are structural abnormality of colonic wall characterized by an outpouchings of the colon at weak points in the circular muscle where blood vessels (vasa recta) penetrate to supply the mucosa [3]. Diverticula per se do not give rise to symptoms; in fact, 80 % of patients with colonic diverticula are asymptomatic, and the mere presence of colonic diverticula is defined as asymptomatic diverticulosis [4]. The term "diverticular disease" (DD) implies that the diverticula have given rise to illness [1]. An acute inflammation of colonic diverticula is defined as acute diverticulitis, while symptomatic uncomplicated diverticular disease is a syndrome characterized by recurrent abdominal symptoms, such as abdominal pain, bloating, and changes in bowel habits, in the absence of macroscopically evident signs of acute inflammation of diverticula [4].

The natural history of DD is poorly understood. Early population-based, retrospective studies showed that patients with diverticulosis had a 10–25 % lifetime

P. Andreozzi • G. Manes (✉)

Department of Gastroenterology and Digestive Endoscopy, G. Salvini Hospital, Viale Forlanini 95, 20024 Garbagnate Milanese and Rho, Milan, Italy

e-mail: gimanes@tin.it

© Springer International Publishing Switzerland 2016   99
E. Grossi, F. Pace (eds.), *Human Nutrition from the Gastroenterologist's Perspective*,
DOI 10.1007/978-3-319-30361-1_7

risk of developing acute diverticulitis. A recent population-based cohort study reappraised the risk of developing diverticulitis; in a survival analysis of 2222 patients with diverticulosis incidentally discovered during colonoscopy, only 95 patients (4.3 %; 6 cases per 1000 patient-years) developed diverticulitis over an 11-year follow-up period [5]. Nevertheless, diverticular disease and its complications are a relevant cause of hospitalization and mortality, particularly in elderly patients, with a significant economic impact on the health-care systems in developed countries [2, 6].

7.2 Pathophysiology of Diverticulosis and Diverticular Disease

Pathogenesis of diverticular disease is not fully understood. When we consider the pathogenesis of diverticular disease, we have to separate the mechanisms underlying the development of diverticula (diverticulosis) from those underlying the onset of symptoms (diverticular disease).

Several mechanisms have been proposed to explain the development of diverticula. It is likely that the pathophysiology of diverticulosis is multifactorial: from this point of view, complex interactions among genetic factors, environmental influences (diet, colonic microbiota), and impairment of colonic motility and weakness may result in their formation [7] (see Fig. 7.1).

The pathological mechanism that causes the development of inflammation in colonic diverticula remains unclear. It has been hypothesized that the obstruction of these diverticula by fecal material causes the abrasion of the mucosa and the access of fecal bacteria into the lamina propria, resulting in an acute inflammation of the mucosa and subsequent extension of inflammation to the mesenteric and pericolic fat [8].

7.3 Diverticular Disease as a Western Disease

Historically, diverticulosis has been considered as a "disease of Western world" because of its high prevalence in developed countries compared with certain parts of Africa and Asia [9]. Indeed, early studies conducted by Painter and Burkitt in the last century showed a lower prevalence of this condition in rural Africa compared to Western countries [10]. Moreover, some features of colonic diverticula were different in Western and underdeveloped countries: in Western countries the diverticula are most common in sigmoid tract and left colon and occur in old people, while in Asian population they are predominantly in the right colon and occur at a younger age [9]. However, data from these postmortem studies were influenced by several problems of sampling bias, including the different life expectancies of the two populations.

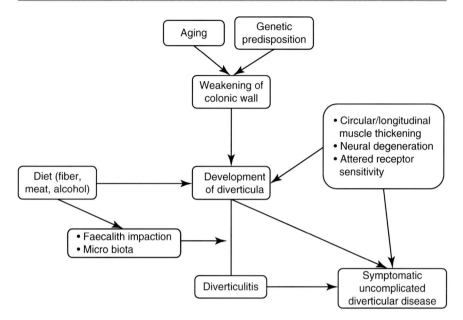

Fig. 7.1 Mechanisms underlying the development of diverticulosis and symptomatic diverticular disease

In the last decades, several studies were performed in migrant populations to evaluate the prevalence of diverticulosis and diverticular disease in different ethnic groups: a UK study observed a lower prevalence of diverticular disease among Indian-subcontinent Asian patients compared with other ethnic groups [11]. Similarly, a Dutch cross-sectional study of 3004 patients undergoing colonoscopy found that diverticulosis was diagnosed significantly more often in immigrant men than in native Dutch [12].

Interestingly, the change of the environment may influence the risk of diverticular disease: in a Swedish study population that prospectively followed a national cohort of four million residents, the authors assessed the risk of hospital admissions and deaths because of diverticular disease and acute diverticulitis from 1991 to 2000 [13]. According to previous studies, they found a lower risk for hospital admissions because of diverticular disease and acute diverticulitis for the non-Western immigrants than for Western immigrants and native Swedes. Interestingly, the risk in immigrant population increased with years of residence in Sweden.

Although the epidemiological data have some limitations, the evidences suggest that diverticular disease is a condition that affects mainly the developed countries. The cause may be attributed to genetics and environmental factors. In particular, the differences in terms of lifestyle factors, including dietary habits, might play a critical role in the etiology of this disease.

7.4   Role of Western Pattern Diet in Diverticular Disease

The higher prevalence of diverticular disease in developed countries and in western-ized migrants suggests that "Western lifestyle" plays a critical role in the development of diverticula and the onset of diverticulitis.

Western diet is characterized by high intakes of refined grains, red meat, and high-fat foods (especially saturated fatty acids) and is low in fiber and micronutrients (vitamins and minerals) [14]. Painter and Burkitt defined diverticular disease as a "civilization disease" caused by a dietary deficiency of fiber, typical of Western patterns diet [10]. Following this hypothesis, many researchers studied the role of fiber and other foods and food components in the pathogenesis of diverticular disease supporting the idea that the typical components of Western diet increased the risk of diverticulosis or symptomatic diverticular disease. However, early studies were often of poor quality; often retrospective or case-control studies and the risk were often not adjusted for other potential confounding variables (age, sex, smoking, physical activity, obesity). In other cases, dietary advices were administered to patients without the reliable evidences supporting them, but based only on expert opinion or on empiricism.

In the last decades, high-quality studies have, at least partially, clarified some aspects about the role of foods in the development of diverticular disease. In many cases, these studies have challenged the common beliefs regarding the development of diverticula and the onset of diverticulitis. However, many gray areas still remain in the understanding the exact role of diet in the pathogenesis of diverticular disease.

7.5   Role of Fiber

Ever since Painter and Burkitt hypothesized that diverticulosis was a fiber-deficiency disease of Western countries caused by the refining of carbohydrate in the diet, several studies focused on the role of fiber in the pathogenesis of diverticular disease. This hypothesis was based on the evidence that diverticulosis was rare in rural Africa but increasingly common in developed countries. The authors attributed the lower prevalence in that area to the differences in dietary fiber intake and hypothesized that a lower content of dietary fiber in the Western countries led to constipation and high-pressure segmentation of the colon that resulted in mucosal herniation through weak sections of the colon wall. The changes in colonic motility were also confirmed by their motility studies that demonstrated higher intra-colonic pressures in patients with diverticulosis compared to controls. In addition, they demonstrated that individuals consuming a Western diet had longer mean colonic transit times and lower mean stool weights compared to Africans [15]. However, the fiber hypothesis was not fully demonstrated, because no direct measurement of fiber intake in the two groups of patients was done. In addition, they did not account for other differences in terms of diet and lifestyle factors between the two areas.

A recent study has challenged this hypothesis. In this study, the authors have evaluated the fiber intake of 2104 subjects who underwent outpatient colonoscopy by a food frequency questionnaire via phone interview [16]. Contrary to the tenets of the fiber hypothesis, the authors found that a high-fiber but not low-fiber intake was associated with a higher prevalence of diverticula. This association was dose dependent and stronger in individuals with more marked diverticulosis (>3 diverticula). However, these results should be carefully interpreted because they could be bedeviled by potential bias: in fact, dietary habits were assessed several years after the colonoscopic diagnosis of diverticulosis. It is reliable that the higher fiber consumption observed in the group of patients with diverticula may be due to changes in dietary habits owing to this finding. Moreover, it is also achievable that increased fiber consumption may be related to the presence of symptoms of undiagnosed diverticular disease (i.e., constipation).

Although the role of dietary fiber in the development of diverticula is still debated, available evidences agreed about the protective role of the fiber in the development of diverticulitis and its complications. In particular, two large prospective cohort studies have demonstrated an inverse association between dietary fiber intake and diverticular complications. The EPIC-Oxford study has evaluated the risk of diverticular disease and its complications in a cohort of 47,033 men and women in England and Scotland [17]. The researchers found that individuals who reported consuming a vegetarian diet had a lower risk of hospitalization or death from diverticular disease. Moreover, the risk of death or hospitalization was inversely correlated to fiber intake; participants in the highest fifth ($\geq$25.5 g/day for women and $\geq$26.1 g/day for men) had a 41 % lower risk compared with those in the lowest fifth (<14 g/day for both women and men) [17]. Similarly, in the Health Professionals Follow-up Study of 47,888 men, the authors found that the adjusted relative risk was 0.58 (95 % CI 0.41–0.83) for symptomatic diverticular disease when comparing highest with the lowest quintiles of fiber intake [18].

7.6 Role of Nut, Corn, Popcorn, and Seeds

The hypothesis that the consumption of foods that leave rough-indigested participles in the stools leads to diverticulitis by obstruction of a narrow-necked diverticulum was very popular in the last century. Consequently, for more than 50 years, physicians advised patients with diverticula to avoid the consumption of certain foods including nuts, corns, and seeds [19].

A recent large prospective cohort study has challenged this belief. Strate et al. demonstrated that the consumption of seeds and nuts is not associated with an increased risk of diverticulitis or its complication. Surprisingly, the consumption of nuts and popcorn was associated to a reduced risk. In fact, subjects who consumed nuts or popcorn at least twice weekly were at a lower risk of diverticulitis than those who consumed these foods less than once a month (adjusted relative risks: 0.80, 95 % CI 0.63–1.01 for nuts; 0.73, 95 % CI 0.56–0.92 for popcorn). In addition, the authors have examined the relationship between strawberry and blueberry consumption and diverticular complications and found no significant association.

Similarly, the protective effects of nut consumption have been observed also in other diseases [20, 21]. The biological mechanisms by which these foods prevent the risk of diverticulitis are unknown. However, the protective effects of these foods may be explained by the richness of nutrients with anti-inflammatory properties such as vitamin E, lutein, α-linolenic acid, and unsaturated fatty acids.

7.7   Role of Meat

The high intake of animal protein is one of the main dietary differences between Western and underdeveloped nations. It has been hypothesized that the increased consumption of animal proteins increases the risk of diverticular disease by altering the metabolism of bacteria in the colon or increasing the intake of fat. However, the evidences supporting this hypothesis are weak and based on small-series studies [22, 23]. Furthermore, the study of this association is very difficult considering that meat consumption is associated with other well-known risk factors of diverticular disease, such as low-fiber intake, smoking, obesity, or physical activity.

In a study of 264 nonvegetarians and 56 vegetarians, the authors found that the prevalence of diverticulosis was higher in the nonvegetarian group compared to vegetarian group [24]. The EPIC-Oxford study has evaluated the associations of meat consumption with risk of diverticular disease [17]. Crowe et al. found a protective effect of vegetarianism compared to meat eating; vegetarians had a 31 % lower adjusted risk (relative risk 0.69, 95 % CI 0.55–0.86) of diverticular disease compared with meat eaters. However, the researchers showed no significant dose-response association between the amount of meat consumed and the incidence of diverticular disease with a similar risk among meat eaters who consumed <50 g/daily versus >100 g/daily. This result reappraises the role of proteins in the development of diverticular disease, and the increased risk may be due to other known risk factors such as low-fiber intake.

7.8   Role of Alcohol Consumption

The consumption of alcohol is very frequent in Western countries. Several diseases have been associated to alcohol consumption, including heart and liver disease. Some evidences have suggested that alcoholic beverages could be associated to the development of diverticula and acute inflammation.

A prospective cross-sectional study in Japan assessed the alcohol consumption in 2164 consecutive patients who underwent colonoscopy. The authors found a significantly higher prevalence of diverticulosis in alcohol drinkers compared to nondrinkers. Furthermore, the relative risk of diverticulosis tended to increase with the amount of alcohol consumed [25].

Similarly, alcohol seems to be associated to an increased risk to develop acute diverticulitis. In a Danish study, it showed that alcoholism is associated to an increased risk of acute diverticulitis. Alcohol drinkers showed a 2.0- and 2.9-fold increase in relative risk for men and women, respectively [26].

7.9 Role of Vitamin D

Vitamin D has been shown to reduce the release of pro-inflammatory cytokines, and changes in vitamin D serum levels have been associated with several inflammatory diseases, such as inflammatory bowel disease (IBD) or rheumatologic disease [27].

Maguire et al. have evaluated the serum levels of vitamin D in 9116 patients with uncomplicated diverticulosis and 922 patients hospitalized with diverticulitis. The researchers found that patients with uncomplicated diverticulosis had significantly higher mean serum levels of vitamin D compared to patients with diverticulitis (29.1 ng/mL vs. 25.3 ng/mL; $p < 0.0001$). In addition, the researchers found lowest levels of vitamin D in subgroups of patients with more severe disease (patients requiring emergent laparotomy or with recurrent diverticulitis) [28].

Hence, low serum levels of vitamin D may explain geographic and seasonal variations in diverticulitis [29]. However, additional study is needed to support the role of oral supplementation in patients with diverticulosis to prevent the development of diverticulitis and its complications.

7.10 Role of Obesity

Obesity is a recognized risk factor for several diseases. Likely, obesity plays a critical role also in the pathogenesis of diverticular disease. Several epidemiological studies supported this hypothesis. Strate et al. studied the relationship between obesity and diverticular disease during an 18-year follow-up. In details, researchers found that men with a BMI ≥ 30 kg/m^2 had an increased risk to develop diverticulitis and diverticular bleeding compared with those with a BMI of <21 kg/m^2 (adjusted relative risk: 1.78, 95 % CI 1.08–2.94 for diverticulitis; 3.19, 95 % CI 1.45–7.00 for diverticular bleeding). Also waist circumference and waist-to-hip ratio were also associated with the risk of diverticular complications when the highest and lowest quintiles were compared. In particular, waist-to-hip ratio showed a better correlation with the risk of diverticulitis and its complications, suggesting that visceral fat, rather than subcutaneous fat, is important in the development of diverticular complications. According with this finding, a Japanese retrospective study has evaluated visceral fat area in patients with colonic diverticula by using CT images and found that the deposition of visceral fat was higher in those who developed diverticulitis than those with asymptomatic diverticulosis, even though their BMI was no different [30].

The mechanisms by which obesity increases the risk of diverticulitis are not understood. It is well known that adipose tissue is not an inert tissue, but it is an "endocrine organ" able to release pro inflammatory cytokines such as TNF-α, IL-6, and leptin. It is possible to hypothesize that the release of those cytokines from active adipocytes might trigger the inflammatory process. In addition, growing evidences support the role of microbiota in several gastrointestinal and extragastrointestinal disorders. It is also well known that intestinal microbiota significantly differs between obese and lean individuals. For this reason, it is achievable that differences in microbiota composition could play a role in the development of the diverticulitis.

7.11　Summary and Conclusions

Colonic diverticula are common in developed countries, and complications of colonic diverticulosis are responsible for a significant burden of disease. In addition the risk of diverticular disease in emigrants from low to high prevalence areas tends to increase with the time. The link between Western diet and diverticulosis has been propagated in many arenas. Historically, the development of diverticula has been associated to Western diet and early studies focused on the role of fibers: low-fiber diets were thought to increase the intraluminal pressure leading to focal herniation of colonic mucosa. Also other nutrients have been thought to be associated to the development of diverticular disease and its complications.

These evidences support the role of lifestyle factors in the pathogenesis of diverticular disease. Early studies focused the attention on the role of dietary habits, in particular the fiber intake. However, recent studies have challenged the conventional beliefs about the role of certain foods in the pathogenesis of diverticular disease. In particular, low-fiber diet could not be associated to an increased prevalence of diverticular disease, whereas the consumption of nut, corn, popcorn, and seeds does not increase the risk of diverticulitis, but, in some cases, a reduced risk was observed (Table 7.1). These evidences seem to reappraise the role of specific foods in the pathogenesis of diverticular disease.

Table 7.1 Role of foods in diverticular disease

Food	Effect	Degree of certainty	Pathogenetic mechanism	References
Fiber	Low-fiber intake: (a) Reduces the risk of diverticulosis (b) Reduces the risk of diverticulitis development	Low High	Low-fiber intake led to constipation and high-ressure segmentation of the colon resulting in mucosal herniation	[15–17]
Nut, popcorn, and seeds	Reduce the risk of diverticulitis or its complication	High	Richness of nutrients with anti-inflammatory properties	[19]
Alcohol	Increases the risk of acute diverticulitis	Low	Pro-inflammatory stimuli	[26]
Vitamin D	Prevents the development of diverticulitis and its complications	Low	Reduction of the release of pro-inflammatory cytokines	[28]

The only relationship between Western diet and diverticular disease seems to be related to the increase of fat deposition. In fact, several studies agreed about association between obesity, in particular visceral obesity, and symptomatic diverticular disease. In addition, diet-induced changes of gut microbiota may play a role in the pathogenesis of diverticular disease.

However, the evidence about the role of foods in diverticular disease is still weak and incomplete. For this reason other studies are needed in order to better clarify the relationship between diet and diverticular disease before recommending dietary changes to patients with asymptomatic diverticulosis and diverticular disease.

References

1. Strate LL, Modi R, Cohen E, Spiegel BM (2012) Diverticular disease as a chronic illness: evolving epidemiologic and clinical insights. Am J Gastroenterol 107:1486–1493
2. Everhart JE, Ruhl CE (2009) Burden of digestive diseases in the United States part II: lower gastrointestinal diseases. Gastroenterology 136:741–754
3. Slack WW (1962) The anatomy, pathology, and some clinical features of diverticulitis of the colon. Br J Surg 50:185–190
4. Cuomo R, Barbara G, Pace F et al (2014) Italian consensus conference for colonic diverticulosis and diverticular disease. U Eur Gastroenterol J 2:413–442
5. Shahedi K, Fuller G, Bolus R et al (2013) Long-term risk of acute diverticulitis among patients with incidental diverticulosis found during colonoscopy. Clin Gastroenterol Hepatol 11:1609–1613
6. Papagrigoriadis S, Debrah S, Koreli A et al (2004) Impact of diverticular disease on hospital costs and activity. Colorectal Dis 6:81–84
7. Humes DJ, Spiller RC (2014) The pathogenesis and management of acute colonic diverticulitis. Aliment Pharmacol Ther 39:359–370
8. Humes D, Simpson J, Spiller RC (2007) Colonic diverticular disease. BMJ Clin Evid. 2007 Aug 15;2007. pii: 0405.
9. Commane DM, Arasaradnam RP, Mills S, Mathers JC, Bradburn M (2009) Diet, ageing and genetic factors in the pathogenesis of diverticular disease. World J Gastroenterol 15:2479–2488
10. Painter NS, Burkitt DP (1971) Diverticular disease of the colon: a deficiency disease of Western civilization. Br Med J 2:450–454
11. Kang JY, Dhar A, Pollok R et al (2004) Diverticular disease of the colon: ethnic differences in frequency. Aliment Pharmacol Ther 19:765–769
12. Loffeld RJ (2005) Diverticulosis of the colon is rare amongst immigrants living in the Zaanstreek region in the Netherlands. Colorectal Dis 7:559–562
13. Hjern F, Johansson C, Mellgren A, Baxter NN, Hjern A (2006) Diverticular disease and migration–the influence of acculturation to a Western lifestyle on diverticular disease. Aliment Pharmacol Ther 23:797–805
14. Cordain L, Eaton SB, Sebastian A et al (2005) Origins and evolution of the Western diet: health implications for the 21st century. Am J Clin Nutr 81:341–354
15. Burkitt DP, Walker AR, Painter NS (1972) Effect of dietary fibre on stools and the transit-times, and its role in the causation of disease. Lancet 2:1408–1412
16. Peery AF, Sandler RS, Ahnen DJ et al (2013) Constipation and a low-fiber diet are not associated with diverticulosis. Clin Gastroenterol Hepatol 11:1622–1627
17. Crowe FL, Appleby PN, Allen NE et al (2011) Diet and risk of diverticular disease in Oxford cohort of European Prospective Investigation into Cancer and Nutrition (EPIC): prospective study of British vegetarians and non-vegetarians. BMJ 343:d4131
18. Aldoori WH, Giovannucci EL, Rimm EB et al (1994) A prospective study of diet and the risk of symptomatic diverticular disease in men. Am J Clin Nutr 60:757–764

19. Strate LL, Liu YL, Syngal S et al (2008) Nut, corn, and popcorn consumption and the incidence of diverticular disease. JAMA 300(8):907–914
20. Jenab M, Ferrari P, Slimani N et al (2004) Association of nut and seed intake with colorectal cancer risk in the European Prospective Investigation into Cancer and Nutrition. Cancer Epidemiol Biomarkers Prev 13:1595–1603
21. Hu FB, Stampfer MJ (1999) Nut consumption and risk of coronary heart disease: a review of epidemiologic evidence. Curr Atheroscler Rep 1:204–209
22. Manousos O, Day NE, Tzonou A (1985) Diet and other factors in the aetiology of diverticulosis: an epidemiological study in Greece. Gut 26:544–549
23. Lin OS, Soon M, Wu S, Chen Y, Hwang K, Triadafilopoulos G (2000) Dietary habits and right-sided colonic diverticulosis. Dis Colon Rectum 43:1412–1418
24. Gear JSS, Fursdon P, Nolan DJ, et al (1979) Symptomless diverticular disease and intake of dietary fibre. Lancet 313:511–514
25. Nagata N, Niikura R, Shimbo T, et al. (2013) Alcohol and smoking affect risk of uncomplicated colonic diverticulosis in Japan. PLoS One 8:e81137
26. Tønnesen H, Engholm G, Moller H (1999) Association between alcoholism and diverticulitis. Br J Surg 86:1067–1068. doi:10.3389/fphys.2014.00244.eCollection2014
27. Wöbke TK, Sorg BL, Steinhilber D (2014) Vitamin D in inflammatory diseases. Front Physiol 5:244
28. Maguire LH, Song M, Strate LE, Giovannucci EL, Chan AT (2013) Higher serum levels of vitamin D are associated with a reduced risk of diverticulitis. Clin Gastroenterol Hepatol 11(12):1631–1635
29. Maguire LH, Song M, Strate LL, Giovannucci EL, Chan AT (2015) Association of geographic and seasonal variation with diverticulitis admissions. JAMA Surg 150(1):74–77
30. Yamada E, Ohkubo H, Higurashi T et al (2013) Visceral obesity as a risk factor for left-sided diverticulitis in Japan: a multicenter retrospective study. Gut Liv 7:532–53

How Much Fat Does One Need to Eat to Get a Fatty Liver? A Dietary View of NAFLD

8

Anna Simona Sasdelli, Francesca Alessandra Barbanti, and Giulio Marchesini

8.1 Introduction

A pathogenic role of diet in liver fat accumulation has long been considered, and it came to the attention of the media and a wider community following the movie "Supersize Me." In that movie, Morgan Spurlock reports his devastating experience with fast-food toxicity. After consuming three meals a day in a fast-food restaurant for 1 month, he increased body weight by nearly 10 kg, and his liver enzymes peaked at 290 U/L (alanine aminotransferase – ALT) from baseline value of 20 U/L [1]. This one-patient experiment was repeated in Sweden a few years later. Healthy subjects consuming at least two fast-food-based meals a day for 4 weeks, doubling the caloric intake and increasing body weight by 5–15 %, reported a remarkable increase in ALT levels (on average from 22 to 97 U/L), and the amount of hepatic triglyceride content, measured by nuclear magnetic resonance spectroscopy (MRS), increased from 1.1 to 2.8 % [2]. This corresponds to a 154 % increase in hepatic fat, in the presence of a mere 18 % increase in total body fat (dual energy X-ray absorptiometry). These values are largely in keeping with data on the relationship between total body fat, abdominal visceral fat, and hepatic fat, calculated by Thomas et al. using tracer isotopes [3].

A.S. Sasdelli • F.A. Barbanti
Department of Medical & Surgical Sciences, "Alma Mater Studiorum" University, S. Orsola-Malpighi Hospital, 9, Via Massarenti, 40138 Bologna, Italy
e-mail: annasimona.sasdelli@gmail.com

G. Marchesini (✉)
Department of Medical & Surgical Sciences, "Alma Mater Studiorum" University, S. Orsola-Malpighi Hospital, 9, Via Massarenti, 40138 Bologna, Italy

Bologna University, Bologna, Italy
e-mail: giulio.marchesini@unibo.it

© Springer International Publishing Switzerland 2016   109
E. Grossi, F. Pace (eds.), *Human Nutrition from the Gastroenterologist's Perspective*,
DOI 10.1007/978-3-319-30361-1_8

In the present review, we shall discuss (a) the evidence linking calorie excess and dietary fat intake with liver fat; (b) the role of individual macronutrients and the antioxidant properties of micronutrients modulating the overall effect; and (c) the recommendations for a healthy diet, in order to prevent and to cure liver fat accumulation. In general, all data should be put in the context of the general balance between calorie intake and calorie expenditure, considering the complementary role of physical activity in fat oxidation and metabolism.

8.2 Macronutrient Intake and Liver Fat

There is strong evidence that some dietary factors are involved in the pathogenesis of hepatic steatosis. According to a few experimental studies [4, 5], approximately 60 % of liver triglycerides are derived from free fatty acids (FFAs) pouring into the liver from adipose tissue, 26 % come from de novo synthesis in the liver, and 15 % are dietary fatty acids that reach the liver via chylomicron uptake and mix with fatty acids already present in the common pool [4, 6]. This explains why dietary fat and carbohydrate (CHO) intake are both detrimental for hepatic triglyceride accumulation and why different clinical studies provided conflicting results, as reported in several reviews [7]. Cortez-Pinto et al., comparing the habitual dietary intake in 45 patients with nonalcoholic steatohepatitis (NASH), with a mean BMI of 31 kg/m^2 (type 2 diabetes mellitus – T2DM, 38 %) vs. 856 healthy subjects (BMI, 27 kg/m^2; T2DM, 7 %) using a food-frequency questionnaire, reported a lower intake of carbohydrate and fiber and an increased intake of total fat and n-6 polyunsaturated fatty acids (PUFAs) in NASH [8]. The detrimental effects of a high-fat diet go well beyond hepatic fat accumulation, being associated with atheroma formation and cardiovascular disease, but a low-fat diet is also considered a pivotal recommendation for the prevention and treatment of NAFLD. Several studies have confirmed that liver fat is modulated by dietary fat content in the short and long term [9–11], and overweight/obese NASH patients have altered fatty acid metabolism and accumulated both total and FFAs, particularly saturated fatty acids (SFAs) and monounsaturated fatty acids (MUFAs) [12] (Fig. 8.1).

The role of dietary carbohydrates is less predictable, but there is evidence that also carbohydrates may activate specific metabolic pathways which turn the excessive dietary carbohydrates, mostly derived from high-glycemic index foods, into fatty acids, i.e., by inducing de novo hepatic lipogenesis and decreasing lipid oxidation. Solga et al. used a standardized food recall questionnaire to calculate total calories and macronutrients intake in 70 obese subjects (90 % with NAFLD; mean age, 44; median body mass index (BMI), 55 kg/m^2) entering a bariatric surgery program, where a liver biopsy was obtained at the time of the surgical procedure [13]. No significant association was found between preoperative total daily calorie or protein intake and the severity of steatosis, fibrosis, or necroinflammation. A higher CHO intake was significantly associated with the severity of hepatic necroinflammation, while a higher fat intake was associated with lower hepatic inflammation. A low-energy, low-CHO diet (approx. 1,000 kcal, 54 % protein, 41 % fat,

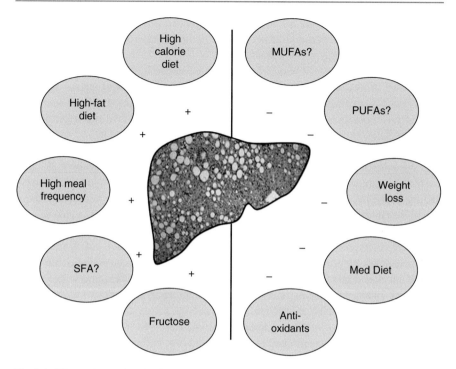

Fig. 8.1 Dietary factors involved in the pathogenesis of nonalcoholic fatty liver disease. Factors favoring steatosis are on the left; factors reducing the risk of steatosis are on the right. *Abbreviations*: *MUFAs* monounsaturated fatty acids, *PUFAs* polyunsaturated fatty acids, *SFAs* saturated fatty acids

5 % CHO) reduced intrahepatic triglyceride content to near zero in a 2-week period [14]. On the contrary, high-CHO, high-SFA, and low-PUFA diets were reported to have a role in NASH and NASH progression [15].

Insulin and triglyceride concentrations are increased in response to large amounts of dietary carbohydrates, particularly in response to simple, unrefined sugars, such as fructose, which may lead to hepatic triglyceride accumulation much more than any dietary fats. Intervention studies in both animals and humans have consistently demonstrated that large doses of fructose might be particularly lipogenic [16, 17], whereas high-fat diets with lower fructose content have detrimental effects on hepatic fat accumulation [18]. Fructose intake was very limited in the human diet before the advent of the processed food industry, because as natural source it was only available in honey and in fruit. Dates, raisins, molasses, and figs have a fructose content higher than 10 % by weight, whereas grapes, raw apples, and persimmons are less rich in fructose (almost 5–10 % by weight). Food preferences have considerably changed in Western countries compared to the healthy, raw food consumption of past generations. More than 50 % of preschool children consume calorie-rich, fructose-sweetened beverages, and prepackaged foods are increasingly replacing fresh foods worldwide. High-fructose corn syrup (HFCS) – a sugar where fructose is in excess of the 50:50 ratio with glucose to form saccharose – is frequently added to processed food because of its low cost, high palatability, and its characteristics favoring prolonged shelf life.

Fructose is not the only reason for hepatic fat accumulation; the overconsumption of soft drinks and processed foods with their high content of sugars, fats, and additives leads to excessive calorie intake. High-calorie intake can lead to increased hepatic fat deposition as much as fructose intake, and overfeeding, regardless of nutrient intake, is responsible for the development of fatty liver [19].

Dietary quality indices assess the quality of a diet according to glycemic index and antioxidant intake and are inversely associated with energy density. A case-control study measuring several indices predicting healthy eating confirmed that the dietary intake in NAFLD patients is generally characterized by poorer dietary habits and higher intake of energy, as well as carbohydrates and fats [20]. The role of antioxidants and the quality of food are thus important in the pathogenesis and progression of NAFLD, in terms of prevention and treatment; oxidative stress, caused by lipid peroxidation, promotes hepatic necroinflammation, which, in turn, is the basis for the development of fibrosis. A low intake of fruits, vegetables, and whole grains and a high intake of carbohydrates and fats are common examples of diets characterized by a low-quality index and increased oxidative stress. Machado et al. reported an impaired glutathione metabolism associated with a reduced antioxidant status in NAFLD, in the presence of high-fat and low-carbohydrate intake [21].

Also protein intake is involved in the general health status, and it also affects liver health. Protein malnutrition, frequently observed after malabsorptive bariatric surgery, is a cause of hepatic steatosis, and refeeding may variably improve liver status. The total amount of proteins, calcium, and vitamin D in the diet is frequently related and is generally assumed as an index of healthy eating; calcium and vitamin D intake may frequently be lower than recommended, particularly in obese subjects, and may contribute to hepatic steatosis favoring insulin resistance and diabetes [22].

Finally, high meal frequency, a common feature in the Western lifestyle, may have negative effects on liver disease [23]; fats and sugars, when consumed in excess and as between-meal snacks, affect hepatic glucose metabolism, due to the continuous flow of nutrients through the portal vein, which stimulates de novo lipogenesis and the accumulation of intrahepatic triglycerides. Education to healthy habits is thus mandatory, particularly among young people, because a higher energy intake during childhood and early adolescence, leading to obesity, is associated with very high risk of NAFLD and future risk of NAFLD progression [24].

8.3   Diet and Liver Fat: The Experimental Evidence

A large body of evidence links dietary modifications to liver fat in experimental animals.

Supplementation of vitamin A, vitamin C, and vitamin E improves liver fat [25], via decreased oxidative stress. The harmful effects of SFAs have been reported in multiple animal models, where diets rich in SFAs have been shown to increase liver fat and promote hepatocyte injury. In recent years attention has been progressively given to the beneficial effects of dietary n-3 and n-6 PUFAs, acting on the mitochondrial citrate carrier (CIC), which brings citrate from mitochondria into cytosol for de novo lipogenesis. PUFAs significantly decrease the activity and the expression of mitochondrial CIC [26], while MUFAs or SFAs do not produce any detrimental effect on CIC activity and expression. More recently, an isocaloric switch from an atherogenic Western-type diet rich in SFAs (cocoa butter) to diets rich in PUFAs (pumpkin seed oil) showed a protective effect in experimental animals, reducing NAFLD development; both refined and virgin pumpkin seed oil improved cholesterol and triglyceride plasma levels, and virgin oil was also shown to reduce systemic and vascular inflammation markers [27], in keeping with the antioxidant properties of the several phytochemicals present in unrefined oils.

Krill oil, fish oil, and olive oil may also be used in order to increase the content of the diet with n-3 fatty acids. Krill oil contains eicosapentaenoic acid (EPA) and docosahexaenoic acid (DHA), i.e., n-3 PUFAs. Also fish oil has a consistent amount of n-3 PUFAs, but in krill oil they are stored as phospholipids rather than triglycerides. Krill oil supplementation leads to a significant reduction in hepatomegaly and steatosis in mice; these beneficial effects are the result of a decreased activity of mitochondrial CIC, reducing de novo lipogenesis and increasing FFAs oxidation [26, 28].

8.4 Trial of Selective Fat Intake, Antioxidants, and Food Quality in the General Population and in NAFLD

The harmful effects of SFAs have also been reported in the general population, and dietary supplementation with MUFAs and/or PUFAs has been investigated as a potential treatment against NAFLD. Progression from pure fatty liver to NASH might again be mediated by oxidative stress [29, 30], but the possibility that the total antioxidant capacity of the diet might modulate the presence or severity of NAFLD has never been confirmed by intervention studies increasing fruit and vegetable intake. The most relevant studies linking selective dietary intake of fat and NAFLD in humans are reported in Table 8.1 [31–43].

The first studies date back to 2006, when Capanni et al. reported that low-dose n-3 PUFAs improved the biochemical and ultrasonographic features of NAFLD. From that time on, a series of pilot studies and underpowered randomized controlled studies and epidemiological evidence were generally in favor of a beneficial effect of PUFAs on circulating triglycerides, with conflicting results on hepatic fat content and liver enzymes. The dose of PUFAs was increased to 4–6 g/day [33, 36], or fish oil (9 g/day) [35], with specific effects on plasma triglycerides.

In the last 2 years, four randomized controlled studies were performed to settle the issue of the beneficial effects of PUFAs in patients with NAFLD. Scorletti et al. tested the effects of DHA plus EPA (Omacor/Lovaza, 4 g/day) on MRS-assessed intrahepatic triglycerides and biomarkers-measured fibrosis [39]. The erythrocyte

Table 8.1 Analysis of the most relevant trials on the effects of dietary fat on NAFLD development or progression

Author, year [Ref]	Type of study No. of cases	Treatment Duration Measurements	Results	Comments
Capanni, 2006 [31]	Pilot study in 56 NAFLD cases	n-3 PUFAs (1000 mg/day) in 42 (14 noncompliant as controls) 12 months US, DPI, biochemistry	Liver enzymes, lipid profile, glucose, US echotexture, and DPI improved on PUFAs; no changes in controls	Dietary PUFAs supplementation improves the biochemical, US, and hemodynamic features of steatosis
Tanaka, 2008 [32]	Pilot trial in 23 biopsy-proven NASH; mean age, 56; BMI, 28 kg/m^2 7 posttrial biopsies	EPA (2700 mg/day) 12 months Biochemistry, liver biopsy	ALT, FFAs, and markers of oxidative stress improved, irrespective of stable body weight Posttreatment biopsy showed improvement of steatosis, fibrosis, ballooning, and lobular inflammation in 6/7 patients	EPA supplementation is safe and efficacious for NASH, because of its anti-inflammatory and antioxidant properties
Zhu, 2008 [33]	RCT 134 NAFLD patients with hyperlipidemia	n-3 PUFAs, 6000 mg/day (n=66) vs. PL (n=68) 6 months US, anthropometry, biochemistry	ALT, TG, and LDL chol improved in PUFA group. No changes in BW. At US, complete NAFLD regression in 20% vs. 7% on PL; partial regression in 53% vs. 35%	Diet supplementation with n-3 PUFAs improves serum lipid levels and partly normalizes the US evidence of NAFLD
Spadaro, 2008 [34]	RCT 40 patients with NAFLD	AHA-recommended diet + PUFAs, 2000 mg/day (n=20) vs. diet (n=20) 6 months US, biochemistry	AST, TG, and TNF-alpha improved on PUFAs. At US, complete NAFLD regression in 33% vs. 0% on PL; partial regression in 50% vs. 28%	PUFAs supplementation of recommended diet improves plasma profile and US features of NAFLD
Vega, 2008 [35]	Sequential design 17 NAFLD patients	4-week PL, then 8-week fish oil (9 g/day) Biochemistry, MRS	Decreased TGs (by 46%) and VLDL + IDL (by 21%). No change in hepatic TG content at MRS	High-dose PUFAs are effective on circulating TGs, with no effect on hepatic TG content

Cussons, 2009 [36]	RCT 25 PCOS women (mean age, 32.7; BMI, 34.8 kg/m²)	n-3 PUFAs (4 g/day) vs. PL 8 weeks Biochemistry, MRS	Reduced plasma TGs and IHTG at MRS vs. PL. The effect was particularly significant in women with steatosis, defined as IHTG >5 %. Reduced systolic and diastolic pressure with PUFAs	n-3 PUFA supplementation has a beneficial effect on hepatic fat and CV risk factors in women with PCOS, including those with hepatic steatosis
Bozzetto, 2012 [37]	RCT of isocaloric dietary intervention 45 T2DM patients (37 men, 8 women), aged 35–70	4 dietary groups: (1) high CHO/high fiber; (2) high CHO/high MUFA; (3) high CHO/high fiber + PA; (4) high MUFA + PA 8 weeks Biochemistry, MRS	Body weight is stable in all groups. IHTG decreased more in MUFAs (−29 %) or MUFA + PA (−25 %) vs. in CHO/fiber (−4 %) or CHO/fiber + PA (−6 %). Repeated measures ANOVA, adjusted for baseline covariates, showed a significant effect on IHTG for diet (P=0.006), not for PA	An isocaloric MUFA-rich diet is better than a diet higher in CHO and fiber, with low glycemic index, on IHTG content, independently of programs of aerobic training
Bjermo, 2012 [38]	RCT of isocaloric dietary intervention 67 obese subjects (15 % with T2DM) ages 30–65. 61 completed the study	Diet high in vegetable n−6 PUFAs (PUFA diet) vs. SFAs mainly from butter (SFA diet) 10 weeks Biochemistry, MRI, MRS	IHTG decreased on PUFA diet not on SFA diet (between-group difference from baseline: MRI, 16 %; P<0.001; MRS, 34 %; P=0.02). Cytokine receptor concentrations lower during the PUFA diet. In compliant subjects, lower insulin and lipid levels on PUFA diet	n−6 PUFAs reduce liver fat and modestly improve metabolic status, without weight loss. The study reported downregulation of PCSK9, a possible mechanism for the effects of PUFAs
Scorletti, 2014 [39] WELLCOME study	RCT 103 NAFLD patients (95 completed the study (55 M, 40 F))	DHA + EPA, 4 g/day (n=51) vs. PL (n=52) 18 months MRS	IHTG marginally reduced on treatment with DHA + EPA (p=0.1). Adherence (tested by DHA + EPA enrichment in erythrocytes) significantly associated with reduced liver fat (p=0.007)	A significant decrease in liver fat might theoretically be achieved by high-dose DHA + EPA treatment in NAFLD
Rosqvist, 2014 [40] LIPOGAIN study	RCT 39 healthy, normal-weight subjects (age, 20–38§; BMI, 18–27 kg/m²; no T2DM)	Muffins with n-6 PUFAs (linoleic acid), or SFAs (palmitic acid) adjusted to a 3 % weight gain 7 weeks Anthropometry, MRI, transcriptomics	Similar weight gain. Liver fat and VAT increased more on SFAs. PUFAs caused a threefold larger increase in lean tissue. Genes regulating energy dissipation, IR, body composition, and fat-cell differentiation differently regulated by diets	Overeating SFAs promotes hepatic and visceral fat storage, whereas PUFAs promote lean tissue accretion in healthy humans

(continued)

Table 8.1 (continued)

Author, year [Ref]	Type of study No. of cases	Treatment Duration Measurements	Results	Comments
Sanyal, 2014 [41]	RCT of EPA-E, a synthetic PUFA 243 NASH subjects with (NAS ≥4); 25% non-completers	Low-dose EPA-E, 1800 mg/day (n=82) vs. high-dose EPA-E, 2700 mg/day (n=86) vs. PL (n=75) 12 months Liver biopsy, biochemistry	Primary end point (NAS reduction, no fibrosis worsening) met in 35–40%, without difference between groups. No effects of EPA-E on histology or biochemistry, but lower TG levels (−6.5 mg/dL vs. +12 in PL; P=0.03)	EPA-E, at doses used in the trial, does not produce any valuable effect on NAFLD CLINICAL
Argo, 2015 [43]	RCT in non-cirrhotic NASH (41 subjects, 34 completers)	n-3 PUFAs (3000 mg/d; n=17) vs. PL (n=17) 1 year Liver biopsy, MRI	No difference between groups for the primary end point (NAS reduction ≥2 points, no fibrosis progression). n-3 PUFAs caused a larger decrease in IHTG in subjects with increased or stable weight. No PUFA effects on liver cell injury or IR	n-3 PUFAs at 3000 mg/day for 1 year do not promote NASH regression or any additional clinically significant improvement, in addition to a marginal decrease in liver fat

Abbreviations: AHA American Heart Association, *ALT* alanine aminotransferase, *ANOVA* analysis of variance, *AST* aspartate aminotransferase, *BMI* body mass index, *BW* body weight, *CHO* carbohydrates, *CV* cardiovascular, *DHA* docosahexaenoic acid, *DPI* Doppler perfusion index, *EPA-E* ethyl-eicosapentaenoic acid, *FFAs* free fatty acids, *IDL* intermediate density lipoproteins, *IHTG* intrahepatic TG content, *IR* insulin resistance, *LDL chol* low-density lipoproteins cholesterol, *MRI* magnetic resonance imaging, *MRS* magnetic resonance spectroscopy, *MUFAs* monounsaturated fatty acids, *NAFLD* nonalcoholic fatty liver disease, *NAS* NAFLD activity score, *NASH* nonalcoholic steatohepatitis, *PA* physical activity, *PCOS* polycystic ovary syndrome, *PCSK9* proprotein convertase subtilisin/kexin type 9, *PL* placebo, *PUFAs* polyunsaturated fatty acids, *RCT* randomized controlled trial, *SFAs* saturated fatty acids, *TGs* triglycerides, *TNF-alpha* tumor necrosis factor-alpha, *T2DM* type 2 diabetes mellitus, *US* ultrasonography, *VAT* visceral adipose tissue, *VLDL* very low-density lipoproteins

DHA and EPA enrichment was also measured as a correlate of treatment adherence. The study reported a trend toward improvement in liver fat percentage on DHA/EPA treatment, but the results were possibly biased by contamination in the placebo group and by a variable adherence in the Omacor group. They concluded that higher doses and/or higher adherence to treatment might possibly confirm a beneficial effect of treatment on the liver.

The LIPOGAIN study compared overfeeding by muffins enriched with n-6 PUFAs (rich in linoleic acid) to overfeeding with similar muffins enriched with SFAs (palmitic acid) and concluded that PUFAs were more effective in promoting lean mass accretion, whereas SFAs promoted liver fat increase. The study also pointed to a regulatory action of different fatty acids on genes regulating energy dissipation and on body composition [40].

Finally, two studies compared PUFAs with placebo on the targets of NASH resolution without any worsening of fibrosis, as agreed by international regulatory agencies for the treatment of NASH. Low- and high-dose synthetic PUFAs were no better than placebo on NASH remission in 243 patients treated for 12 months, but produced a significant reduction of plasma triglycerides [41]. The study was powered to exclude a significant type 2 error, also considering dropouts and the higher-than-expected effect obtained by placebo. These negative results were confirmed by a smaller study in non-cirrhotic NASH, where 1-year treatment did not produce any significant histological advantage over placebo, with the exception of a marginal decrease in liver fat [43].

Olive oil, the cornerstone of the Mediterranean diet, contains oleic acid, an n-9 MUFA.

A few studies have tested the possible beneficial effects of fats associated with the Mediterranean diet. A high-MUFA diet was reported to be effective on intrahepatic triglyceride content in subjects with T2DM, independent of any program of physical activity [37]. More recently, the effects of the Mediterranean diet were compared with a low-fat/high-CHO diet (LF/HCD), in a crossover comparison of 6 weeks. The two diets did not produce any significant weight loss, but intrahepatic triglycerides were remarkably reduced in response to the Mediterranean diet, as measured by MRS [44]. In 73 consecutive NAFLD patients, the adherence to Mediterranean diet significantly correlated with the severity of steatosis; NASH patients reported significantly lower values in the Mediterranean diet score, an index of adherence to a Mediterranean dietary pattern, measured on 11 typical elements [45]. In particular, the intake of fat from dairy sources, a significant component of the Mediterranean diet, might play a role on low liver fat accumulation, favoring glucose tolerance and insulin sensitivity [42].

8.5   Recommendation for a Healthy Diet

All medical associations have long issued formal recommendations to highlight the importance of weight loss as the most effective treatment for NAFLD prevention and treatment. As detailed above, diet and lifestyle can significantly affect the clinical features of NAFLD, but motivation to change lifestyle habits, particularly in the area of physical activity, is frequently insufficient to produce significant effects [46]. The long-term risk of poor outcome is increased by unhealthy diets low in antioxidants, such as vitamin C, vitamin A, vitamin E, and selenium; the plasma levels of these micronutrients are frequently low in NAFLD compared with levels in healthy subjects [20, 47]. Adherence to healthy lifestyle recommendations is low in most patients with NAFLD, and prolonged programs of cognitive-behavioral treatment are probably needed to improve patients' adherence and long-term outcome [48]. Healthy eating should become the most favorable option in the population, and current recommendations may be summarized as follows:

(a) *Calorie restriction.* Calorie restriction per se seems beneficial regardless of macronutrient composition. In order to obtain a reasonable weight loss, the overall calorie intake should be restricted to 1,200–1,500 kcal/day for women and 1,500–1,800 kcal/day for men, to produce an energy defect of 500–750 kcal/day. This calorie gap is expected to generate a weight loss in the range of 0.5–1.0 kg/week, also depending on the amount of physical activity, which becomes mandatory in order to achieve long-term weight loss maintenance. The macronutrient composition of the calorie-restricted diet should however be tailored to the patients' preferences in order to favor long-term adherence.

(b) *Carbohydrate intake.* The amount of carbohydrates should be controlled and maintained above 50 % of the total energy, choosing whole grains and low-glycemic index foods. Simple, unrefined sugars, such as fructose, should be banned. They may lead to hepatic triglyceride accumulation, favoring de novo hepatic lipogenesis.

(c) *Protein intake.* High-protein diets do not remarkably increase weight loss under strictly controlled conditions [49], as is the case of rehabilitation in-hospital programs for severe obesity. In overweight or grade 1 obesity, a moderate increase in protein content may help maintain a less severe energy defect, restricting the amount of lipid and carbohydrates.

(d) *Lipid intake.* The ability of high-fat diets in inducing fatty liver is questionable. Dietary fats, in the absence of calorie excess, are unlikely to become a major driver for NAFLD, but not all fat is alike, and some fats appear to be more deeply involved in the pathogenesis of NAFLD. The recommended amount of energy from dietary fats should be maintained below 30–35 % of the total daily energy intake, with large preference for MUFAs and PUFAs, whereas SFAs should be maintained below 7 % of total energy. There is also some evidence that dairy fat may have beneficial effects on liver fat accumulation.

(e) *Mediterranean diet.* Diets supplemented with extra-virgin olive oil or nuts have been shown to decrease the markers of oxidative stress, and there is evidence that the Mediterranean diet, associated with physical activity and cognitive behavior therapy, may have an important role in the prevention and treatment of NAFLD [50]. Also moderate alcohol consumption is a component of the Mediterranean diet; there is evidence that alcohol, namely, wine drinking, below the cutoffs of alcohol abuse (20 g/day in males, 10 g in females), may have a protective effect on liver fat accumulation [51]. Similarly, no harmful effects of coffee intake on NAFLD have ever been reported [52].

Conclusion

There is no answer to the title question; there is no definite limit to the amount of fat in the diet to reduce the risk of NAFLD. The evidence from the literature supports the concept that NAFLD is determined by a hypercaloric dietary intake, independently of macronutrients composition, and some kind of fats may only indirectly contribute to increase/reduce the risk of hepatic fat accumulation. In general, a variable diet, rich in fruits and vegetables, with moderate amounts of unrefined carbohydrate and low SFAs, no fructose-enriched soft drinks and processed foods, and moderate alcohol intake, represents the optimal dietary intake to combat the majority of metabolic diseases. This diet will also help prevent cardiovascular diseases and a variety of degenerative disorders [53]. We need concerted actions from institutions, health authorities, and the whole community to favor healthy lifestyles and to halt the obesity epidemics responsible for most metabolic disorders.

References

1. Marchesini G, Ridolfi V, Nepoti V (2008) Hepatotoxicity of fast food? Gut 57:568–570
2. Kechagias S, Ernersson A, Dahlqvist O, Lundberg P, Lindstrom T, Nystrom FH (2008) Fast-food-based hyper-alimentation can induce rapid and profound elevation of serum alanine aminotransferase in healthy subjects. Gut 57:649–654
3. Thomas EL, Hamilton G, Patel N, O'Dwyer R, Dore CJ, Goldin RD et al (2005) Hepatic triglyceride content and its relation to body adiposity: a magnetic resonance imaging and proton magnetic resonance spectroscopy study. Gut 54:122–127
4. Donnelly KL, Smith CI, Schwarzenberg SJ, Jessurun J, Boldt MD, Parks EJ (2005) Sources of fatty acids stored in liver and secreted via lipoproteins in patients with nonalcoholic fatty liver disease. J Clin Invest 115:1343–1351
5. Jacome-Sosa MM, Parks EJ (2014) Fatty acid sources and their fluxes as they contribute to plasma triglyceride concentrations and fatty liver in humans. Curr Opin Lipidol 25:213–220
6. Green CJ, Hodson L (2014) The influence of dietary fat on liver fat accumulation. Nutrients 6:5018–5033
7. McCarthy EM, Rinella ME (2012) The role of diet and nutrient composition in nonalcoholic Fatty liver disease. J Acad Nutr Diet 112:401–409
8. Cortez-Pinto H, Jesus L, Barros H, Lopes C, Moura MC, Camilo ME (2006) How different is the dietary pattern in non-alcoholic steatohepatitis patients? Clin Nutr 25:816–823
9. Utzschneider KM, Bayer-Carter JL, Arbuckle MD, Tidwell JM, Richards TL, Craft S (2013) Beneficial effect of a weight-stable, low-fat/low-saturated fat/low-glycaemic index diet to reduce liver fat in older subjects. Br J Nutr 109:1096–1104
10. van Herpen NA, Schrauwen-Hinderling VB, Schaart G, Mensink RP, Schrauwen P (2011) Three weeks on a high-fat diet increases intrahepatic lipid accumulation and decreases metabolic flexibility in healthy overweight men. J Clin Endocrinol Metab 96:E691–E695
11. Westerbacka J, Lammi K, Hakkinen AM, Rissanen A, Salminen I, Aro A et al (2005) Dietary fat content modifies liver fat in overweight nondiabetic subjects. J Clin Endocrinol Metab 90:2804–2809

12. de Almeida IT, Cortez-Pinto H, Fidalgo G, Rodrigues D, Camilo ME (2002) Plasma total and free fatty acids composition in human non-alcoholic steatohepatitis. Clin Nutr 21:219–223

13. Solga S, Alkhuraishe AR, Clark JM, Torbenson M, Greenwald A, Diehl AM et al (2004) Dietary composition and nonalcoholic fatty liver disease. Dig Dis Sci 49:1578–1583

14. Browning JD, Davis J, Saboorian MH, Burgess SC (2006) A low-carbohydrate diet rapidly and dramatically reduces intrahepatic triglyceride content. Hepatology 44:487–488

15. Toshimitsu K, Matsuura B, Ohkubo I, Niiya T, Furukawa S, Hiasa Y et al (2007) Dietary habits and nutrient intake in non-alcoholic steatohepatitis. Nutrition 23:46–52

16. Moore JB, Gunn PJ, Fielding BA (2014) The role of dietary sugars and de novo lipogenesis in non-alcoholic fatty liver disease. Nutrients 6:5679–5703

17. Fakhoury-Sayegh N, Trak-Smayra V, Khazzaka A, Esseily F, Obeid O, Lahoud-Zouein M et al (2015) Characteristics of nonalcoholic fatty liver disease induced in wistar rats following four different diets. Nutr Res Pract 9:350–357

18. Marina A, von Frankenberg AD, Suvag S, Callahan HS, Kratz M, Richards TL et al (2014) Effects of dietary fat and saturated fat content on liver fat and markers of oxidative stress in overweight/obese men and women under weight-stable conditions. Nutrients 6:4678–4690

19. Gonzalez C, de Ledinghen V, Vergniol J, Foucher J, Le Bail B, Carlier S et al (2013) Hepatic steatosis, carbohydrate intake, and food quotient in patients with NAFLD. Int J Endocrinol 2013:428542

20. Hashemi Kani A, Alavian SM, Esmaillzadeh A, Adibi P, Azadbakht L (2013) Dietary quality indices and biochemical parameters among patients with Non Alcoholic Fatty Liver Disease (NAFLD). Hepat Mon 13:e10943

21. Machado MV, Ravasco P, Jesus L, Marques-Vidal P, Oliveira CR, Proenca T et al (2008) Blood oxidative stress markers in non-alcoholic steatohepatitis and how it correlates with diet. Scand J Gastroenterol 43:95–102

22. Targher G, Bertolini L, Scala L, Cigolini M, Zenari L, Falezza G et al (2007) Associations between serum 25-hydroxyvitamin D3 concentrations and liver histology in patients with non-alcoholic fatty liver disease. Nutr Metab Cardiovasc Dis 17:517–524

23. Koopman KE, Caan MW, Nederveen AJ, Pels A, Ackermans MT, Fliers E et al (2014) Hypercaloric diets with increased meal frequency, but not meal size, increase intrahepatic tri-glycerides: a randomized controlled trial. Hepatology 60:545–553

24. Anderson EL, Howe LD, Fraser A, Macdonald-Wallis C, Callaway MP, Sattar N et al (2015) Childhood energy intake is associated with nonalcoholic fatty liver disease in adolescents. J Nutr 145:983–989

25. Oliveira CP, Gayotto LC, Tatai C, Della Nina BI, Lima ES, Abdalla DS et al (2003) Vitamin C and vitamin E in prevention of Nonalcoholic Fatty Liver Disease (NAFLD) in choline deficient diet fed rats. Nutr J 2:9

26. Ferramosca A, Zara V (2014) Modulation of hepatic steatosis by dietary fatty acids. World J Gastroenterol 20:1746–1755

27. Morrison MC, Mulder P, Stavro PM, Suarez M, Arola-Arnal A, van Duyvenvoorde W et al (2015) Replacement of dietary saturated fat by PUFA-rich pumpkin seed oil attenuates non-alcoholic fatty liver disease and atherosclerosis development, with additional health effects of virgin over refined oil. PLoS One 10:e0139196

28. Tandy S, Chung RW, Wat E, Kamili A, Berge K, Griinari M et al (2009) Dietary krill oil sup-plementation reduces hepatic steatosis, glycemia, and hypercholesterolemia in high-fat-fed mice. J Agric Food Chem 57:9339–9345

29. Koek GH, Liedorp PR, Bast A (2011) The role of oxidative stress in non-alcoholic steatohepa-titis. Clin Chim Acta 412:1297–1305

30. Georgoulis M, Fragopoulou E, Kontogianni MD, Margariti A, Boulamatsi O, Detopoulou P et al (2015) Blood redox status is associated with the likelihood of nonalcoholic fatty liver disease irrespectively of diet's total antioxidant capacity. Nutr Res 35:41–48

31. Capanni M, Calella F, Biagini MR, Genise S, Raimondi L, Bedogni G et al (2006) Prolonged n-3 polyunsaturated fatty acid supplementation ameliorates hepatic steatosis in patients with non-alcoholic fatty liver disease: a pilot study. Aliment Pharmacol Ther 23:1143–1151

32. Tanaka N, Sano K, Horiuchi A, Tanaka E, Kiyosawa K, Aoyama T (2008) Highly purified eicosapentaenoic acid treatment improves nonalcoholic steatohepatitis. J Clin Gastroenterol 42:413–418

33. Zhu FS, Liu S, Chen XM, Huang ZG, Zhang DW (2008) Effects of n-3 polyunsaturated fatty acids from seal oils on nonalcoholic fatty liver disease associated with hyperlipidemia. World J Gastroenterol 14:6395–6400

34. Spadaro L, Magliocco O, Spampinato D, Piro S, Oliveri C, Alagona C et al (2008) Effects of n-3 polyunsaturated fatty acids in subjects with nonalcoholic fatty liver disease. Dig Liver Dis 40:194–199

35. Vega GL, Chandalia M, Szczepaniak LS, Grundy SM (2008) Effects of N-3 fatty acids on hepatic triglyceride content in humans. J Invest Med 56:780–785

36. Cussons AJ, Watts GF, Mori TA, Stuckey BG (2009) Omega-3 fatty acid supplementation decreases liver fat content in polycystic ovary syndrome: a randomized controlled trial employing proton magnetic resonance spectroscopy. J Clin Endocrinol Metab 94: 3842–3848

37. Bozzetto L, Prinster A, Annuzzi G, Costagliola L, Mangione A, Vitelli A et al (2012) Liver fat is reduced by an isoenergetic MUFA diet in a controlled randomized study in type 2 diabetic patients. Diabetes Care 35:1429–1435

38. Bjermo H, Iggman D, Kullberg J, Dahlman I, Johansson L, Persson L et al (2012) Effects of n-6 PUFAs compared with SFAs on liver fat, lipoproteins, and inflammation in abdominal obesity: a randomized controlled trial. Am J Clin Nutr 95:1003–1012

39. Scorletti E, Bhatia L, McCormick KG, Clough GF, Nash K, Hodson L et al (2014) Effects of purified eicosapentaenoic and docosahexaenoic acids in nonalcoholic fatty liver disease: results from the Welcome* study. Hepatology 60:1211–1221

40. Rosqvist F, Iggman D, Kullberg J, Cedernaes J, Johansson HE, Larsson A et al (2014) Overfeeding polyunsaturated and saturated fat causes distinct effects on liver and visceral fat accumulation in humans. Diabetes 63:2356–2368

41. Sanyal AJ, Abdelmalek MF, Suzuki A, Cummings OW, Chojkier M, Group E-AS (2014) No significant effects of ethyl-eicosapentanoic acid on histologic features of nonalcoholic steato-hepatitis in a phase 2 trial. Gastroenterology 147(377–384):e371

42. Kratz M, Marcovina S, Nelson JE, Yeh MM, Kowdley KV, Callahan HS et al (2014) Dairy fat intake is associated with glucose tolerance, hepatic and systemic insulin sensitivity, and liver fat but not beta-cell function in humans. Am J Clin Nutr 99:1385–1396

43. Argo CK, Patrie JT, Lackner C, Henry TD, de Lange EE, Weltman AL et al (2015) Effects of n-3 fish oil on metabolic and histological parameters in NASH: a double-blind, randomized, placebo-controlled trial. J Hepatol 62:190–197

44. Ryan MC, Itsiopoulos C, Thodis T, Ward G, Trost N, Hofferberth S et al (2013) The Mediterranean diet improves hepatic steatosis and insulin sensitivity in individuals with non-alcoholic fatty liver disease. J Hepatol 59:138–143

45. Kontogianni MD, Tileli N, Margariti A, Georgoulis M, Deutsch M, Tiniakos D et al (2014) Adherence to the Mediterranean diet is associated with the severity of non-alcoholic fatty liver disease. Clin Nutr 33:678–683

46. Centis E, Moscatiello S, Bugianesi E, Bellentani S, Fracanzani AL, Calugi S et al (2013) Stage of change and motivation to healthier lifestyle in non-alcoholic fatty liver disease. J Hepatol 58:771–777

47. Musso G, Gambino R, De Michieli F, Biroli G, Premoli A, Pagano G et al (2007) Nitrosative stress predicts the presence and severity of nonalcoholic fatty liver at different stages of the development of insulin resistance and metabolic syndrome: possible role of vitamin A intake. Am J Clin Nutr 86:661–671

48. Marchesini G, Petta S, Dalle Grave R (2015) Diet, weight loss, and liver health in NAFLD: patho-physiology, evidence and practice. Hepatology. doi:10.1002/hep.28392. [Epub ahead of print]

49. Dalle Grave R, Calugi S, Gavasso I, El Ghoch M, Marchesini G (2013) A randomized trial of energy-restricted high-protein versus high-carbohydrate, low-fat diet in morbid obesity. Obesity (Silver Spring) 21:1774–1781

50. Abenavoli L, Milic N, Peta V, Alfieri F, De Lorenzo A, Bellentani S (2014) Alimentary regimen in non-alcoholic fatty liver disease: Mediterranean diet. World J Gastroenterol 20:16831–16840
51. Moriya A, Iwasaki Y, Ohguchi S, Kayashima E, Mitsumune T, Taniguchi H et al (2015) Roles of alcohol consumption in fatty liver: a longitudinal study. J Hepatol 62:921–927
52. Saab S, Mallam D, Cox GA 2nd, Tong MJ (2014) Impact of coffee on liver diseases: a systematic review. Liver Int 34:495–504
53. Estruch R, Ros E, Salas-Salvado J, Covas MI, Corella D, Aros F et al (2013) Primary prevention of cardiovascular disease with a Mediterranean diet. N Engl J Med 368:1279–1290

Tasters, Supertasters, Genes and Environment: How Dietary Choices Influence Our Health

9

Hellas Cena and Clio Oggioni

9.1 Physiology of Taste

9.1.1 Five Tastes

Taste is one of the essential senses and plays such a crucial role for nutrition and health, providing information about food and preventing the ingestion of toxic substances.

Yet, taste should not be confused with flavour. Taste includes only gustatory sensations that originate in organs of the oral cavity – taste buds – and are elicited by water-soluble compounds interacting with the epithelial cells of taste buds. In contrast, flavour reveals the combined sensory experience of olfaction and gustation and is generated by the integration of taste and smell signals in the orbitofrontal and other areas of the cerebral cortex to generate flavours and mediate food recognition [1].

The taste system consents the distinction of five basic tastes: salty, sour, sweet, bitter and umami. Each of these tastes represents different nutritional or physiological requirements. Salty taste senses intake of Na+ and other minerals, which play a central role in maintaining body's water balance and blood circulation. Sour taste detects the presence of acids, avoiding the ingestion of spoiled foods. Sweet taste signals sugars and carbohydrates, usually indicate high-energy food. Umami taste, elicited by L-glutamate and a few other L-amino acids, reveals the protein content in

H. Cena (✉) • C. Oggioni
Department of Public Health, Experimental and Forensic Medicine – Unit of Human Nutrition, University of Pavia, Pavia, Italy
e-mail: hellas.cena@unipv.it; clio.oggioni@gmail.com; clio.oggioni@unimi.it

© Springer International Publishing Switzerland 2016   123
E. Grossi, F. Pace (eds.), *Human Nutrition from the Gastroenterologist's Perspective*,
DOI 10.1007/978-3-319-30361-1_9

food. Finally, bitter taste may protect against some food toxins and poisoning [2]. Recent evidences support a role for fat detection in humans, and fat taste has been proposed as an additional taste essential in sensing the presence of fatty acids in foods [3].

9.1.2 Signalling

The signalling for taste is mediated by taste receptor cells (TRCs), which are organised in taste buds located within gustatory papillae. In humans, there are about 5,000 taste buds in the oral cavity, situated on the superior surface of the tongue, on the palate and on the epiglottis. There is a long-held misconception that the tongue has specific zones for each flavour. Tastes can actually be sensed by all parts of the tongue. Merely the sides of the tongue are more sensitive than the middle. This is always true except for the bitter taste that is being sensed more in the back of our tongue. This might be protective so anyone can spit out any poisonous or spoiled food or substance before being swallowed [4]. Four types of papillae have been described: fungiform papillae, mostly located on the dorsal surface in the anterior two-thirds of the tongue; foliate papillae, present on lateral margins towards the posterior part of the tongue; circumvallate papillae, arranged in a V-shaped row at the back of the tongue and filiform papillae, which are found all over the surface of the tongue and do not contain taste buds. These are considered to have a mechanical function and not to be directly involved in taste sensation (Fig. 9.1).

TRCs project microvilli to the apical surface of the taste bud, where they form the 'taste pore'; this is the site of interaction with tastants [4].

Recently [5] extra-oral taste receptors have been identified in the GI tract and even in the skeletal muscle, brain, respiratory tract. Sperm also expresses taste receptors. The exact role of these receptors in regions other than the mouth needs to be further elucidated. Doing so will lead to a better understanding of human physiology and integration of neuronal activity and metabolism.

9.1.3 Nervous System Connections

TRCs make contact with other neurons at synapses with primary sensory axons that run in the three cranial nerves, VII (facial), IX (glossopharyngeal) and X (vagus), which innervate the taste buds. The central axons of these primary sensory neurons, in the corresponding cranial nerve ganglia, project to the nucleus of the solitary tract in the medulla. Gustatory information is then transferred from the nucleus of the solitary tract to the thalamus and next to gustatory areas of the cortex. This wide taste information representation in the brain probably serves to integrate it with interoceptive (hunger, satiety, appetites) and exteroceptive (vision, olfaction, somatosensation) signals and to generate behavioural responses to taste stimuli (Fig. 9.2) [6].

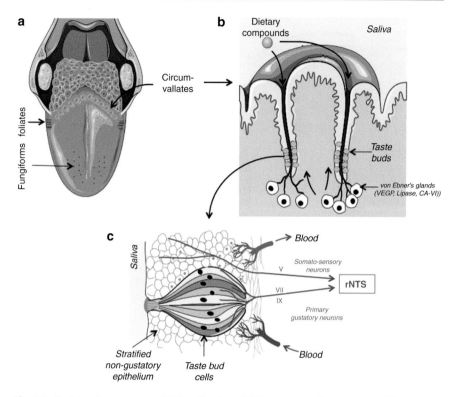

Fig. 9.1 Peripheral taste system. (**a**) Localisation of different types of gustatory papillae onto the human tongue. (**b**) Sagittal section of a circumvallate papillae (CVP) showing its typical dome-shaped structure and the anatomical relationship with the von Ebner's glands. (**c**) Schematic representation of a taste bud. *CA-VI* carbonic anhydrase, *rNTS* rostral nucleus of solitary tract, *VEGP* von Ebner's gland protein, *V* trigeminal endings, *VII* afferent fibres of the chorda tympani nerve; *IX* afferent fibres of the glossopharyngeal nerve (Source: *Taste of fat: a sixth taste modality?* Philippe Besnard, Patricia Passilly-Degrace, and Naim A. Khan. Physiologie de la Nutrition & Toxicologie, U. 866 INSERM/Université de Bourgogne, Franche Comté/AgroSup. Dijon, Dijon, France [3])

9.2   Supertaster

9.2.1   Taster Classification

Blakeslee first studied the variability in testing a bitter thiourea compound, phenylthio-carbamide (PTC) [7]. He hypothesised that the physiologic role of taste variability could be related to evolutionary adaptation to specific environments to recognise substances either potentially dangerous or necessary for biological functions. From there on scientists have phenotypically classified the human population into three categories: insensitive, sensitive and hypersensitive to bitterness [8]. The term supertaster was given referring to individuals who belong to the latter category [9]. Due to the toxicity

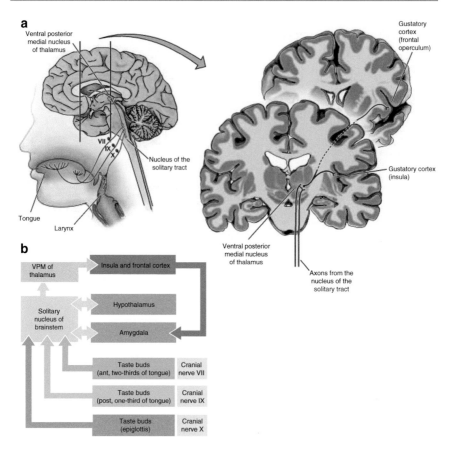

Fig. 9.2 Organisation of the human taste system. (**a**) The relationship between the gustatory system and the nucleus of solitary tract and cortex in the brain. (**b**) Diagram of taste information pathways [6]

of PTC, the safer chemical PROP (6-n-propylthiouracil) has been afterwards used in human experimental studies to determine bitter taster status [10]. The use of PROP/NaCl ratio has been suggested to discriminate medium tasters from supertasters [11].

Miller and Reedy first discovered anatomic differences between non-tasters and tasters using dyes (including blue food colouring) that differentially stain structures on the tongue [12]. Dyes fail to stain fungiform papillae as well as taste pores, so they can be respectively counted and viewed under magnification. More studies were performed, and scientists found that PROP tasters had more taste pores than non-tasters did [11, 13]. Later Bartoshuk et al. extended their observations to supertasters; supertasters are showing more fungiform papillae and taste pores [14]. The association between the number of fungiform papillae and bitterness of PROP has been further supported by other studies. Given that females have more fungiform papillae and thus more taste pores than males do, it follows that females are more likely than males to be supertasters [15].

9.2.2   Genetics

The perception of sweet, umami and bitter tastes is all mediated via G-coupled protein receptors, encoded by the TAS1R and TAS2R taste receptor gene families, while salty and sour tastes are transduced via ion channels [16]. Many genetic studies have been conducted, and it is now recognised that the variance of the phenotypic distribution is explained by the haplotypes generated by three polymorphisms in the TAS2R38 gene on chromosome 7 accounting for 55–85 % of the variance in PTC sensitivity [17].

9.2.3   Taste and Food Preferences

The influence of genetics in food preferences is controversial. Many studies have been conducted on this subject with different results.

The non-tasters tended to consume more sweet foods, while supertasters tended to avoid them. PROP tasters avoid food and beverages with a strong bitter component, such as broccoli, kohlrabi, turnips and alcohol [18, 19]. Further research has revealed that PROP tasters also dislike energy-dense, high-fat food [20]. However, the data on food preferences and fat intake vary across studies, with no clear association between taster status and food preferences or body weight [10]. There are studies showing no association [21] or even the opposite association, between PROP tasters and fat intake [22, 23] as well as between these subjects and their higher body fat composition.

Research on children has shown similar results. Hedge and Sharma studied a group of 500 children ages 8–12 years old. Body mass index (BMI) was calculated. The supertasters appeared to remain thinner than both their non-taster counterparts and medium tasters. The non-tasters tended more to obesity [24]. Moreover Keller and Tepper assessed weight differences revealing different results in eating habits and body weight in boys who were non-tasters compared to general population as well as medium- and supertasters reporting also a higher protein intake [25].

9.3   Origin of Taste Preferences and Genetic Determinants

Sweet, sour, salty, bitter, umami or savoury taste preferences have a strong innate component [26, 27]. Sweet, umami and salty substances are innately preferred, whereas bitter and many sour substances are innately rejected. Nevertheless, these innate tendencies can be modified by pre- and postnatal experiences.

The development of the human senses is linked to that of the central nervous system during the first weeks of gestation. In fact, the first taste buds appear in the embryonic phase, and as soon as the foetus starts swallowing, the aromatic compounds contained in the amniotic fluid stimulate taste receptors [28, 29] and cause at a central level, among other reflexes, the movements of the tongue and the salivary secretion [30, 31].

The amniotic sac, in which foetuses grow and develop, is susceptible to sensory changes received by maternal nutrition and food choices that flavour amniotic fluid [32]. The foetus swallows about 200–760 ml of amniotic fluid per day (depending on the stage of development) and is therefore exposed to a large amount of different flavours, including various simple sugars, like glucose and fructose, fatty acids, amino acids, proteins and salts [33]. The composition of amniotic fluid changes during foetal development also with the foetus urine output. Later on during gestation, facial expression changes have been reported in response to taste receptor stimuli, especially for bitter taste, with subsequent changes in the frequency of swallowing.

In this way, children can experience taste and different flavours before birth.

These early sensory experiences lead to develop preferences after birth for the same flavours that have become somehow 'familiar' during uterine life, thanks to the transmission from the mother's diet to the amniotic fluid [27, 33, 34]. In newborns taste is the most developed of all senses; different studies have shown an innate preference for sweet taste and a high dislike for sour taste and for bitter ones, although reaction changes for the bitter ones have been reported within the first months of life [28] (Table 9.1).

From an evolutionary standpoint sweet taste preference can be explained either by the automatic recognition of safety and the high nutritional value perceived [35]. However, recent studies have demonstrated that sweet taste preferences are partly inherited. Chromosome 16p11.2 may harbour genetic variations that affect the consumption of sweet foods. Keskitalo et al. reported that a 40–50 % of the variation in these traits might be explained by inherited mechanisms, unlike the salty intensity and pleasantness ratings that are mostly not inherited [36].

Despite this sweet taste innate preference, the degree of liking for sweetness varies greatly among individuals depending on both environmental backgrounds and genetics. Indeed results obtained from twin studies suggest that approximately half of the variation in liking for sweet solution and frequency of sweet foods may be explained by genetic factors, whereas the rest of the variation may be due to environmental factors unique to each twin individual [37].

Taste development continues after birth as babies are exposed to breast milk or commercial infant formulas and later on to new solid foods. Breast-milk taste changes 1–2 h post-maternal consumption of foods like garlic or vanilla [28] and can influence breast-milk intake of the infants.

Table 9.1 Innate reactions to taste compounds

Basic taste	Innate reaction	Development
Sweet	Positive	Prenatally
Sour	Negative/ rejecting	Uncertain prenatally
Salty	Positive	At the age of 4–6 months
Bitter	Negative/ rejecting	Prenatally

From:http://www.eufic.org/article/en/artid/how-taste-preferences-develop/
Source Mela [35]

Beauchamp et al. have demonstrated that there is a sensitive learning period in the first several months of life during which unpalatable flavours (to those not familiar with them) can be rendered palatable [27] providing strong evidence for both a dosing and a timing effect [38] and highlighting that what they experienced in early life is 'imprinted' and influences taste preferences during weaning in addition to persist as a preference for a considerable time.

This is particularly true and has been demonstrated in breastfed infants who may live different taste experiences depending on the foods and beverages that their mothers consume, influencing the infants' subsequent liking and acceptance of these flavours in solid foods later on. Several studies have shown that maternal exposure to particular foods does influence food choices in children who had been breastfed [28], as well as specific preferences have been observed in subjects who had been formula milk fed [39].

Beauchamp et al. suggest that breast milk may therefore be considered as a 'bridge' between the in utero experiences with flavours in amniotic fluid to those in solid foods at weaning and beyond. These experiences interact with genetic differences in flavour perception [40], and together genes and experience play a central role in establishing food likes and dislikes thereby impacting on the health and wellness of the infant, the child and the adult.

These experiences set the stage for later food choices and are important in establishing lifelong food habits. A better understanding of the early factors that determine taste development and food choices will add evidence-based knowledge to identify strategies to enhance healthy eating across the lifespan.

9.4   Food Choices

The way people eat influences their health in many ways. Diabetes, overweight, obesity, hypertension, dyslipidaemia are just some of the diseases related to inadequate dietary intake, as well as some cancers. Food choices seem to be changing partially due to socio-environmental factors including economic, social and cultural status as genetics and the physiology of human body: taste, hunger and satiety [41].

Sensory perception, cost, comfort, health, symbolism and taste define the value from which food choices originate (Figs. 9.2 and 9.3).

Many studies [43–45] have shown how socioeconomic factors, and especially family lifestyle, influence both dietary habits and lifestyle choices.

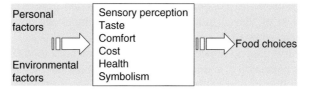

Fig. 9.3 Factors determining food choices (Source. Allegri et al. [41]. Modified from Furst et al. [42])

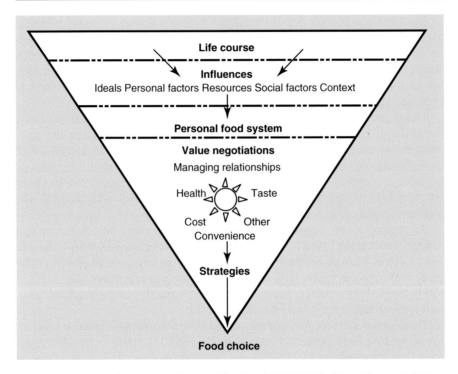

Fig. 9.4 Food choice determinants (Source: Allegri et al. [41]. Modified from Furst et al. [42])

The interactions of all these factors influence the characteristics of food choices that individuals make [41].

Since food choices have an enormous impact on health, it is necessary that all the variables that determine them should be considered: personal and environmental factors, sensory perception, taste, comfort, cost, health and symbolism (Fig. 9.4).

Inappropriate eating habits, particularly among younger countries both in developed and in developing ones, has led to the development of new chronic degenerative diseases defined as 'comfort' diseases, increasingly common and disabling [41] with early onsets.

Food choices and taste preferences towards energy-dense foods, high in sugars and fats and low in other nutrients, as desserts, may be linked to positive feedback due to associations with positive social events, although studies on animal models have shown that rats would rather choose energy-dense foods than lower-energy ones, probably thanks to post-digestive positive reaction experiences [46]. This effect referred to as 'flavour-nutrient learning' has important similarities to that observed in humans too [47].

In children it is easy to notice a higher like of these tasty foods high in energy sugars and fats compared to less tasty ones like vegetables that they are often forced to eat; however flavour-nutrient learning (FNL) could be an effective mechanism to change their preferences [48].

A good example is the development of preference towards bitter taste like coffee by mere exposure. The repeated exposure to such a drink with the frequent addition of milk or sugar to make it less bitter will transform a natural dislike in an acquired taste that will influence through experience and regular consumption preferences.

Many studies have looked into the effectiveness of repeated taste exposure for increasing vegetable acceptance in children with conflicting results [49]. Repeated exposure might not be successful for those children who have an increased sensitivity to bitter taste [49], while associative conditioning, that is pairing novel or disliked foods, like bitter vegetables, with liked flavours repeatedly, was more effective than exposure in increasing liking [50].

Food preferences are the result of numerous factors such as taste conditioning, adaptation and biological factors. However, family has a particularly high-standing role in what is called 'taste education' process. Family produces a great social facilitation of food preferences and intake [51], and from the very beginning parents can influence taste preferences over time. Although preferences and aversions are highly individual and neophobia phases are physiological, family context plays a key role in the development of taste preferences and may contribute to future healthy food choices [30].

9.5   Food and Environment

Popkin and colleagues have profusely studied changes in dietary and activity patterns in modern society and its implication in developing non-communicable diseases. Obesity is nowadays an epidemic illness, and it has, among the others, environmental causes. Popkin imputes rapid variations in the levels and composition of dietary and activity/inactivity patterns in transitional societies to different socioeconomic and demographic conditions [52]. The shift towards a diet higher in fat and meat and lower in carbohydrates and fibre, together with the shift towards less-intense physical activity, leads to nutritional and health effects [53]. As matter of fact, there are huge differences between eating patterns in urban areas and rural settings, particularly regarding the consumption of food prepared and consumed away from home. Therefore, it is clear that evolution of society and globalisation play a key role in addressing food choices.

Moreover it is well established that lower-income families have lower-quality diets [54] and that environmental factors may either reduce or strengthen the influence of the genetic predisposition that mediates food preferences. The role of the 6-n-propylthiouracil (PROP) taste phenotype on eating behaviour and food choices across life stages is the most-studied one in taste research [55].

However, this is not the only genetic taste factor involved in food preference, eating behaviour and therefore weight status. The involvement of the PROP taste phenotype in body weight status is controversial especially in children, and data suggest that PROP status may have a greater influence on body weight later in the life cycle, particularly in the context of a sedentary lifestyle [55] since in children it may be influenced by fat mass and obesity-related gene on adiposity development.

Taste genetic factors participate in the food linking and disliking process as well as in food preference and selection furthermore in body weight [37, 55, 56]. A deeper understanding of their function and role as well as the discovery of other genes and phenotypes along with environmental and behavioural factors affecting food intake will allow a better comprehension of weight maintenance and obesity development in childhood.

9.6   Causes and Consequences of Taste Loss

The sense of taste is a very important one, although its loss is considered less important compared to the vision or hearing loss that humans might experiment [27].

Luckily, a complete loss of gustation is rare; besides taste and smell are the only sensory systems that have the capacity to regenerate after damage, so some recovery of function is usually possible. Unfortunately partial taste loss as the ability to detect sweet, sour, salty, bitter or umami is a relatively common problem that has a tremendous impact on quality of life [57].

Although individuals can often compensate for partial loss, when it does occurs, eating and nutrition is regularly severely compromised, and the subsequent behaviours, particularly food choice and intake, are among the most important ones in terms of the health issues reported in developed and developing societies [58].

Most of what is considered a deficit of taste is usually due to an olfactory deficit. Taste is influenced by food smell, texture and temperature and even tongue movements that increase distribution of the food in the mouth and therefore on the taste buds.

The major determinants of taste loss may be classified in physiological, pathological and iatrogenic causes.

Among the first ones, we include age and gender [59]. Taste modifications in the elderly are mainly related to smell loss and are more conspicuous in men. Infections of the middle ear can partially damage the sense of taste. Normal ageing produces taste loss due to changes in taste cell membranes involving altered function of ion [60] channels and receptors rather than taste-bud loss. In women hormonal changes in pregnancy and menopause may also influence taste perception. Smoking, alcohol and substance abuse may cause taste modification too.

Among the second ones, we count all the oral cavity disorders including oral inflammations, infections, poor oral hygiene, dentures or other palatal prostheses that may impair sour and bitter perception.

Other than smell dysfunction, the most frequent causes of taste dysfunction are prior viral upper respiratory tract infections (URTIs), head trauma and idiopathic causes.

Heartburn or gastric reflux is another common cause of loss of taste. Reflux and regurgitation of gastric acid produce hypogeusia and frequently dysgeusia resulting in the perception of acidic or metallic taste.

Nutritional deficiencies mainly caused by undernutrition, malabsorption, alcoholism and vitamin and mineral deficiencies may lead to taste disturbances.

Table 9.2 Vitamin and mineral deficiencies and oral cavity disorders

Nutrient	Disorder
Vitamin B_{12} or cobalamin	Angular stomatitis
Vitamin B_3 or niacin	Atrophy of lingual papillae
Vitamin C or ascorbic acid	Ulcerations
Vitamin B_2 or riboflavin	Cheilosis
Vitamin B_3 or niacin	Glossitis
Vitamin B_9 or folates	
Vitamin B_{12} or cobalamin	
Vitamin B_2 or riboflavin	Magenta tongue
Vitamin B_1 or thiamin	Taste receptor damage
Vitamin A	Taste receptor damage
Zinc	Hypogeusia/ageusia
Copper	
Nickel	

Nutritional impairment due to chronic renal failure, liver disease including cirrhosis, cancer and acquired immunodeficiency syndrome is a less common cause of taste disturbances (Table 9.2).

Endocrine disorders also are involved in taste disorders. Diabetes mellitus, hypogonadism, Sjögren's syndrome and pseudohypoparathyroidism may decrease taste sensation, while hypothyroidism and adrenal cortical insufficiency may increase taste sensitivity [57].

Taste disorders have been described also in Cushing's syndrome, panhypopituitarism, pseudohypoparathyroidism, Kallmann's syndrome and Turner's syndrome [61].

Neoplasia or lesions associated with taste pathways as oral cavity cancer and malignancies of the head and neck, but also of other sites, are associated with decreased appetite and loss of taste perception as well as radiation treatment of head and neck that damages taste receptors and decreases salivary flow, altering taste perception.

Many other diseases can affect gustation like lichen planus, aglycogeusia, Sjögren syndrome and erythema multiform, as well as direct nerve or CNS damage, as in multiple sclerosis, facial paralysis and thalamic or uncal lesions [58].

Gustatory aura has been reported in epilepsy and migraine headache, and psychiatric conditions such as depression and eating disorders show taste disorders.

Toxic chemical exposure to benzene, benzol, butyl acetate, carbon disulphide, chlorine, ethyl acetate, formaldehyde, hydrogen selenide, paint solvents, sulfuric acid, trichloroethylene and industrial agent exposure to chromium, lead and copper have shown taste alterations.

Among the iatrogenic causes, surgical manipulation on the oral cavity may alter taste decreasing the number of taste buds, but also otologic surgery, stretching or transection of the chorda tympani nerve, may result in temporary dysgeusia.

Bariatric surgery as Roux-en-Y gastric bypass has shown sensory changes in taste in almost three-thirds of the patients investigated [62].

Prescription medications can be responsible for taste loss and should be evaluated in all patients with taste disturbance. Angiotensin-converting enzyme inhibitors may cause hypogeusia and a strongly metallic, bitter or sweet taste [63], while medications like anticholinergics, antidepressants and antihistamines may cause excessive dryness of the oral cavity as common side effects with consequent taste perception alteration [61].

Finally, as reported earlier in the chapter, the taste is influenced by biological factors like genetics and familiarity. Studies have shown that the ability to taste phenylthiourea (bitter) and other compounds with an –N–C= group is an autosomal dominant trait and that phenylthiourea tasters sense saccharin, potassium chloride (KCl) and caffeine as more bitter [58].

Type I familial dysautonomia (i.e. Riley-Day syndrome) causes severe hypogeusia or ageusia because of the absence of taste-bud development. It is a rare hereditary disorder caused by mutations within the gene that encodes for I-к-B kinase complex-associated protein (IKAP) [64], and it occurs more often in subjects of Eastern European Jewish ancestry.

This disorder is characterised by a smooth tongue devoid of fungiform papillae and of taste buds and is clinically associated with poor taste discrimination [65].

Taste disorders, although rare, are usually not considered critical to life and insignificant compared to other specialised senses loss. However, they affect daily living and may cause loss of appetite and poor food choices as well as impaired detection of potential spoiled or contaminated food. Most taste defects are due to smell defects that alter the perception of flavour and should be assessed and treated accordingly. Moreover, some people refer to taste disturbances not as for defects or losses of flavour perception but for distortions or painful sensations such as bad taste, acid, metallic or rancid taste or even burning. This condition known as dysgeusia can increase with age or can be due to drug therapy side effects and lead to major quality of life issues and health risk profiles, including increased or decreased susceptibility to certain diseases.

Treatments of taste dysfunctions are often difficult and slow to achieve benefits or complete symptomatic remission; therefore support is one of the most important aspects of treatment as well as dietary recommendations for improving the overall food experience through optimising food texture, aroma, temperature and colour, when taste is compromised.

Conclusions

The spread of inappropriate eating habits has led to the development of chronic degenerative diseases defined as 'comfort' diseases [41], which raise health issues and increase risk of several conditions such as diabetes mellitus, metabolic syndrome, cardiovascular and pulmonary disorders and cancer. The increasing gap between nutritional science findings and the food choices coincides with the spread of obesity epidemic and other food-related diseases.

Undergoing research will help evaluate and better understand the relationships between taste, palatability and taste receptors in the tongue, in extra-oral sites and in the brain besides their hormonal involvement in taste perception and hedonic responses to food [66].

9.6.1 Questions for the Future

A full understanding of taste sense and flavour perception is central to preventing such diseases that are strongly impacted by how much we like some foods and dislike others regulating their acceptability and modulating their intake.

Deeper comprehension of the role of the receptors for high salt, sour taste and for non-canonical tastes such as fatty acids are awaited [67] as well as molecular understanding of taste plasticity and evaluation of food texture.

Electrophysiological response patterns have been shown to code for taste quality in humans [68], and results that postulate evidence for a link between taste-related decision-making and the predictive value of these brain response patterns are just beginning to be provided.

Future responses on the identification of the extra-oral taste receptor roles [69] may lead to insights into the integration of neuronal activity and metabolism. The expression of a functional sweet taste receptor reported in numerous extragustatory tissues has been proposed to regulate metabolic processes [70]. This newly recognised role offers the opportunity to study this receptor as a potential novel therapeutic target for the treatment of obesity and related metabolic dysfunctions, such as diabetes and hyperlipidemia.

References

1. Small DM, Prescott J (2005) Odor/taste integration and the perception of flavor. Exp Brain Res 166:345–357
2. Chaudhari N, Roper SD (2010) The cell biology of taste. J Cell Biol 190:285–296
3. Besnard P, Passilly-Degrace P, Khan NA (2016) Taste of fat: a sixth taste modality? Physiol Rev 96:151–176
4. Schmidt RL, Lang F, Heckmann M (2011) Physiologie des Menschen: mit Pathophysiologie. Springer, Heidelberg
5. Depoortere I (2014) Taste receptors of the gut: emerging roles in health and disease. Gut 63:179–190
6. Purves DA, George J, Fitzpatrick D, Katz LC, LaMantia A-S, McNamara JO, Williams SM (2001) The organization of the taste system. Neuroscience, 2nd edn. Sinauer Associates, Sunderland
7. Blakeslee AF (1932) Genetics of sensory thresholds: taste for phenyl thio carbamide. Proc Natl Acad Sci U S A 18:120–130
8. Blakeslee AF, Salmon TN (1935) Genetics of sensory thresholds: individual taste reactions for different substances. Proc Natl Acad Sci U S A 21:84–90
9. Bartoshuk LM (1991) Sweetness – history, preference, and genetic-variability. Food Technol Chic 45:108
10. Herbert C, Platte P, Wiemer J, Macht M, Blumenthal TD (2014) Supertaster, super reactive: oral sensitivity for bitter taste modulates emotional approach and avoidance behavior in the affective startle paradigm. Physiol Behav 135:198–207

11. Bartoshuk LM, Duffy VB, Miller IJ (1994) Ptc/prop tasting – anatomy, psychophysics, and sex effects. Physiol Behav 56:1165–1171
12. Miller IJ Jr, Reedy FE Jr (1990) Variations in human taste bud density and taste intensity perception. Physiol Behav 47:1213–1219
13. Essick GK, Chopra A, Guest S, McGlone F (2003) Lingual tactile acuity, taste perception, and the density and diameter of fungiform papillae in female subjects. Physiol Behav 80:289–302
14. Bartoshuk LM (2000) Comparing sensory experiences across individuals: recent psychophysical advances illuminate genetic variation in taste perception. Chem Senses 25:447–460
15. Prutkin J, Fisher EM, Etter L et al (2000) Genetic variation and inferences about perceived taste intensity in mice and men. Physiol Behav 69:161–173
16. Feeney E, O'Brien S, Scannell A, Markey A, Gibney ER (2011) Genetic variation in taste perception: does it have a role in healthy eating? Proc Nutr Soc 70:135–143
17. Kim UK, Jorgenson E, Coon H, Leppert M, Risch N, Drayna D (2003) Positional cloning of the human quantitative trait locus underlying taste sensitivity to phenylthiocarbamide. Science 299:1221–1225
18. Duffy VB (2007) Variation in oral sensation: implications for diet and health. Curr Opin Gastroenterol 23:171–177
19. Eldeghaidy S, Marciani L, McGlone F et al (2011) The cortical response to the oral perception of fat emulsions and the effect of taster status. J Neurophysiol 105:2572–2581
20. Goldstein GL, Daun H, Tepper BJ (2005) Adiposity in middle-aged women is associated with genetic taste blindness to 6-n-propylthiouracil. Obes Res 13:1017–1023
21. Catanzaro D, Chesbro EC, Velkey AJ (2013) Relationship between food preferences and PROP taster status of college students. Appetite 68:124–131
22. Yackinous C, Guinard JX (2001) Relation between PROP taster status and fat perception, touch, and olfaction. Physiol Behav 72:427–437
23. Yackinous CA, Guinard JX (2002) Relation between PROP (6-n-propylthiouracil) taster status, taste anatomy and dietary intake measures for young men and women. Appetite 38:201–209
24. Hedge AM, Sharma A (2008) Genetic sensitivity to 6-n-propylthiouracil (PROP) as a screening tool for obesity and dental caries in children. J Clin Pediatr Dent 33:107–111
25. Keller KL, Tepper BJ (2004) Inherited taste sensitivity to 6-n-propylthiouracil in diet and body weight in children. Obes Res 12:904–912
26. Beauchamp GK, Mennella JA (2009) Early flavor learning and its impact on later feeding behavior. J Pediatr Gastroenterol Nutr 48(Suppl 1):S25–S30
27. Beauchamp GK, Mennella JA (2011) Flavor perception in human infants: development and functional significance. Digestion 83(Suppl 1):1–6
28. Beauchamp GK, Mennella JA (1996) Early feeding and the acquisition of flavor preferences. Nestle Nutr Works Ser 36:163–177
29. Manz F, Manz I (2005) Sinnesentwicklung und Sinnesausprägung beim Föten und Säugling. In: v. Engelhardt D, Wild R. (Hg.): Geschmackskulturen. Vom Dialog der Sinne beim Essen und Trinken, Frankfurt/New York 2005.
30. Tastes differ – how taste preferences develop. Available at http://www.eufic.org/article/en/artid/how-taste-preferences-develop/ Accessed January 2016.
31. Haubrich S (2006) Einfluss von hypoallergener Säuglingsnahrung auf die Entwicklung von Geschmackspräferenzen. Hochschule für Angewandte Wissenschaften Hamburg, Hamburg
32. Mennella JA, Johnson A, Beauchamp GK (1995) Garlic ingestion by pregnant-women alters the odor of amniotic-fluid. Chem Senses 20:207–209
33. Mennella JA, Jagnow CP, Beauchamp GK (2001) Prenatal and postnatal flavor learning by human infants. Pediatrics 107:e88
34. Schaal B, Marlier L, Soussignan R (2000) Human foetuses learn odours from their pregnant mother's diet. Chem Senses 25:729–737
35. Mela D (2001) Development and acquisition of food likes. In: Frewer LJ, Risvik E, Schifferstein H (eds) A European perspective of consumers' food choices. Springer, Berlin, pp 9–21
36. Keskitalo K, Knaapila A, Kallela M et al (2007) Sweet taste preferences are partly genetically determined: identification of a trait locus on chromosome 16. Am J Clin Nutr 86:55–63

37. Keskitalo K, Tuorila H, Spector TD et al (2007) Same genetic components underlie different measures of sweet taste preference. Am J Clin Nutr 86:1663–1669
38. Mennella JA, Griffin CE, Beauchamp GK (2004) Flavor programming during infancy. Pediatrics 113:840–845
39. Haller R, Rummel C, Henneberg S, Pollmer U, Koster EP (1999) The influence of early experience with vanillin on food preference later in life. Chem Senses 24:465–467
40. Mennella JA, Pepino MY, Reed DR (2005) Genetic and environmental determinants of bitter perception and sweet preferences. Pediatrics 115:e216–e222
41. Allegri C, Turconi G, Cena H (2011) Dietary attitudes and diseases of comfort. Eat Weight Disord-St 16:E226–E235
42. Furst T, Connors M, Bisogni CA, Sobal J, Falk LW (1996) Food choice: a conceptual model of the process. Appetite 26:247–265
43. Bellisari A (2008) Evolutionary origins of obesity. Obes Rev 9:165–180
44. Hanson MD, Chen E (2007) Socioeconomic status and health behaviors in adolescence: a review of the literature. J Behav Med 30:263–285
45. Reed DR, Tanaka T, McDaniel AH (2006) Diverse tastes: genetics of sweet and bitter perception. Physiol Behav 88:215–226
46. Birch LL, Fisher JA (1995) Appetite and eating behavior in children. Pediatr Clin N Am 42:931–953
47. Yeomans MR (2012) Flavour-nutrient learning in humans: an elusive phenomenon? Physiol Behav 106:345–355
48. de Wild VW, de Graaf C, Jager G (2013) Effectiveness of flavour nutrient learning and mere exposure as mechanisms to increase toddler's intake and preference for green vegetables. Appetite 64:89–96
49. Keller KL (2014) The use of repeated exposure and associative conditioning to increase vegetable acceptance in children: explaining the variability across studies. J Acad Nutr Diet 114:1169–1173
50. Capaldi-Phillips ED, Wadhera D (2014) Associative conditioning can increase liking for and consumption of brussels sprouts in children aged 3 to 5 years. J Acad Nutr Diet 114:1236–1241
51. Decastro JM (1994) Family and friends produce greater social facilitation of food-intake than other companions. Physiol Behav 56:445–455
52. Popkin BM (2001) Nutrition in transition: the changing global nutrition challenge. Asia Pac J Clin Nutr 10(Suppl):S13–S18
53. Popkin BM (2001) The nutrition transition and obesity in the developing world. J Nutr 131:871S–873S
54. Drewnowski A, Kawachi I (2015) Diets and health: how food decisions are shaped by biology, economics, geography, and social interactions. Big Data 3:193–197
55. Oftedal KN, Tepper BJ (2013) Influence of the PROP bitter taste phenotype and eating attitudes on energy intake and weight status in pre-adolescents: a 6-year follow-up study. Physiol Behav 118:103–111
56. Keskitalo K, Tuorila H, Spector TD et al (2008) The three-factor eating questionnaire, body mass index, and responses to sweet and salty fatty foods: a twin study of genetic and environmental associations. Am J Clin Nutr 88:263–271
57. What the numbers mean: an epidemiological perspective on taste and smell. Availble at http://www.nidcd.nih.gov/health/statistics/smelltaste/Pages/smelltastenumbers.aspx Accessed January 2016
58. Cullen MM, Leopold DA (1999) Disorders of smell and taste. Med Clin N Am 83:57
59. Schiffman SS (1997) Taste and smell losses in normal aging and disease. JAMA-J Am Med Assoc 278:1357–1362
60. Boesveldt S, Lindau ST, McClintock MK, Hummel T, Lundstrom JN (2011) Gustatory and olfactory dysfunction in older adults: a national probability study. Rhinology 49:324–330
61. Bromley SM (2000) Smell and taste disorders: a primary care approach. Am Fam Physician 61:427–436

62. Graham L, Murty G, Bowrey DJ (2014) Taste, smell and appetite change after Roux-en-Y gastric bypass surgery. Obes Surg 24:1463–1468
63. Ackerman BH, Kasbekar N (1997) Disturbances of taste and smell induced by drugs. Pharmacotherapy 17:482–496
64. Norcliffe-Kaufmann L, Kaufmann H (2012) Familial dysautonomia (Riley-Day syndrome): when baroreceptor feedback fails. Auton Neurosci Basic Clin 172:26–30
65. Tokita N, Sekhar HK, Sachs M, Daly JF (1978) Familial dysautonomia (Riley-Day syndrome). Temporal bone findings and otolaryngological manifestations. Ann Otol Rhinol Laryngol Suppl 87:1–12
66. Calvo SS, Egan JM (2015) The endocrinology of taste receptors. Nat Rev Endocrinol 11:213–227
67. Liman ER, Zhang YV, Montell C (2014) Peripheral coding of taste. Neuron 81:984–1000
68. Crouzet SM, Busch NA, Ohla K (2015) Taste quality decoding parallels taste sensations. Curr Biol: CB 25:890–896
69. Behrens M, Meyerhof W (2010) Oral and extraoral bitter taste receptors. Results Probl Cell Differ 52:87–99
70. Laffitte A, Neiers F, Briand L (2014) Functional roles of the sweet taste receptor in oral and extraoral tissues. Curr Opin Clin Nutr Metab Care 17:379–385

From Food Map to FODMAP in Irritable Bowel Syndrome

10

Pasquale Mansueto, Aurelio Seidita, Alberto D'Alcamo, and Antonio Carroccio

10.1 Introduction

Irritable bowel syndrome (IBS) is one of the most common gastrointestinal diseases in the general population, with a prevalence ranging from 12 % to 30 %, mainly affecting younger patients (i.e., <50 years of age) and women [1]. As in other chronic functional gastrointestinal disorders, abdominal discomfort or pain, abnormal bowel habits, and often bloating and abdominal distension are the main clinical features. Their diagnosis is based on symptom patterns (i.e., the Rome III criteria), which also allow categorization in diarrhea-predominant (D-IBS), constipation-predominant (C-IBS), mixed diarrhea and constipation (M-IBS), and unclassified (U-IBS) IBS [2]. Symptom severity ranges from tolerable to severe, both between different patients and in the same patient, affecting patients' quality of life considerably as in some major chronic diseases [3]. Depending on whether diarrhea or constipation is the predominant disorder, antispasmodics, antidepressants, and medications modifying bowel habit represent the main conventional IBS treatments. Unfortunately, most patients report long-term inadequacy of current drug therapy and a tendency to seek a variety of alternative remedies, especially of a dietary nature (up to 65 % of them attribute their symptoms to adverse food reactions) [4]. However, the relationship between IBS symptoms and diet is still controversial,

P. Mansueto • A. Seidita • A. D'Alcamo
Biomedical Department of Internal Medicine and Specialities,
DiBiMIS University of Palermo, Palermo, Italy

A. Carroccio (✉)
Biomedical Department of Internal Medicine and Specialities,
DiBiMIS University of Palermo, Palermo, Italy

Internal Medicine, Giovanni Paolo II Hospital (ASP Agrigento), Sciacca, Italy

Palermo University, Palermo, Italy
e-mail: antonio.carroccio@unipa.it; acarroccio@hotmail.com

© Springer International Publishing Switzerland 2016
E. Grossi, F. Pace (eds.), *Human Nutrition from the Gastroenterologist's Perspective*,
DOI 10.1007/978-3-319-30361-1_10

because of research quality and low number of scientific studies [5]. This represents a glaring gap that needs to be addressed.

10.2   IBS Pathogenesis

Development and maintenance of IBS symptoms has been attributed to multiple factors, such as altered small bowel and/or colonic motility (slow, fast, or uncoordinated), visceral hypersensitivity ("visceral hyperalgesia"), imbalance in neurotransmitters, genetic factors, infections, inflammation, and psychological dysfunction [6].

A correlation between IBS and the microorganisms that reside in physiological or pathological conditions in the gut has been stressed in some subgroups. In particular, small intestinal bacterial overgrowth (SIBO) could be responsible for increased fermentation and gas production in the small intestine, leading to symptoms [7]. To date authors do not agree on the possible pathogenic mechanisms of postinfectious IBS, but the evidence of persistent low-grade mucosal inflammation in some patients could explain how enteric infections affect gut physiology [8].

Similar histological abnormalities have also been found in colon mucosal biopsies of patients with IBS who did not describe any preexisting acute infectious gastroenteritis, suggesting a more general "inflammatory hypothesis" for IBS [9]. Increased numbers of jejunum and terminal ileal mucosa mast cells – a clue for a role for food allergy in an IBS subgroup [10], eosinophils [10], T lymphocytes (T helper [T_H]2 and T_H17) [11], B lymphocytes, and plasma cells [12] – characterize this inflammation. This composite infiltrate interacts with the intestinal nerve plexus and nociceptive structures [13]. Further evidence of the inflammatory theory of IBS lies in the increased IgE, tryptase, eosinophil cationic protein, and eosinophil protein X fecal levels [14]. Either exogenous factors, including food antigens and changes in the resident microbial flora, or endogenous chemical irritants, such as bile salts, might be responsible for mucosal inflammation and local activation of the immune system. In particular, mucosal immune cell activation results in changes in the function of submucosal and myenteric neurons, linking these two effector systems in the genesis of gastrointestinal function disorders [15].

These pathogenic hypotheses might apparently conflict with the classical one that IBS represents a disturbance of the "brain-gut axis." In this context female gender, family history of IBS, history of physical or sexual abuse, and comorbid psychiatric disorders are strong IBS risk factors [16]. Some studies sustain that either stressful early life events or psychiatric comorbidity or both mediate low-level inflammation as well as lymphocytes and mast cell infiltration of the bowel. Thus, an increasing number of researchers promote the idea of a three-way relationship between IBS, mood disturbance, and immune dysregulation [17].

10.3   The Facts: Diet in IBS Patients

Most IBS patients assign a significant role to diet in their symptom onset or persistence, and over 60 % of them would like to know what kind of foods should be avoided [5, 6]. Unfortunately, only 1–3 % of them are diagnosed as suffering from food allergy using current medical methods. The discrepancy between self-perception and diagnostic tools is a major source of frustration both for patients and health care professionals, who are unable to provide reliable answers and support [18]. Several studies agree that 60 % of IBS patients experience worse symptoms following food ingestion, 28 % within 15 min after eating, and 93 % within 3 h. The most common foods singled out are wheat products (pasta, bread, pizza), cow's milk and milk-derived products, tomato, eggs, certain meats, fish/shellfish, cabbage, peas/beans, onion, hot spices, garlic, apple, peach, citrus, fried food, smoked products, fats, food additives, nuts, hazelnuts, chocolate, alcohol, and caffeine [14, 19].

Böhn et al. examined a cohort of 197 adult IBS patients with food allergy/intolerance, IBS symptoms, somatic symptoms, depression and general anxiety, and gastrointestinal-specific anxiety, using quality of life questionnaires. Eighty-four percent of subjects reported symptoms related to at least one food, and over 70 % noted symptoms after intake of food items with incompletely absorbed carbohydrates (i.e., fermentable oligo-, di-, and monosaccharides and polyols, FODMAPs) such as dairy products, beans/lentils, apple, flour, and plum. Noteworthy, self-reported food intolerance was associated with reduced quality of life (sleep, physical status, and social interactions) [20]. A Norwegian population-based cross-sectional study reported that 70 % of IBS subjects perceived a food intolerance (mean 4.8 food items), 62 % limited or excluded foods from their diet (mean 2.5 food items), and 12 % drastically modified daily intake causing nutritional deficiencies in the long run [21]. Data emerging from many studies is the lower consumption of spaghetti, pasta, couscous, and rice in IBS than in controls. The first three products are made using durum wheat, which tends to be high in gluten and FODMAPs, while the last tends to be low [22]. Similarly, lactose is considered one of the main causes of IBS symptoms. Therefore, these patients have a lower consumption of milk and other dairy products often self-inducing important nutritional deficits. Furthermore, IBS patients have been reported to have a significantly lower intake of retinol (vitamin A) equivalent, β-carotene, and magnesium, due to a lower consumption of certain vegetables (tomatoes, raw vegetables, etc.). Controversially, they report a higher consumption of pears, peach, grapes, melon, mango, and plums, which are rich in FODMAPs and documented as possible trigger factors of symptoms [22].

Finally, 12 % of IBS patients either limit or avoid alcohol intake due to self-reported intolerance [19].

In conclusion, IBS patients try to avoid certain food items rich in gluten and FODMAPs, even though the higher consumption of some FODMAP-rich fruits and vegetables remains questionable. The total calories, carbohydrates, proteins, and fat intake does not seem to differ from the general population, but such dietary restrictions could be responsible for their low calcium, phosphorus, vitamin B2, and vitamin A intake.

10.4   A Possible Role for Food Allergy and Intolerance

The large amount of evidence on dietary components causing IBS symptoms has not clarified the possible pathogenic mechanisms underlying this relationship. Physicians have suggested a possible role for food allergy or food intolerance.

"Food allergy" (or sensitivity or hypersensitivity) is defined as "reproducible adverse reaction arising from specific immune responses occurring on exposure to specific food antigens." Whenever similar reactions occur without evidence of immunological mechanisms, they are named "food intolerance" [23].

The role of IgE-mediated and non-IgE-mediated allergic response in IBS has been studied for a long time, producing only conflicting data and no consistent evidence. The first studies evaluated that possible association are from the mid-1980s, but several have been conducted more recently [5, 24]. The results of these recent studies are reported in Tables 10.1 and 10.2. Authors mainly focused on the conventional methods (total serum IgE test, skin prick test (SPT), radioallergosorbent test (RAST), search for IgE fragment crystallizable (FC) in fecal extracts, elimination diets, and rechallenges) to diagnose IgE-mediated allergies in patients reporting IBS-like symptoms [5, 25]. The main discrepancy found in these studies is between self-perceived food intolerance and the positive results of diagnostic tests [25]. Two hypotheses were proposed to explain these results: (1) low serum-specific IgE levels and (2) inadequate allergenic preparations used for SPT and ImmunoCAP. These hypotheses would explain the low prevalence of wheat IgE-mediated enteropathy, including food allergy in IBS patients [26].

Inadequacy of the conventional methods (SPT and serum food allergen-specific IgE levels) to identify IgE-mediated responses in IBS patients led us to evaluate the efficacy of flow cytometric cellular allergen stimulation test (FLOW-CAST) in the diagnosis of food allergy in 120 consecutive IBS patients [27]. We concluded that this diagnostic test might supplement or better replace routine allergy tests [27].

The substantial lack of agreement on the role of typical IgE-mediated allergic reactions in IBS pathogenesis has led physicians to explore alternative hypotheses. In particular, hypersensitivity reactions induced by a different antibody class (i.e., IgG) seem to be of some importance (Table 10.3).

10.4.1 IBS and Food Intolerance

Other physicians instead focused nonimmunologic responses to food antigens (i.e., food intolerances), but questionable outcomes have been seen both due to issues surrounding diagnostic tools and difficulties in projecting well-designed dietary trials. Triggers for symptom onset or worsening have been historically identified in caffeine, alcohol, fiber, and fats, although strong evidence is conflicting in some and lacking in most. Correct identification of symptom-inducing foods is difficult to achieve both because meals are complex mixtures of dietary components and the timing of symptom onset can vary, both with different foods and with the same food in different patients [19]. However, most evidence identifies foods as the triggering factors of symptom onset rather than as a cause of the condition [28].

The role of dietary components in inducing IBS symptoms has been better explored, with some studies reporting how certain food components can contribute to causing carbohydrate malabsorption [28, 29]. In the last decade, several authors have approached the study and management of suspected food intolerance in IBS,

Table 10.1 Systemic IgE-mediated allergic response in IBS patients

Authors	Year of publication	Populations	Techniques	Results
Petitpierre M et al.	1985	24 IBS patients, 12 atopic and 12 nonatopic	Total serum IgE test, SPT and RAST to various food antigens, 3-week-long low-allergenic diet followed by open challenge, blind dietary provocation test	Fourteen patients identified one or more foods and food additives able to evoke typical IBS symptoms. Nine of these, all from the atopy group, had elevated total serum IgE and positive SPT, suggesting a systemic IgE-mediated food allergy
Zwetchkenbaum J et al.	1988	10 IBS patients with atopy	SPT and open elimination diet	A significant cutaneous reaction was found in 6, whose symptoms improved on elimination diet. Subsequent rechallenge with the offending food allergens failed to produce IBS symptoms
Barau E et al.	1990	Seventeen children with clinical IBS symptoms	Urinary elimination of lactulose and mannitol in fasting condition then after specific food ingestion (selected on a suggestive clinical history or positive SPT or RAST)	Nine had modification of intestinal permeability; all had a personal and/or family history of allergy and/or high total IgE and responded to food exclusion
André et al	1995	312 food allergy patients diagnosed on history, positive SPT and RAST. 95 healthy subjects	Search of IgE FC in fecal extracts	236/312 food allergy patients (73 %) found positive, whereas none of 95 controls were positive. Subgroup analysis showed that 32/312 patients satisfied IBS criteria; 22 of them (68.8 %) were found to have detectable IgE FC in feces
Bischoff SC et al.	1996	375 adult patients of a gastroenterology outpatient clinic	Preliminary selection by clinical signs of atopic disease, elevated IgE (total and/or specific against food antigens), eosinophilia, and responsiveness to DSCG therapy. Confirmation test by endoscopic allergen provocation and/or elimination diet and rechallenge	32 % of subjects complained of abdominal symptoms as a consequence of an adverse food reaction. 14.4 % of them were suspected of suffering from a food allergy. 3.2 % were confirmed as suffering from food allergy

(continued)

Table 10.1 (continued)

Authors	Year of publication	Populations	Techniques	Results
Dainese R et al.	1999	128 consecutive IBS patients	SPT for foods	80/128 (62.5 %) patients self-reported adverse reactions to foods. SPTs were positive in 67/128 patients (52.3 %). Significant differences were proven between the reported foods and sensitization tests
Soares RL et al.	2004	43 subjects divided in group I (IBS), group II (functional dyspepsia), and group III (healthy controls)	SPT for 9 food allergens	SPT was positive in 19.4 % of group I, 2.3 % of group II, and 4 % of group III, with significant differences between group I and the others. However, none of the volunteers with IBS reported intolerance to any isolated food
Jun DW et al.	2006	105 subjects divided in 3 different groups: IBS treated group, IBS untreated group, and control group	SPT for foods and inhalant allergens	SPT was positive in 38.6 % of treated IBS patients, 16.1 % of untreated IBS patients and 3.3 % of controls ($p < 0.01$). The more frequently identified foods were saury, rice, mackerel, buckwheat, sweet potatoes, celery, onions, and trumpet shell; on the contrary, patients reported to be intolerant to dairy products, raw foods, spicy foods, coffee, and alcohol
				Thus, no correlation could be proven between patients' intolerance and SPT results
Uz E et al.	2007	53 C-IBS, 19 D-IBS, and 28 M-IBS and 25 healthy controls	Total IgE, SPT for 11 common allergens, and ECP and eosinophil counts	SPT positivity, mean IgE and ECP levels were higher in patients than in controls, but there was no statistically significant difference among IBS subgroup. Foods rich in dietary fibers, gas-producing agents, or foods containing significant amounts of carbohydrates were the main responsible for SPT positivity

C-IBS constipation-predominant IBS, D-IBS diarrhea-predominant IBS, DSCG disodium cromolyn glycate, ECP eosinophil cationic protein, IBS irritable bowel syndrome, FC fragment crystallizable, M-IBS mixed diarrhea and constipation IBS, RAST radioallergosorbent test, SPT skin prick test

Table 10.2 Local IgE-mediated allergic response in IBS patients

Authors	Year of publication	Populations	Techniques	Results
Santos J et al.	1999	8 patients with food allergy and 7 healthy volunteers	Jejunal food challenge. Closed-segment perfusion technique was used to investigate the effects on luminal release of tryptase, histamine, prostaglandin D(2), eosinophil cationic protein, peroxidase activity, and water flux	A rapid increase in intestinal release of tryptase, histamine, prostaglandin D(2), and peroxidase activity was found, whereas no increase of eosinophil cationic protein could be detected. Release of these mediators notably increase water secretory response
Arslan G et al.	2002	20 patients (7 patients with food allergy and 13 with food intolerance)	Duodenal mucosa challenge with allergen extracts via a nasoduodenal tube. Endosonography was used to identify the response	Increased mucosal thickness was found in 11 patients, but no significant difference was found between the allergic and the intolerance group
Arslan G et al.	2005	32 patients with chronic abdominal complaints self-attributed to food hypersensitivity/allergy	Duodenal mucosa challenge with allergen extracts via a nasoduodenal tube. External ultrasound was used to identify the response	14 (44 %) of the 32 patients had a sonographic response (increased wall thickness, diameter, peristalsis, and/or luminal fluid) after challenge. A positive sonographic response was significantly related to a positive SPT and DBPCFC
Coëffier M et al.	2005	25 patients with food allergy and 14 control patients	Analysis by real-time RT-PCR of the levels of epsilonGT, IL-4, IL-13, IFN-gamma, IL-4Ralpha, STAT6 and FcepsilonRIalpha mRNA on cecum biopsies	EpsilonGT and IL-4 expression were increased in food allergy patients, whereas IL-13, IFN-gamma, IL-4Ralpha, STAT6 and FcepsilonRIalpha were not altered
Lidén M et al.	2008	21 patients with primary Sjögren's syndrome and 18 healthy controls	Rectal challenge with CMP using the mucosal patch technique to measure nitric oxide production and myeloperoxidase release	A post-challenge inflammatory response was identified in 38 % of patients as a sign of CMP sensitivity not linked to serum IgE or IgG/IgA antibodies to milk proteins. All CMP-sensitive patients suffered from IBS, diagnosed according to Rome III criteria

CMP cow's milk proteins, *DBPCFC* double-blind placebo-controlled food challenge, *IBS* irritable bowel syndrome, *IL* interleukin, *RT-PCR* real-time polymerase chain reaction, *SPT* skin prick test

Table 10.3 Non-IgE-mediated allergic response in IBS patients

Authors	Year of publication	Populations	Techniques	Results
El Rafei A et al.	1989	25 patients with suspected food allergy	DBPCFC, specific IgG4 and IgE levels dosage	Increased serum IgG4 or IgE levels were found in 63 % of patients with a positive history of food allergy. IgG4 or IgE increased in 91 % DBPCFC-positive patients
Niec AM et al.	1998	7 clinical trials	Meta-analysis	15–71 % response rate to exclusion diet; the most commonly incriminated foods were milk, wheat, eggs, potatoes, and celery. All studies suffered from limitations in their trial designs
Atkinson W et al.	2004	150 IBS patients	Patients received either an elimination diet based on IgG positivity or a sham diet for 12 weeks, excluding the same number of foods but not those to which they had antibodies	IBS symptom severity score showed a 10 % greater reduction in the IgG-based elimination diet. Patients with a greater number of sensitivities, as determined by the IgG test, reported a greater reduction in symptoms
Zar S et al.	2005	25 IBS patients	Analysis of food-specific IgG4 antibody-guided exclusion diet on symptoms and rectal compliance	Patients reported significant improvement in pain severity and frequency, bloating severity, satisfaction with bowel habits, and overall quality of life. Rectal compliance increased significantly, but the thresholds for urge to defecate/ discomfort were unchanged
Zar S et al.	2005	108 IBS patients (52 D-IBS, 32 C-IBS, and 24 M-IBS) and 43 controls	SPT, IgG4, and IgE against common food antigens	IgG4 titers to wheat, beef, pork, and lamb were significantly higher in IBS patients than controls. In addition, IgE titers had no significant difference between the groups, and SPT was positive for only a single antigen in 5 of 56 patients. Authors concluded that no correlation could be found between the IgG4 antibody elevation and patients' symptoms
Drisko J et al.	2006	20 IBS patients	Response to food-specific IgG-based elimination diet	All patients reported significant improvement in symptoms, stool frequency, and quality of life

Zuo XL et al.	2007	37 IBS patients and 20 controls	Serum IgG and IgE antibody titers to 14 common foods	Higher titers for some food-specific IgG antibodies (crab, egg, shrimp, soybean, and wheat) were found in IBS patients, but there was no significant correlation between symptom severity and IgG antibody titers
Guo H et al.	2012	77 D-IBS patients and 26 controls	Preliminary dosage of food-specific IgG, followed by a 12-week IgG-based elimination diet	39 (50.65 %) patients with D-IBS compared with four (15.38 %) controls were positive to food-specific IgG. All symptom scores decreased after elimination diet
Ligaarden SC et al.	2012	269 subjects with IBS and 277 control subjects	Food- and yeast-specific IgG and IgG4 antibodies	After correction for subject characteristics and diet, no significant differences of food-specific IgG and IgG4 antibody levels were found between groups
Aydınlar EI et al.	2013	21 patients with migraine and IBS	Preliminary IgG antibody tests against 270 food allergens. Evaluation of patients at baseline (usual diet), after a first diet (elimination or provocation diets), and after a second diet (interchange of elimination or provocation diets)	Food elimination based on IgG antibodies effectively reduced symptoms with a positive impact on the quality of life

C-IBS constipation-predominant IBS, *DBPCFC* double-blind placebo-controlled food challenge, *D-IBS* diarrhea-predominant IBS, *IBS* irritable bowel syndrome, *M-IBS* mixed diarrhea and constipation IBS, *SPT* skin prick test looking at FODMAPs with increasing interest, focusing on the effects of a low FODMAP diet [28, 30–34]. More recently, a new clinical entity – non-celiac gluten sensitivity (NCGS) – has burst into this complex "world," and it has been suggested that it may be important in a subgroup of IBS patients [35–37], although contradictory data seem to deny the role of a gluten-free diet in the treatment of these patients [38].

10.5   What Are FODMAPs?

Several studies have explored the changes in dietary composition during the last few decades, in particular how it could have been modified by urbanization. Reports conflict about whether sugar intake has increased, but agree on the same focus point: the proportion of sugar intake made up of fructose is increasing. In this context, the intakes of fruit juices as well as the use of high-fructose corn syrup (which contains 42–55 % fructose) as sweeteners in many manufactured foods seem to play the leading role [39]. However, no direct studies of time trends in fructan ingestion are available, but indirect evidence indicates changes in their consumption patterns. Pasta and pizza intake, major sources of fructans, has increased exponentially, and at the same time, the type of fructans in the diet is changing. Similarly, even if no direct data is available about intake of polyols, it is likely that their use as food additives to produce "sugar-free" products has led to increased consumption [39].

Poorly absorbed, short-chain carbohydrates and polyols (lactose, fructose, and sorbitol) were tested throughout the 1980s and 1990s (especially observational cohort studies), to identify their role as symptom inducer in functional bowel disorders and IBS. Authors agree they act in a dose-dependent manner and that a dietary restriction of all three together could bring symptomatic relief [30, 31, 34]. However, international literature about the biochemistry and physiology of digestion denotes how other carbohydrates are involved in IBS-like symptom onset. Fructo-oligosaccharides (fructans or FOS) and galacto-oligosaccharides (galactans or GOS) are short-chain carbohydrates incompletely absorbed in the human gastrointestinal tract. In particular, patients report worsening of symptoms whenever these sugars are consumed in combination (e.g., lactose with fructans, fructose with sorbitol, etc.), indicating their additive effects [33, 40]. Other potential culprits seem to be incompletely absorbed polyols, i.e., mannitol, maltitol, and xylitol, used as artificial sweeteners, but also found naturally in foods [41]. In 2005, a team of Australian researchers theorized that foods containing these poorly absorbed, short-chain carbohydrates worsen the symptoms of some digestive disorders and coined the acronym FODMAPs, grouping them all together according to their chain length [42]. Characteristics shared by all these short-chain highly osmotic carbohydrates are the poor absorption in the small intestine and the rapid fermentation by gut bacteria. These specific features are responsible for increased gas production, bowel distension, bloating, cramping, and diarrhea – all symptoms of IBS, triggered in association with intrinsic visceral hypersensitivity [43].

FODMAP intake varies across ethnic and dietary groups due to different dietary behavior. Fructose and fructans are most widespread in the North American and Western European diets; therefore, they should be considered the ones to which nearly all patients with IBS are exposed in their everyday diet.

10.6   Possible Mechanisms of FODMAP Triggering of IBS Symptoms

How FODMAPs exert their effects on IBS patients is still uncertain, but some researchers are studying the matter. The poor absorbability of FODMAPs in the small intestine has been considered a possible starting point, as shown using an ileostomy model. Carbohydrates increase water content in the output from the stoma, mainly because of an osmotic effect. This effect could easily explain diarrhea in some individuals [29]. Undseth et al. used magnetic resonance imaging to study the osmotic effect of FODMAPs by the analysis of small bowel water content (SBWC). Fructose, lactulose, inulin, or mannitol meals but not a glucose meal increase water content in patients suffering from D-IBS but not in healthy volunteers [44].

Other authors focused on gas production after FODMAP fermentation in the gut. Ong et al. designed a single-blind, crossover, short-term, interventional study to assess gas production during low and high FODMAP diets in IBS patients and healthy volunteers. The high FODMAP diet produced higher levels of breath hydrogen in both groups; interestingly, IBS patients were found to have higher levels during each dietary period than the controls. The latter reported just increased flatus production on a high FODMAP diet, whereas IBS patients complained of rapid onset of gastrointestinal symptoms and lethargy. Conversely on a low FODMAP diet, breath hydrogen production (and consequently symptom score in IBS patients) was reduced both in healthy volunteers and in patients. This study confirms the additive bacterial fermentative nature of the short-chain carbohydrates (with production of short-chain fatty acids [SCFA], including butyrate, and gases such as carbon dioxide, hydrogen, and in some people methane) and their role in causing gastrointestinal symptoms [33]. In the context of bacterial fermentation, Brighentini et al. found that the speed of hydrogen production is inversely proportional to FODMAP chain length [45], and Clausen et al. indicated the fermentative rather than osmotic effect of short-chain carbohydrates after entering the colon [46].

Another research line points to FODMAP effects on gastrointestinal motility [47]. To assess such effects on gastrointestinal motility, Madsen et al. evaluated 11 healthy volunteers in a double-blind crossover investigation. The subjects ingested a glucose solution or a mixture of fructose and sorbitol, in random order, marked with (99m) Tc-diethylenetriaminepentaacetic acid. The mouth-to-cecum transit of the radiolabeled marker was faster, and the percentage content of the marker in the colon was higher after ingestion of the fructose-sorbitol mixture than after ingestion of glucose [48]. Both the osmotic effect of FODMAPs and a contemporary activation of neural feedback pathways and/or hormonal changes from SCFA production, secondary to FODMAP bacterial fermentation, might be responsible for this increased gut motility [49].

In addition, in animal models (rats), fructo-oligosaccharides were responsible for injury of the colonic epithelium and increased intestinal permeability [50].

FODMAP ingestion effects go beyond the gastrointestinal tract, being responsible for systemic effects. Mild depression has been reported in women with IBS, after fructose and lactose intake [51], improving when free fructose is eliminated from the diet.

FODMAPs also affect the intestinal flora of these patients. Patients with IBS have fewer *Lactobacillus* spp. and *Bifidobacterium* spp. in their intestinal flora than healthy individuals. These bacteria bind to epithelial cells, inhibit pathogen adhesion, and enhance barrier function; in addition, they do not produce gas upon fermenting carbohydrates, an effect which is amplified as they also inhibit *Clostridium* spp. growth. Bacteria such as *Clostridium* spp. break down FODMAPs, induce gas production, and cause large intestine distension, with abdominal discomfort and pain [52].

All this evidence could lead us to think that all the different carbohydrates making up the large family of FODMAPs have similar physiological effects and therefore should be considered together. That is true only to a limited extent. Although all exert an osmotic effect, this varies according to the molecular weight and rapidity of absorption of the specific carbohydrate. Absorption across the small intestinal wall varies according to the dose and speed of intestinal transit and for fructose the luminal glucose content (glucose facilitates fructose absorption) and individual absorptive capacity via fructose-specific transporters. Thus, fructose and polyols have a greater osmotic effect than fructans and galacto-oligosaccharides, whereas their luminal concentration will fall more distally because of their slow absorption as opposed to no absorption for oligosaccharides. Conversely, oligosaccharides will have greater fermentative effects since they are not absorbed [53].

These hypotheses are consistent with current knowledge of IBS pathogenesis, among which, visceral hypersensitivity is the most important. Gut distention, due to increased gas production and other mechanisms, abnormally stimulates the enteric nervous system, which reacts by altering its motility patterns. The brain analyzes such changes and interprets them as bloating, discomfort, and pain. Dietary components that could stimulate this mechanism should have the following features: (a) poorly absorbed in the proximal small intestine, (b) composed of small molecules (i.e., osmotically active), (c) rapidly fermented by bacteria (potentially they should be fermented both by small intestinal and cecal bacteria, expanding, at the same time, the bacterial population, i.e., a "prebiotic" effect), and (d) associated with hydrogen production. All these seem to describe dietary FODMAPs. In others words, to better highlight an abovementioned concept, FODMAPs do not cause IBS [30], but represent possible triggers for symptom onset, and their intake reduction might reduce patient complaints.

10.7   Low FODMAP Diet Benefits for IBS Patients

Diets based on fructose, with or without sorbitol, and lactose restriction, have been used for a long time, in the management of patients suffering from functional gut symptoms and IBS. Unfortunately, conflicting results have been reported in literature [30, 31, 34]. The very limited success of this approach is the probable cause of the slow spread of this kind of diet. Noteworthy, limited FODMAP restriction ignores the evidence that there is potentially a great amount of FODMAPs in the everyday diet, all of which have similar end-effects in the bowel. Recently, authors have embraced the "FODMAP concept" or approach: a global FODMAP restriction should have a far greater and more consistent effect than a limited one. Thus, reduction of the intake of all poorly absorbed short-chain carbohydrates should be more effective in preventing luminal distension (and consequently symptom onset) than merely concentrating on one of these [54].

A research trial designed as a retrospective uncontrolled audit by Shepherd et al. was the first to confirm the role of a low FODMAP diet in managing gastrointestinal complaints. Patients with IBS and fructose malabsorption underwent a low fructose/fructan (and polyol, if the patients noted symptom induction) diet. Seventy-four percent of patients reported abdominal symptom improvement, with a durable efficacy closely related to dietary compliance. However, this study suffers from a significant weakness in its retrospective approach that greatly undermines its reliability, especially in a field where "placebo effect" is particularly widespread [34]. To resolve this issue and prove the efficacy of a low FODMAP diet, the same author designed a randomized, double-blind, placebo-controlled, quadruple arm crossover, rechallenge trial with fructose, fructans, fructose plus fructans, and glucose (as placebo) at varying doses (low, medium, or high). Twenty-five patients with IBS, who had documented fructose malabsorption as well as a previously demonstrated durable (3–36 months) symptomatic response to reduction of dietary FODMAPs, were enrolled in the study. Abdominal symptoms recurred in 70–80 % of patients, in a dose-dependent way, when fed with pure forms of FODMAPs, especially with fructose plus fructans; this proved an additive effect, especially if compared to 15 % complaining of the same abdominal symptoms when fed a similar diet spiked with placebo [28]. Although conducted according to the strictest scientific rules, this study has the weakness of being carried out in a single center in Australia. This specific feature has made other studies necessary to confirm these preliminary observations.

In 2012, Staudacher et al. performed a randomized, controlled, non-blinded trial in 41 United Kingdom patients with IBS. Physicians investigated the effects of fermentable carbohydrate restriction on gastrointestinal symptoms, luminal microbiota, and SCFA. Patients were randomly assigned to intervention diet or habitual diet group for 4 weeks. Patients in the intervention group more frequently reported symptom reduction compared with controls. In addition, even though the total luminal bacteria at follow-up did not differ between groups, when adjusted for baseline, the intervention group had lower concentrations of bifidobacteria. Finally, no difference in total or individual fecal SCFA could be found between groups. Unfortunately, this study also had several other weaknesses: small sample size, use of a "habitual" diet, which varied from patient to patient, the lack of a standardized low FODMAP diet, and differences in patient-provider contact time [40]. In 2014, going back to Australia, a randomized, placebo-controlled, single-blind, crossover study, evaluated the effect of different diets in a group of 30 patients with IBS and 8 healthy individuals. Subjects were randomly assigned to groups receiving 21 days of either a diet low in FODMAPs or a typical Australian diet, followed by a washout period of at least other 21 days, before crossing over to the alternate diet. IBS patients effectively reduced symptoms on the low FODMAP diet. Noteworthy, with no difference in IBS subgroup, patients reported the greatest symptom improvement within the first 7 days. No significant changes were found between diets in healthy controls. Although better designed than prior studies, the crossover design, the use of a "typical" Australian diet, and the small sample size make it difficult to apply the results of this study to all IBS patients [32]. In the same period, Pedersens et al. conducted a randomized, controlled, unblinded trial in 123 IBS patients [55]. Patients underwent one of the following diets for 6 weeks: low in FODMAPs, high *Lactobacillus rhamnosus* GG, and a normal Danish/Western diet. At week 6, a statistically significant reduction in the IBS severity score system was observed in the low FODMAP group and *Lactobacillus rhamnosus* GG group compared to the normal Danish/Western diet group. However, adjusted linear regression analysis showed a statistically significant improvement of IBS severity score in the low FODMAP diet group vs. normal Danish/Western diet group, but not in *Lactobacillus rhamnosus* GG group vs. normal Danish/Western diet group. Finally, quality of life was not significantly altered in any of the three groups. Analysis of IBS subgroups showed the results were significant for the D-IBS and M-IBS subtypes, but not for the C-IBS subtype, in both low FODMAP and *Lactobacillus rhamnosus* GG treatment groups. The unblinded design and absence of both a placebo capsule group and a standardized prepreared low FODMAP diet make it difficult to interpret this study [56].

Other studies comparing effects of a low FODMAP diet to normal diets are reported in Table 10.4.

10.8   Diagnosis of FODMAP "Malabsorption"

The clinical and pathophysiological features of FODMAPs are not yet clear, and the difficulty of establishing a diagnosis of FODMAP malabsorption is even more trying. Usually, after an accurate clinical history, including dietary and lifestyle assessment, with a focus on potential food intolerance, patients undergo clinical investigations in accordance with local/national guidelines. The most frequently required investigations are blood and fecal tests, endoscopy and/or radiological imaging to rule out any organic disease. In the absence of organic disease or food allergy, patients are diagnosed as suffering from a functional gastrointestinal disorder. Unfortunately to date diagnosis of food intolerance in most areas is still impossible, and only a few tests are clinically useful to identify specific food intolerance. Breath hydrogen levels provide a reliable measure of sugar absorption. A significant rise in breath hydrogen following test sugar intake demonstrates poor absorption with subsequent fermentation by intestinal microflora [57]. Positivity to a breath test could allow the identification of carbohydrates responsible of symptom onset and whose exclusion from the diet could reduce intestinal discomfort. In contrast, a

Table 10.4 FODMAP diet comparative studies

Authors	Year of publication	Study design	Populations	Intervention	Results
Staudacher HM et al.	2011	Nonrandomized comparative study	82 consecutive patients with IBS	Standard (i.e., National Institute for Health and Clinical Excellence, NICE, dietary guidelines, which include either use of probiotics or exclusion diets or increasing fiber intake or decreasing fiber intake) versus FODMAP dietary advice	To assess symptom reduction, all the patients compiled specific standardized questionnaires, which pointed out more satisfaction in the low FODMAP group, with significant improvements in bloating, abdominal pain, and flatulence
Chumpitazi BP et al.	2015	Double-blind crossover intervention	35 children with Rome III IBS	Patients were randomized, after a 1-week baseline diet period, to a low FODMAP diet or typical American childhood diet, followed by a 5-day washout period before crossing over to the other diet	Compared to baseline, children had fewer daily abdominal pain episodes on a low FODMAP diet and more episodes on the typical American childhood diet. Children who responded to the low FODMAP diet would have a different microbiome composition and associated microbial metabolic capacity compared to those who did not respond
Ong DK et al.	2010	Single-blind crossover intervention	15 IBS patients and 15 healthy subjects	Low (9 g/day) or high (50 g/day) FODMAP diet for 2 days	In IBS patients, the high FODMAP diet increased gastrointestinal symptoms and lethargy, whereas in healthy volunteers only flatus production increased. Both groups had increased production of breath hydrogen on a high FODMAP diet, but IBS patients had higher levels than the controls. Breath methane did not increase in patients with IBS on the high FODMAP diet, but was reduced in healthy subjects

(continued)

Table 10.4 (continued)

Authors	Year of publication	Study design	Populations	Intervention	Results
De Roest RH et al.	2013	Prospective observational study	90 IBS patients	Dietary advices regarding the low FODMAP diet	All the patients experienced a beneficial effect in symptom control; in particular larger symptomatic improvement was proven in subjects with fructose malabsorption compared to the others
Mazzawi T et al.	2013	Prospective observational study	46 IBS patients	Dietary advices regarding the low FODMAP diet	Patients had to complete 4 questionnaires prior to and 3 months after receiving a dietary interview. IBS symptom score decreased once the patients had received dietary guidance. The total score for quality of life increased significantly after dietary guidance sessions. No statistical differences were pointed out in calories, carbohydrate, fiber, protein, fat, or alcohol intake following the dietary interview. Consumption of certain fruits and vegetables that were rich in FODMAPs, as well as insoluble fibers, decreased
Pedersen N et al.	2014	Prospective observational study	19 IBS patients	Six weeks free diet followed by 6 weeks low FODMAP diet	Patients were asked to record their symptoms on a web application. A significant improvement in disease activity was observed during both the control and low FODMAP diet periods, IBS quality of life changed significantly only during the second
Huamán JW et al.	2015	Prospective observational study	30 IBS patients	Low FODMAP diet for 2 months	At the end of the study period, more than 70 % of patients reported a positive impact of the low FODMAP diet in controlling overall symptoms and specific symptoms, such as functional abdominal bloating, flatulence, abdominal pain, diarrhea, and fatigue. By contrast, constipation was controlled in only 48 % of patients

Author	Year	Study type	Patients	Intervention	Results
Ostgaard H et al.	2012	Retrospective observational study	36 IBS patients, 43 IBS patients who had received dietary guidance 2 years earlier, and 35 healthy controls	Dietary advices versus free diet	IBS patients voluntarily avoided certain foods, some of which belong to FODMAPs, but at the same time, they had a higher consumption of other foods rich in FODMAPs. In addition, they avoided other foods that are crucial for their health. The group of IBS patients who had received dietary advices avoided all FODMAP-rich foods, consumed more foods with probiotic supplements, and did not avoid food sources that were crucial to their health. These patients, compared to unguided IBS patients, had improved quality of life and reduced symptoms
Zubek J et al.	2012	Case series	40 IBS patients who underwent low FODMAP diet	Low FODMAP diet for 4–12 weeks	Patients reported a statistically significant reduction for bloating, abdominal pain, and diarrhea
O'Meara C et al.	2013	Case series	27 symptomatic IBS patients	Instruction on avoidance of dietary FODMAPs and individually tailored nutritional advices	14/27 patients were revalued after receiving dietary advices; 13/14 had satisfactory relief of global IBS symptoms; 10/12 patients reported an improvement in abdominal pain; 13/14 an improvement in bloating; 11/12 an improvement in flatulence; 10/13 an improvement in fecal urgency
MCgeoch V et al.	2014	Case series	80 IBS patients on low FODMAP diet	Low FODMAP diet	46/80 patients were enrolled (other patients did not present at follow-up visit); patients reported a lower incidence of each IBS symptom. The biggest improvements were reported for bloating (93 %) and flatulence (92 %)

(continued)

Table 10.4 (continued)

Authors	Year of publication	Study design	Populations	Intervention	Results
Rao SS et al.	2015	Systematic review	Adult patients with IBS on low FODMAP diet	NA	Authors found only 6 eligible studies on FODMAP-restricted diets, whose heterogeneity and methodological quality did not allow them to perform a meta-analysis. Overall IBS symptoms improved in 4/4 studies, C-IBS symptoms in 1/3 studies, and 3 studies did not meet inclusion criteria
Marsh A et al.	2015	Meta-analysis	Adult patients with IBS on low FODMAP diet	NA	A significant decrease in IBS symptom severity scores and increase in IBS quality of life scores was found for individuals on a low FODMAP diet in RCTs and nonrandomized interventions. In addition, a low FODMAP diet significantly reduced severity of both overall symptoms and specific symptoms such as abdominal pain and bloating in the RCTs. Similar results were pointed out in nonrandomized interventions

C-IBS constipation-predominant IBS, *IBS* irritable bowel syndrome, *RCT* randomized controlled trials negative breath test proves complete absorption of the sugar suggesting that intake of that specific carbohydrate should not influence patient symptoms. Therefore, breath hydrogen testing to define absorption of a fructose and/or lactose load is very useful as it can reduce the extent of the necessary dietary restriction [57]. Routinely, to diagnose FODMAP malabsorption, fructose (testing dose of 35 g), lactose (testing dose of 25–50 g), and sorbitol (testing dose of 10 g) breath tests are performed. Nevertheless, physicians should remember that there are three other FODMAPs (fructans, galactans, and mannitol) acting as potential triggers of IBS symptoms. No specific breath test is available for fructans and galactans, since they are always malabsorbed and fermented, whereas mannitol breath test is rarely performed, as it is not a widespread component in the diet and can be investigated as a trigger through simple dietary elimination and rechallenge [57].

However, breath tests have a moderate degree of false positivity. As an example, IBS patients suffering from SIBO, diagnosed by lactulose breath test, a reliable and noninvasive test for the diagnosis of this condition, might have falsely abnormal breath tests for fructose, lactose, and sorbitol [58].

10.9 Tables of the FODMAP Content of Foods: Strengths and Weaknesses

A number of studies offer more specific knowledge about food composition, in particular, FODMAP content, which allows us to better modify the dietary regimens of IBS patients. The broader range of FODMAPs, including FOS, GOS, and mannitol, in addition to fructose, lactose, and sorbitol, forces us to avoid all these carbohydrates in low FODMAP diets, with elimination of an extended spectrum of foods. Such large restrictions are required to publish tables of food composition on fruits, vegetables, breads, and cereals [59]. The impact of dietary modification of FODMAPs can have on functional gut symptoms should shift the focus to the possibility of simply and accurately assessing FODMAP intake in individuals and specific populations. In this context, administration of food frequency questionnaires (FFQs) is a simple and useful assessment. The Monash University Comprehensive Nutrition Assessment Questionnaire (CNAQ), a 297-item comprehensive, semi-quantitative FFQ, has shown its efficacy in estimating intake of macro- and micronutrients, FODMAPs, and glycemic index/load, in an Australian population. Barret et al. validated this FFQ proving how this tool allows patients to identify a wide range of low FODMAP foods and manage their IBS with less restrictive diets [60].

One of the most important limits to the spread of a low FODMAP diet is the development of tables assessing FODMAP-rich and FODMAP-poor foods. To date, published lists of food composition report only a limited description of FODMAP content. The recent development of FODMAP content measuring methodologies, together with a systematic examination of fruits, vegetables, and cereals, partially overcome this issue. However, the strongest limitation is the absence of a unique and widely approved cutoff level indicating a food as "high" or not in FODMAPs. This is further complicated by the direct relationship between the total amount of

FODMAPs ingested and whether symptoms will be induced or not. Several studies have tried to assess possible cutoff levels to avoid symptom induction [34, 59]. The preliminary results hint that the total dose for therapeutic benefit in IBS population should be less than 0.5 g FODMAPs per sitting or less than 3 g FODMAPs per day. Unfortunately, CNAQ showed that these values are considerably lower than the amount obtainable through a strict diet [34].

10.10   Practical Low FODMAP Diet Management

The efficacy shown by a low FODMAP diet allows its use as a potentially effective treatment option for IBS patients, under the monitoring of an expert dietitian. A preliminary step, because of the variability of response to diet and the possible coexistence of a food allergy, is to identify the predictors of both of these different conditions. Reports of atopic history, symptoms related to mast cell activation, or concurrent systemic manifestations, such as urticaria or asthma, should direct our focus to an IgE-mediated food allergy.

Considering the different nature of each FODMAP, it is not surprising that not all of these carbohydrates will be symptom triggers for all patients. Malabsorbed FODMAPs due to altered gut flora, visceral hypersensitivity, and motility disorders, typical of IBS patients, are the ones most likely to play a major role in inducing symptoms [33]. Noteworthy, fructans and galactans are always malabsorbed and fermented by intestinal microflora. The remaining FODMAPs will induce symptoms only in the proportion of IBS patients that malabsorbs them. In this regard, lactose and fructose malabsorption in white IBS patients is estimated to be 25 % and 45 %, respectively [30]. Finally, polyols are incompletely absorbed, but their low amounts found naturally in foods as well as in sugar-free products and medications is usually well tolerated in most people [30].

Breath tests should be considered useful diagnostic tools helping physicians to implement personalized specific low FODMAP diet, but they cannot be considered mandatory. Where breath tests cannot be performed, a trial of a full low FODMAP diet can be conducted, followed by challenge with each carbohydrate (fructose, lactose, sorbitol, and mannitol) initially avoided. As a final step, small amounts of fructans and galactans may be tested to assess the level of tolerance, even though they are associated with gas-induced symptoms, even in healthy subjects [33].

Nowadays, the low FODMAP diet has been mainly evaluated as a dietician-delivered diet. A one-to-one patient-dietitian setting, together with the use of written educational material and recipe books, has been used, but some group education sessions have been tested with apparent success and cost reduction [61].

Noteworthy, some patients report using instructions and diet sheets by themselves to manage their symptoms. Physicians should be cautious of this approach, discouraging patients to continue without a dietician's consultation, due to the lack of sufficient ad hoc studies and the possible dietary self-induced imbalance. Rao et al. tried to create a systematic approach to patients at the first consultation. (1) Define patient's lifestyle and alimentary behavior. Physicians should address patients with direct questioning and ask them to compile pre-completed food record diaries (for at least a 7-day period). This approach allows the identification of daily FODMAP intake. (2) Explain the scientific basis of FODMAP physiopathology in IBS. Patients must be aware of the role of FODMAPs to increase the likelihood of lasting diet compliance. (3) Provide specific dietary instructions. (4) Discuss techniques to avoid unintentional FODMAP intake. Patients often report great difficulty handling situations where food preparation cannot be controlled. (5) Instruct patients about the need for a strict and long-term diet. Patients sensitive to FODMAPs often observe symptom improvement within the first week of a restricted diet. However, it has been found that there is a clear increase in efficacy over the first 6 weeks, so it is recommended to attempt strict adherence for at least 6–8 weeks. If the diet has shown little efficacy after 8 weeks, it may be discontinued [62].

These preliminary steps allow physicians to assess symptom response on a strict FODMAP diet. Obviously such a limited diet cannot be continued for long; thus, it should be a must to define individual tolerance. Single carbohydrate reintroduction allows this process ensuring maximum variety in the diet, to avoid overrestrictions and reduce the risk of nutritional inadequacy. Rechallenge must be taken separately for each carbohydrate with food as simple as possible to avoid overlaps. Whenever patients report inadequate response to the diet, specific questioning is required to determine the adherence and modify any deficiency. If adherence is indicated, attention should be paid to reduce intake of resistant starch and both insoluble and soluble fiber [43].

Adherence to a low FODMAP diet has been found to be relatively high, in particular after adequate instruction. Unwillingness to undertake dietary recommendations, difficulties accessing and increased expense of wheat-free foods, and dislike of the taste represented the main barriers to adherence [34].

10.11 Limitations and Potential Concerns of the Low FODMAP Diet in IBS Patients

The presented data show that a low FODMAP diet could lead to symptom control in specific subclasses of IBS patients, but it is far from being effective in all of them. Foods represent just the trigger of symptom onset, and since diets do not influence the pathophysiological substrate of IBS, intermittent symptoms remain in many patients, albeit at a tolerable level [32].

Requiring further and better definition is the security of long-term low FODMAP diets; such a restrictive diet is at risk of being nutritionally inadequate. In this context, some preliminary data come from Staudacher et al. who reported that a strict 4-week-long low FODMAP diet reduced total carbohydrate intake, including both total sugars and starches; however, total energy, protein, fat, and non-starch polysaccharide levels did not change. In addition, authors found a reduction of total calcium intake in patients following a restricted diet for more than 4 weeks [40]. However, a restricted low FODMAP diet should not compromise nutritional adequacy, eliminating whole categories of food. Expert dietician consultation is important in food substitution with suitable alternatives from the same food group. The greatest difficulties are with legumes (including chickpeas, baked beans, red kidney beans, and lentils), since these all contain fructans and galactans. Fortunately, in a low FODMAP diet, foods such as seeds, nuts, and quinoa are encouraged, as well as eating legumes in small amounts [43]. As reported by Staudacher et al. [40], reduction in fiber intake might be a consequence of the restriction of wheat-based products, so patients should be advised, as part of dietary counseling, to ensure adequate intake of resistant starch and non-starch polysaccharides. In addition, FODMAPs (particularly oligosaccharides, such as inulin) are prebiotic, increasing growth of bacteria with known health benefits (especially *Bifidobacterium* spp.), and precursors for SCFA production, known to be important for colonic health. Thus, it is likely that a low FODMAP diet would counteract the prebiotic actions of FODMAPs and reduces SCFA production [59]. In this context, 26 IBS patients and 6 healthy subjects were randomly allocated in one of two dietetic regimens differing only in FODMAP content and then crossed over after a washout period. Participants collected a 5-day fecal sample during their habitual diet and after 17 days of a low FODMAP diet and Australian diet. Analysis of stool found greater microbial diversity, reduced total bacterial abundance, higher fecal pH, but similar SCFA concentrations during the low FODMAP diet compared with the Australian diet. Prebiotic bacteria, namely, *Bifidobacterium* spp., concentrations were similar in the two diets, but total bacterial abundance decreased on low FODMAP diet. On the contrary, the Australian diet increased relative abundance of butyrate-producing *Clostridium* cluster XIVa and mucus degrading-associated *Akkermansia muciniphila* and reduced mucus degrading-associated *Ruminococcus torques*. This study indicates that FODMAP reduction is not "antiprebiotic." Noteworthy, even if no reduced prebiotic effect by FODMAPs was found, there was a reduction in total bacterial abundance. The functional and health implications of such changes need further studies, to exclude possible adverse effects in the long term [63]. Hence, it is important to emphasize that patients receiving this dietary restriction should be monitored for long-term effects on health, and more data are needed regarding benefits vs. harms [58].

For all the abovementioned reasons, a strict long-term low FODMAP diet must be discouraged. Reintroduction of FODMAP foods should be instituted as soon as possible after achieving a good symptomatic response. This will allow identification of the cutoff level of food restriction that each patient requires to adequately control symptoms without encountering nutritional imbalances [42].

10.12 IBS and NCGS

Having assessed the role of food as a possible trigger for symptom onset in IBS patients, we must recognize a role of primary importance for wheat, the basis of most popular diets in the Western world [35–37, 64]. Several reasons have been proposed to explain its role as symptom inducer: (1) high fructans content, as member of the family of FODMAPs; (2) autoimmune disorder trigger; and (3) high IgE and non-IgE-mediated allergenicity.

Extending the perspective over the longtime encoded disorders, researchers' attention is shifting to non-celiac gluten sensitivity (NCGS) [65].

The NCGS is a syndrome characterized by intestinal and extraintestinal symptoms related to the ingestion of gluten-containing food, in subjects that are not affected by either celiac disease (CD) or wheat allergy (WA) [37, 64, 65]. In 2013, Biesiekierski et al. tested 37 subjects with IBS, based on Rome III criteria, and NCGS. Authors aimed to investigate if IBS symptoms were related to gluten intake rather than FODMAPs. Participants were randomly assigned to groups given a 2-week gluten-free and reduced FODMAP diet and were then placed on a high-gluten diet (16 g/day), a low-gluten diet (2 g/day), or placebo diet (no gluten), for 1 week. After a washout period of at least 2 weeks, patients were randomized to the second arm and, then, again after a 2-week-long washout period, to the third arm. During the diet challenges, a visual analogue scale was used to assess symptoms. Twenty-two participants then crossed over to groups given gluten or control diets for 3 days. In all participants, gastrointestinal symptoms consistently and significantly improved during reduced FODMAP intake, but significantly worsened when their diets included gluten or whey protein. However, gluten-specific effects were observed in only 8 % of participants, and the worsening of symptoms across dietary arms was thought to be due to stress put on the patients due to the need for frequent clinic visits rather than due to diet differences [38]. According to these results, the authors concluded that NCGS does not exist and that the symptoms in the self-reported gluten-sensitive patients were due to the FODMAP content in the wheat. However, looking at the study's supplemental file, it emerged that among 149 patients initially recruited, only 40 were included in the study, and more than two-thirds of the patients were excluded since they had the DQ2 or the DQ8 alleles or an increase in duodenal mucosa lymphocytes. It is well known that both of these are very frequent characteristics in NCGS patients. By excluding these patients, the Australian colleagues introduced a selection bias, and we suggest that they have studied another kind of NCGS patients, preselecting only those without any immunologic activation [38].

In NCGS, patients complain of IBS-like symptoms, often related to extraintestinal manifestations, which disappear on a gluten-free diet. This evidence, however, has not eliminated all doubts about what is actually responsible for the clinical manifestations of this new disease (gluten or other components of wheat), thus we suggested the term "non-celiac wheat sensitivity" (NCWS) [66]. With a prevalence ranging from 0.55 % to 6 % of the general United States population, NCWS represents an extremely widespread problem [65]. Usually, it affects females (male to female ratio ranging between 1:2.5 and 1:4) [37, 65] in the third-fourth decades of life [37].

Unfortunately, to date physicians have not managed to identify a specific marker for this disease, so it is mainly defined by "negative" criteria: (1) lack of the key CD criteria (e.g., autoimmunity and histology), (2) no evidence of IgE-mediated wheat allergy, and (3) response to wheat elimination diet (implemented in a blinded fashion to avoid a possible placebo/nocebo effect) [64, 67]. Clinical manifestations usually occur soon after wheat ingestion, improving or disappearing (within hours or few days) on gluten elimination diet and relapsing following its reintroduction. Gastrointestinal disorders and systemic manifestations are complexly weaved in NCWS, but they can also occur separately [36, 64]. Gastrointestinal involvement consists of IBS-like symptoms, such as abdominal pain, bloating, and bowel habit abnormalities, whereas systemic manifestations are extremely variable: fatigue, foggy mind, headache, depression, joint and muscle pain, leg or arm numbness, dermatitis (from skin rash to eczema), anemia, and several others [37, 65]. The very frequent presence of extraintestinal symptoms is an important argument to exclude FODMAPs as the cause of NCGS. Furthermore, as a confirmation of a prevalent or exclusive immunologic pathogenesis of NCGS, there is the recent evidence that higher proportions of patients with NCWS develop autoimmune disorders (mainly Hashimoto's thyroiditis), have an elevated frequency of antinuclear antibodies (ANA) in the serum, and showed DQ2/DQ8 haplotypes compared with patients with IBS [68].

In any case, NCWS pathogenesis is still largely undetermined and debated [64]. Proposed pathogenic mechanisms are (1) non IgE-mediated wheat allergy [37, 65], (2) activation of the innate immunity mechanisms by amylase-trypsin inhibitors (ATIs) [65], and (3) gastrointestinal neuromuscular abnormalities induced by the gliadin, leading to smooth muscle hyper-contractility and indirectly to increase in luminal water content [69]. At the current level of knowledge, researchers agree that there is a reasonable overlap between NCWS and IBS, and NCWS and IBS patients might easily crossover.

10.13 Low FODMAP Diet or Gluten-Free Diet in NCWS? This Is the Question

The coexistence of gluten and fructans in wheat has recently raised the question of which of the two evidence-based dietary approaches, gluten-free diet or low FODMAP diet, physicians should advise to IBS patients [59]. A consistent number of patients increasingly recognize an association between gut symptoms and/or fatigue and ingestion of wheat products, such as pasta and bread. An Australian survey of 1,184 IBS adults reported that 8 % avoid wheat or consume a gluten-free diet to relieve their symptoms [70].

Even if a low FODMAP diet, being more restrictive, offers a higher chance of symptomatic response, a gluten-free diet could remove a specific pathogenic factor. To date, no consensus has been reached. A gluten-free diet might be used if the clinic is geared toward an exclusion diet followed by DBPC rechallenge, especially in patients with biomarkers suggesting gluten-related relevant pathogenic events: circulating antibodies to whole gliadin, high in vitro basophil activation, increased fecal eosinophil cationic protein and tryptase, and increased duodenal IEL density (>25/100 enterocytes) with or without eosinophil infiltration. Non-responder subjects should be tested with a low FODMAP diet. Alternatively, a low FODMAP diet might be used as the first approach, and in those with insufficient response, gluten could be removed as the second step. If an adequate response occurs, then non-wheat-based FODMAP intake can be cautiously increased [53].

Conclusion

Emerging evidence argues with increasing insistence for the role of food intolerance in the management of IBS symptoms. Food components should be considered not as etiological elements of IBS, but as symptom triggers. Thus, changes in dietary intake might allow consistent improvement in symptoms and quality of life even if they do not represent a cure and don't influence the pathogenic mechanisms. To date, physicians are focusing on the role of a low FODMAP diet in symptom improvement in many patients suffering from IBS. The increasing evidence for this dietary approach supports the hypothesis that it should be the first dietary modification in patients suffering from IBS. However promising, this dietary approach still leaves many questions unanswered, including the evaluation of possibly significant nutritional concerns. This point must be stressed, and patients should be discouraged from undertaking a low FODMAP diet without adequate support from a dietitian. To further complicate the extended framework of IBS triggers, there are many other food components besides carbohydrates worthy of being studied. Among these, dietary fats might change visceral hypersensitivity, whereas naturally occurring chemicals, widespread in foods, could interact with gut receptors or have direct actions on the enteric nervous system and mast cells. Finally, the role of wheat and gluten in IBS is far from being completely understood, and physicians should always consider the possible use of a sequential dietetic approach (low FODMAP/gluten-free diet).

Funding   This study was supported by a grant from the University of Palermo (project 2012-ATE-0491 – "Gluten-sensitivity e sindrome del colon irritabile").

Conflicts of Interest Statement   None.

References

1. Ford AC, Moayyedi P, Lacy BE, Lembo AJ, Saito YA, Schiller LR et al (2014) Task Force on the Management of Functional Bowel Disorders. American College of Gastroenterology monograph on the management of irritable bowel syndrome and chronic idiopathic constipation. Am J Gastroenterol 109(Suppl 1):S2–S26
2. Rome Foundation (2006) Guidelines – Rome III diagnostic criteria for functional gastrointestinal disorders. J Gastrointest Liver Dis 15:307–312
3. Mönnikes H (2011) Quality of life in patients with irritable bowel syndrome. J Clin Gastroenterol 45(Suppl):S98–S101
4. Spanier JA, Howden CW, Jones MP (2003) A systematic review of alternative therapies in the irritable bowel syndrome. Arch Intern Med 163:265–274
5. Bischoff SC, Mayer JH, Manns MP (2000) Allergy and the gut. Int Arch Allergy Immunol 121:270–283
6. Barbara G, De Giorgio R, Stanghellini V, Cremon C, Salvioli B, Corinaldesi R (2004) New pathophysiological mechanisms in irritable bowel syndrome. Aliment Pharmacol Ther 20(Suppl 2):1–9

7. Grace E, Shaw C, Whelan K, Andreyev HJ (2013) Review article: small intestinal bacterial overgrowth – prevalence, clinical features, current and developing diagnostic tests, and treatment. Aliment Pharmacol Ther 38:674–688
8. Rhodes DY, Wallace M (2006) Post-infectious irritable bowel syndrome. Curr Gastroenterol Rep 8:327–332
9. Camilleri M, Lasch K, Zhou W (2012) Irritable bowel syndrome: methods, mechanisms, and pathophysiology. The confluence of increased permeability, inflammation, and pain in irritable bowel syndrome. Am J Physiol Gastrointest Liver Physiol 303:G775–G785
10. Walker MM, Warwick A, Ung C, Talley NJ (2011) The role of eosinophils and mast cells in intestinal functional disease. Curr Gastroenterol Rep 13:323–330
11. Ortiz-Lucas M, Saz-Peiró P, Sebastián-Domingo JJ (2010) Irritable bowel syndrome immune hypothesis. Part one: the role of lymphocytes and mast cells. Rev Esp Enferm Dig 102:637–647
12. Vicario M, González-Castro AM, Martínez C, Lobo B, Pigrau M, Guilarte M et al (2015) Increased humoral immunity in the jejunum of diarrhoea-predominant irritable bowel syndrome associated with clinical manifestations. Gut 64:1379–1388
13. Barbara G, Stanghellini V, De Giorgio R, Cremon C, Cottrell GS, Santini D et al (2004) Activated mast cells in proximity to colonic nerves correlate with abdominal pain in irritable bowel syndrome. Gastroenterology 126:693–702
14. Carroccio A, Brusca I, Mansueto P, Soresi M, D'Alcamo A, Ambrosiano G et al (2011) Fecal assays detect hypersensitivity to cow's milk protein and gluten in adults with irritable bowel syndrome. Clin Gastroenterol Hepatol 9:965–971
15. Ishihara S, Tada Y, Fukuba N, Oka A, Kusunoki R, Mishima Y et al (2013) Pathogenesis of irritable bowel syndrome – review regarding associated infection and immune activation. Digestion 87:204–211
16. Surdea-Blaga T, Băban A, Dumitrascu DL (2012) Psychosocial determinants of irritable bowel syndrome. World J Gastroenterol 18:616–626
17. Andreasson AN, Jones MP, Walker MM, Talley NJ, Nyhlin H, Agréus L (2013) Prediction pathways for innate immune pathology, IBS, anxiety and depression in a general population (the PopCol study). Brain Behav Immun 32, e46
18. Rona RJ, Keil T, Summers C, Gislason D, Zuidmeer L, Sodergren E et al (2007) The prevalence of food allergy: a meta-analysis. J Allergy Clin Immunol 120:638–646
19. Simren M, Mansson A, Langkilde AM, Svedlund J, Abrahamsson H, Bengtsson U et al (2001) Food-related gastrointestinal symptoms in the irritable bowel syndrome. Digestion 63:108–115
20. Böhn L, Störsrud S, Törnblom H, Bengtsson U, Simrén M (2013) Self-reported food-related gastrointestinal symptoms in IBS are common and associated with more severe symptoms and reduced quality of life. Am J Gastroenterol 108:634–641
21. Monsbakken KW, Vandvik PO, Farup PG (2006) Perceived food intolerance in subjects with irritable bowel syndrome – etiology, prevalence and consequences. Eur J Clin Nutr 60:667–672
22. Ostgaard H, Hausken T, Gundersen D, El-Salhy M (2012) Diet and effects of diet management on quality of life and symptoms in patients with irritable bowel syndrome. Mol Med Rep 5:1382–1390
23. Boettcher E, Crowe SE (2013) Dietary proteins and functional gastrointestinal disorders. Am J Gastroenterol 108:728–736
24. Petitpierre M, Gumowski P, Girard JP (1985) Irritable bowel syndrome and hypersensitivity to food. Ann Allergy 54:538–540
25. Soares RL, Figueiredo HN, Maneschy CP, Rocha VR, Santos JM (2004) Correlation between symptoms of the irritable bowel syndrome and the response to the food extract skin prick test. Braz J Med Biol Res 37:659–662
26. Simonato B, De Lazzari F, Pasini G, Polato F, Giannattasio M, Gemignani C et al (2001) IgE binding to soluble and insoluble wheat flour proteins in atopic and non-atopic patients suffering from gastrointestinal symptoms after wheat ingestion. Clin Exp Allergy 31:1771–1778

27. Carroccio A, Brusca I, Mansueto P, Pirrone G, Barrale M, Di Prima L et al (2010) A cytologic assay for diagnosis of food hypersensitivity in patients with irritable bowel syndrome. Clin Gastroenterol Hepatol 8:254–260
28. Shepherd SJ, Parker FC, Muir JG, Gibson PR (2008) Dietary triggers of abdominal symptoms in patients with irritable bowel syndrome: randomized placebo-controlled evidence. Clin Gastroenterol Hepatol 6:765–771
29. Barrett JS, Gearry RB, Muir JG, Irving PM, Rose R, Rosella O et al (2010) Dietary poorly absorbed, short-chain carbohydrates increase delivery of water and fermentable substrates to the proximal colon. Aliment Pharmacol Ther 31:874–882
30. Barrett JS, Irving PM, Shepherd SJ, Muir JG, Gibson PR (2009) Comparison of the prevalence of fructose and lactose malabsorption across chronic intestinal disorders. Aliment Pharmacol Ther 30:165–174
31. Gudmand-Höyer E, Riis P, Wulff HR (1973) The significance of lactose malabsorption in the irritable colon syndrome. Scand J Gastroenterol 8:273–278
32. Halmos EP, Power VA, Shepherd SJ, Gibson PR, Muir JG (2014) A diet low in FODMAPs reduces symptoms of irritable bowel syndrome. Gastroenterology 146:67–75
33. Ong DK, Mitchell SB, Barrett JS, Shepherd SJ, Irving PM, Biesiekierski JR et al (2010) Manipulation of dietary short chain carbohydrates alters the pattern of gas production and genesis of symptoms in irritable bowel syndrome. J Gastroenterol Hepatol 25:1366–1373
34. Shepherd SJ, Gibson PR (2006) Fructose malabsorption and symptoms of irritable bowel syndrome: guidelines for effective dietary management. J Am Diet Assoc 106:1631–1639
35. Biesiekierski JR, Newnham ED, Irving PM, Barrett JS, Haines M, Doecke JD et al (2011) Gluten causes gastrointestinal symptoms in subjects without celiac disease: a double-blind randomized placebo-controlled trial. Am J Gastroenterol 106:508–514
36. Carroccio A, Mansueto P, D'Alcamo A, Iacono G (2013) Non-celiac wheat sensitivity as an allergic condition: personal experience and narrative review. Am J Gastroenterol 108:1845–1852
37. Carroccio A, Mansueto P, Iacono G, Soresi M, D'Alcamo A, Cavataio F et al (2012) Non-celiac wheat sensitivity diagnosed by double-blind placebo-controlled challenge: exploring a new clinical entity. Am J Gastroenterol 107:1898–1906
38. Biesiekierski JR, Peters SL, Newnham ED, Rosella O, Muir JG, Gibson PR (2013) No effects of gluten in patients with self-reported non-celiac gluten sensitivity after dietary reduction of fermentable, poorly absorbed, short-chain carbohydrates. Gastroenterology 145:320–328
39. Nielsen SJ, Siega-Riz AM, Popkin BM (2002) Trends in energy intake in US between 1977 and 1996; similar shifts seen across age groups. Obes Res 10:370–378
40. Staudacher HM, Lomer MC, Anderson JL, Barrett JS, Muir JG, Irving PM et al (2012) Fermentable carbohydrate restriction reduces luminal bifidobacteria and gastrointestinal symptoms in patients with irritable bowel syndrome. J Nutr 142:1510–1518
41. Yao CK, Tan HL, van Langenberg DR, Barrett JS, Rose R, Liels K et al (2014) Dietary sorbitol and mannitol: food content and distinct absorption patterns between healthy individuals and patients with irritable bowel syndrome. J Hum Nutr Diet 27(Suppl 2):263–275
42. Muir JG, Gibson PR (2013) The low FODMAP diet for treatment of irritable bowel syndrome and other gastrointestinal disorders. Gastroenterol Hepatol 9:450–452
43. Gibson PR, Shepard SJ (2012) Food choice as a key management strategy for functional gastrointestinal symptoms. Am J Gastroenterol 107:657–666
44. Hoad CL, Marciani L, Foley S, Totman JJ, Wright J, Bush D et al (2007) Non-invasive quantification of small bowel water content by MRI: a validation study. Phys Med Biol 52:6909–6922
45. Brighenti F, Casiraghi MC, Pellegrini N, Riso P, Simonetti P, Testolin G (1995) Comparison of lactulose and inulin as reference standard for the study of resistant starch fermentation using hydrogen breath test. Ital J Gastroenterol 27:122–128
46. Clausen MR, Jorgensen J, Mortensen PB (1998) Comparison of diarrhea induced by ingestion of fructooligosaccharide Idolax and disaccharide lactulose: role of osmolarity versus fermentation of malabsorbed carbohydrate. Dig Dis Sci 43:2696–2707

47. Piche T, Zerbib F, Varannes SB, Cherbut C, Anini Y, Roze C et al (2000) Modulation by colonic fermentation of LES function in humans. Am J Physiol Gastrointest Liver Physiol 278:G578–G584
48. Madsen JL, Linnet J, Rumessen JJ (2006) Effect of nonabsorbed amounts of a fructose-sorbitol mixture on small intestinal transit in healthy volunteers. Dig DisSci 51:147–153
49. El-Salhy M, Gilja OH, Gundersen D, Hatlebakk JG, Hausken T (2014) Interaction between ingested nutrients and gut endocrine cells in patients with irritable bowel syndrome (review). Int J Mol Med 34:363–371
50. Ji S, Park H, Lee D, Song YK, Choi JP, Lee SI (2005) Post-infectious irritable bowel syndrome in patients with Shigella infection. J Gastroenterol Hepatol 20:381–386
51. Ledochowski M, Widner B, Sperner-Unterweger B, Propst T, Vogel W, Fuchs D (2000) Carbohydrate malabsorption syndromes and early signs of mental depression in females. Dig Dis Sci 45:1255–1259
52. Kassinen A, Krogius-Kurikka L, Mäkivuokko H, Rinttilä T, Paulin L, Corander J et al (2007) The fecal microbiota of irritable bowel syndrome patients differs significantly from that of healthy subjects. Gastroenterology 133:24–33
53. De Giorgio R, Volta U, Gibson PR (2015) Sensitivity to wheat, gluten and FODMAPs in IBS: facts or fiction? Gut. doi:10.1136/gutjnl-2015-309757
54. Fernández-Bañares F, Rosinach M, Esteve M, Forné M, Espinós JC, Maria Viver J (2006) Sugar malabsorption in functional abdominal bloating: a pilot study on the long-term effect of dietary treatment. Clin Nutr 25:824–831
55. Pedersen N, Ankersen DV, Felding M, Vegh Z, Burisch J, Munkholm P (2014) Mo1210: low FODMAP diet reduces irritable bowel symptoms and improves quality of life in patients with inflammatory bowel disease in a randomized controlled trial. Gastroenterology 146:S-587
56. Pedersen N, Andersen NN, Végh Z, Jensen L, Ankersen DV, Felding MS et al (2014) Ehealth: low FODMAP diet vs Lactobacillus rhamnosus GG in irritable bowel syndrome. World J Gastroenterol 20:16215–16226
57. Braden B (2009) Methods and functions: breath tests. Best Pract Res Clin Gastroenterol 23:337–352
58. Nucera G, Gabrielli M, Lupascu A, Lauritano EC, Santoliquido A, Cremonini F et al (2005) Abnormal breath tests to lactose, fructose and sorbitol in irritable bowel syndrome may be explained by small intestinal bacterial overgrowth. Aliment Pharmacol Ther 21:1391–1395
59. Biesiekierski JR, Rosella O, Rose R, Liels K, Barrett JS, Shepherd SJ et al (2011) Quantification of fructans, galacto-oligosaccharides and other short-chain carbohydrates in processed grains and cereals. J Hum Nutr Diet 24:154–176
60. Barrett JS, Gibson PR (2010) Development and validation of a comprehensive semi-quantitative food frequency questionnaire that includes FODMAP intake and glycemic index. J Am Diet Assoc 110:1469–1476
61. Whigham L, Joyce T, Harper G, Irving PM, Staudacher HM, Whelan K et al (2015) Clinical effectiveness and economic costs of group versus one-to-one education for short-chain fermentable carbohydrate restriction (low FODMAP diet) in the management of irritable bowel syndrome. J Hum Nutr Diet. doi:10.1111/jhn.12318
62. Rao SS, Yu S, Fedewa A (2015) Systematic review: dietary fibre and FODMAP-restricted diet in the management of constipation and irritable bowel syndrome. Aliment Pharmacol Ther 41:1256–1270
63. Halmos EP, Christophersen CT, Bird AR, Shepherd SJ, Gibson PR, Muir JG (2015) Diets that differ in their FODMAP content alter the colonic luminal microenvironment. Gut 64:93–100
64. Mansueto P, Seidita A, D'Alcamo A, Carroccio A (2014) Non-celiac gluten sensitivity: literature review. J Am Coll Nutr 33:39–54
65. Sapone A, Bai JC, Ciacci C, Dolinsek J, Green PH, Hadjivassiliou M et al (2012) Spectrum of gluten-related disorders: consensus on new nomenclature and classification. BMC Med 10:13
66. Carroccio A, Rini G, Mansueto P (2014) Non-celiac wheat sensitivity is a more appropriate label than non-celiac gluten sensitivity. Gastroenterology 146:320–321

67. Catassi C, Bai JC, Bonaz B, Bouma G, Calabrò A, Carroccio A et al (2013) Non-celiac gluten sensitivity: the new frontier of gluten related disorders. Nutrients 5:3839–3853
68. Carroccio A, D'Alcamo A, Cavataio F, Soresi M, Seidita A, Sciumè C et al (2015) High proportions of people with nonceliac wheat sensitivity have autoimmune disease or antinuclear antibodies. Gastroenterology 149:596–603
69. Verdu EF, Huang X, Natividad J, Lu J, Blennerhassett PA, David CS et al (2008) Gliadin-dependent neuromuscular and epithelial secretory responses in gluten-sensitive HLA-DQ8 transgenic mice. Am J Physiol Gastrointest Liver Physiol 294:G217–G225
70. Golley S, Corsini N, Topping D, Morell M, Mohr P (2015) Motivations for avoiding wheat consumption in Australia: results from a population survey. Public Health Nutr 18:490–499

The Role of Diet in Counteracting Gastroparesis

11

Riccardo Marmo, Antonella Santonicola, and Paola Iovino

11.1 Gastroparesis

Gastroparesis is a syndrome characterized by delayed gastric emptying in the absence of mechanical obstruction. The most common symptoms associated with gastroparesis are early satiety, postprandial fullness, nausea, and vomiting, but also abdominal discomfort and bloating [1]. Nausea, vomiting, early satiety, and postprandial fullness correlate better with delayed gastric emptying than upper abdominal pain and bloating [2]. The symptoms of gastroparesis may overlap with those of other conditions, including gastritis secondary to *Helicobacter pylori* infection, peptic ulcer, and functional dyspepsia.

The most frequent causes of gastroparesis include diabetes (29 %), postsurgical issues (13 %), and idiopathic-related factors (36 %) [2]. Other potential etiologies include Parkinson's disease (7.5 %), collagen vascular disorders (4.8 %), intestinal pseudoobstruction (4.1 %), and other rare causes (6 %) [3]. A subset of patients with gastroparesis refers to the onset of symptoms after a viral prodrome, suggesting a potential viral etiology; this condition is defined as "postinfectious gastroparesis" [4]. The prevalence of gastroparesis is unknown due to the absence of an easy diagnostic test that could be widely applied. It has been demonstrated [5] that "definite gastroparesis" (defined as typical symptoms plus confirmed delayed gastric emptying by scintigraphy) had a prevalence of 24.2 per 100,000 inhabitants, and an incidence of 6.3 per 100,000 persons per year, but some authors hypothesized a "gastroparesis iceberg" with a real prevalence of about 2 % in the general population

R. Marmo (✉)
Gastroenterology Unit, L.Curto Hospital, Polla, SA 84035, Italy
e-mail: ricmarmo1@virgilio.it

A. Santonicola • P. Iovino
Gastrointestinal Unit, Department of Medicine and Surgery, University of Salerno,
Salerno 84081, Italy

© Springer International Publishing Switzerland 2016
E. Grossi, F. Pace (eds.), *Human Nutrition from the Gastroenterologist's Perspective*,
DOI 10.1007/978-3-319-30361-1_11

[3]. The presence of gastroparesis is associated with significantly lower age- and sex-specific survival expected from the general population.

11.2 Gastroparesis Subtypes

- *Diabetic gastroparesis.* In most cases the onset of diabetic gastroparesis is characterized by continuous nausea; 80% of patients also report bloating and 60% early satiety [6]. The prevalence of gastroparesis among diabetic patients is about 5–12% [7]. Women, obese patients with poor glycemic control, and patients with long-standing diabetes or concomitant microvascular complications (i.e., retinopathy, neuropathy, nephropathy) have a higher risk [6]. The relationship between type and severity of symptoms and delayed gastric emptying has not been clearly demonstrated [8]; furthermore, the correlation between glycated hemoglobin (HbA1c) levels and severity of gastroparesis has also to be elucidated [9].
- *Idiopathic gastroparesis* refers to gastroparesis of an unknown cause, without detectable underlying abnormality for the delayed gastric emptying [10]. Most patients with idiopathic gastroparesis are young or middle-aged women; the typically referred symptoms are nausea (34%), vomiting (19%), and pain (23%) [11]. Symptoms of idiopathic gastroparesis overlap with those of functional dyspepsia [12]. It has been demonstrated that 86% of patients with idiopathic gastroparesis met the Rome III criteria for diagnosis of functional dyspepsia [11]. Abdominal pain is more frequently reported by patients with functional dyspepsia, whereas nausea and vomiting are more characteristics of idiopathic gastroparesis [13].
- *Postsurgical gastroparesis* [PSG] represents the third most common etiology of gastroparesis [1]. A delayed gastric emptying may be the consequence of different surgical procedures that can cause a vagal injury, such as surgeries for peptic ulcer disease or gastric malignancy: laparoscopic fundoplication procedure or bariatric surgeries, especially Roux-en-Y gastric bypass and sleeve gastrectomy; esophagectomy; and pancreatoduodenectomy [12].

11.3 Pathophysiology

Ingestion of nutrients induces profound changes in motility, secretion, and release of hormones that coordinate the digestive process and depend on the nature and composition of the ingested nutrients. Normal gastrointestinal motor function depends on a complex coordination between smooth muscles of the gastric fundus, antrum, pylorus, and duodenum under the control of the enteric and autonomic nervous system [14]. During fasting, the proximal gastric tone is maintained by constant cholinergic input from the vagus nerve. During the meal a rapid drop in the intragastric pressure (IGP) through the intrinsic and vago-vagal reflex pathways occurs. This "accommodation" response allows the meal to be stored without increasing, and it is followed by a gradual recovery of IGP that is closely correlated with the occurrence of satiation [15]. The proximal stomach transfers the food from the midstomach to the gastric antrum, where high amplitude contractions break the food into particles of about 1–2 mm, that pass through the pylorus [16]. The emptying speed of a meal is inversely correlated with its caloric content and also depends on the acidity, osmolarity, and viscosity of the meal. During gastric emptying the role of the gastric phase to food intake diminishes, and the intestinal phase with intestinal exposure of the nutrients will dominate physiological control mechanisms. Most of these influences are controlled by a myriad of duodenogastric negative-feedback mechanisms which are mediated through vago-vagal reflexes and hormonal signals to delay the arrival of acidic, hyperosmotic, or calorie-rich gastric contents into the duodenum. For example, lipids stimulate the release of several peptides that synergistically contribute to inhibition of gastric acid secretion, induce gastric relaxation, and the stimulation of pancreatic enzyme secretion. The presence of lipids induces sensations of satiety at low concentrations and occurrence of nausea at higher concentrations. The latter occur at least in part with the release of cholecystokinin (CCK), which also stimulates the gallbladder. Otherwise, the responses to protein are slower with the onset of motor and hormonal signals and, unlike lipid and carbohydrates, are not associated with increased sensitivity to gastric distension.

Gastroparesis has been associated with abnormalities of certain complex mechanisms: impaired gastric accommodation, antral hypomotility, pylorospasm, duodenal dysmotility, autonomic dysfunction, and visceral hypersensitivity [17].

11.4   Diagnosis

The diagnosis of delayed gastric emptying can be performed using one of the following tests: scintigraphy, breath testing, and wireless motility capsule (WMC) [18]. For any type, patients should discontinue drugs that may affect gastric emptying, such as metoclopramide, domperidone, and erythromycin, for at least 2–3 days before testing. Because hyperglycemia (glucose level >200 mg/dl) can determine a delayed gastric emptying, it is recommended to reach a fasting blood glucose of <275 mg/dl in diabetic patients before performing the test [1].

11.4.1 Scintigraphy

Gastric-emptying scintigraphy (GES) of a solid phase meal is considered the standard for diagnosis of gastroparesis [1], as it quantifies the emptying of a physiologic caloric meal. GES should be performed after exclusion of mechanical or structural causes of abnormal gastric emptying. According to both the Society of Nuclear Medicine and Molecular Imaging and the American Neurogastroenterology and Motility Society, a standardized protocol is adopted [19]. A low-fat meal [i.e., a 99 m Tc sulfur colloid labeled egg sandwich] is used to perform the solid phase with standard imaging at 0, 1, 2, and 4 h [19]. Shorter duration solid emptying or sole liquid emptying by scintigraphy is associated with lower diagnostic sensitivity [20]. Dual-isotope labeling of solid and liquid phases may also be performed to increase the test sensitivity [1]. However, the clinical significance of selectively delayed gastric emptying of liquids has not been assessed.

11.4.2 Breath Testing

Breath tests using 13C-labeled substrates, typically 13C-octanoic acid or 13C-spirulina platensis (blue-green algae), have been proposed as alternatives to scintigraphy for determining gastric emptying [21]. These techniques measure $13CO^2$ in exhaled breath samples after duodenal processing of the consumed substrate; the provided results correlate well with those of gastric-emptying scintigraphy [22, 23]. However, breath test results may be unreliable in individuals with conditions that impair digestive, absorptive, or pulmonary function [12].

11.4.3 Wireless Motility Capsule (WMC)

The wireless motility capsule (WMC) can be an alternative diagnostic method to scintigraphy. Gastric emptying is determined when there is a significant increase in pH value as the capsule passes from the antrum to the duodenum. There is a good correlation between the gastric residence time of the WMC and the T-90 % of gastric-emptying scintigraphy (i.e., the time when only 10 % of the meal remains in the stomach), suggesting that the gastric residence time of the WMC represents a time near the end of the emptying of a solid meal [24].

Both WMC and breath testing require further validation before they can be considered as alternates to scintigraphy for diagnosis of gastroparesis.

On the basis of the complex pathophysiological mechanisms underlying gastroparesis, the measurement of overall gastric emptying is unable to distinguish among the subtler forms of dysmotility within different regions of the stomach that could explain better the relationship with symptoms. For example, there are other sophisticated methodologies such the *gastric barostat* that selectively measures proximal tone function and its relationships with symptoms [25, 26]. In fact, it has been used in diabetes and in less common connective tissue disorders such as scleroderma (SSc). A strong association between total autonomic score and gastric compliance has been demonstrated in SSc patients. Moreover, a significant positive correlation was found between cumulative perception scores and gastric compliance suggesting that the proximal stomach could play a role in eliciting gastroparesis-related symptoms [27].

11.5   Dietary Management

Many patients with gastroparesis, from the symptoms arising as a consequence, had reduced oral intake, including macronutrient calories, vitamins (A, B, C, K), minerals (iron, potassium, and zinc) leading to weight loss, vitamin deficiency, and dehydration [28].

Thus the general principles for treating symptomatic gastroparesis are to (1) reduce symptoms; (2) correct and prevent fluid, electrolyte, and nutritional deficiencies; and (3) identify and treat the underlying comorbidities. There is limited scientific evidence for nutritional management strategies due to the limited randomized controlled studies; indeed, the majority of recommendations are based on clinical experience, observational studies, taking into consideration the underlying cause such as postsurgical process or underlying chronic disease course, and on known emptying characteristics of food or nutrients.

The nutritional therapies are oriented to improve the gastric motility compliance and to reduce the symptoms. The gastroparesis severity classification [13] can facilitate the selection of patients that can be treated as outpatients. Mild gastroparesis is characterized by intermittent, easily controlled symptoms with maintenance of weight and nutritional status and is treated with dietary modification and avoidance of medications that slow emptying. Compensated gastroparesis is characterized by moderately severe symptoms with infrequent hospitalizations that are treated with combined prokinetic and antiemetic agents. Gastric failure gastroparesis patients are medication unresponsive, cannot maintain nutrition or hydration, and require frequent emergency department or inpatient care. Individuals with grade 3 gastroparesis may need intermittent intravenous fluids and medications, enteral or parenteral nutrition, and endoscopic or surgical therapy. Patients with unintentional weight loss >5–10 % of usual bodyweight over 3–6 months, repeated hospitalizations for refractory gastroparesis, inability to meet weight goals set by doctor or dietician, or who benefit from gastric decompression or medication have diabetic ketoacidosis, cyclic nausea and vomiting, and poor quality of life due to gastroparesis symptoms that could initiate enteral nutrition supplementation.

A dietary history should be recorded in order to adapt the information obtained to dietary habits correcting those inappropriate and increasing the useful ones focusing on the size of meals, frequency, type, consistency of foods tolerated, and content. An evaluation of weight and anthropometric measurements, glycemic control, and the presence of any vitamin and mineral deficiency is also needed [29].

11.5.1 Meal Volume and Frequency

Gastric-emptying time for larger volume meals is slower. Thus a reduction in meal size is a relevant factor in the dietary management of patients with gastroparesis reducing also the risk of gastroesophageal reflux that enhances nausea and vomiting. The exact meal size will need to be individualized in accordance with the patient response; the meal numbers will need to be increased to compensate for reduced meal volume and ensure adequate nutritional intake.

In the fasting period, the interdigestive migrating motor complex (MMC) has a cyclical contraction sequence of average duration of approximately 7 min spreading through the stomach and small intestine on average about every 90 min and is interrupted by feeding. With ingestion of a meal, the proximal stomach accommodates food by reduction of its tone, and there is an increase in proximal and distal stomach volume without an increase in pressure. The distension of the stomach interrupts

MMC, and the physicochemical composition of the meal determines the duration of disruption. During feeding in the regions in contact with food, the MMC is replaced by contractions of variable amplitude and frequency, which enable mixing and digestion. The duration of these contractions is about 1 h for each 200 kcal ingested [30].

The time required from meal ingestion to commencement of gastric emptying of solid particles through the pylorus (lag time) depends on the particle size. The stomach normally grinds food to particles <2 mm in size, and this action is associated with the lag phase of gastric emptying. In patients with type 1 diabetes and gastroparesis, the administration of a small particle meal consisting of minced and baked beef and pasta and boiled carrots mixed together in a food processor for 3 min significantly increases the gastric-emptying rate and reduce postprandial blood glucose. The meal remaining in the stomach in the diabetic subjects after the small particle meal was significantly less ($p = 0.018$) than that after the large particle meal after 120 min [T_{120}] ($29.7 \pm 5.4\%$ vs. $72.4 \pm 4.5\%$). A significant difference ($p = 0.018$) remained at T_{180} between the meals. The difference was present also in the healthy group: the retention at T_{120} was $17.3 \pm 4.3\%$ after the small particle compared to $45.8 \pm 6.3\%$ after the large particle meal ($p = 0.018$).

The upper gastrointestinal symptoms considered to be the key symptoms of gastroparesis, i.e., nausea/vomiting, postprandial fullness, early satiety, and bloating, had a significantly greater reduction in severity in diabetic patients receiving advice to eat foods with small particle size or food items that could easily be processed into small particle size defined as "the food should be easy to mash with a fork into small particle size, e.g., mealy potatoes" [31].

In the study, the gastric-emptying rate tended to improve more after 20 weeks with the small particle size diet than in the control group, but this was not related to the improvement in symptoms. The authors suggest that symptom improvement is probably more related to the direct effect of the meal rather than via a permanent effect of the diet on gastric emptying/motility. It is likely that gastric emptying is increased in the group receiving low particle size meals as a consequence of bypassing the lag phase of gastric emptying.

Simple measures to reduce particle size, such as adequately chewing food, eating slowly, and using a food processor, may improve symptoms in patients with mild symptoms. Reducing the meal volume could impact on the total calories consumed so that small and frequent meals (six to eight meals, there are no data on how many) may enable patients to tolerate food and achieve adequate calorie intake. By using the gravity effect, after the meal, sitting upright for 1–2 h or by even going for a gentle walk could play a role in helping patients to reduce their symptoms.

11.5.2 Content and Consistency of Foods

In patients in which the nutritional strategy of small particle size and increasing the frequency of the meals do not reach the goal, the next step is to introduce a more liquid-pureed-based meal or have alternate days with some solid food and then consume more liquid-type meals as the symptoms progress and the feeling of fullness increases. During the solid-emptying period, there is a positive correlation between emptying of solids and antral motility, while no relation exists between antral motility and emptying of the liquid phase of the meal. The liquid component disperses rapidly throughout the stomach and empties after a minimal lag period. The half-emptying time of nonnutrient liquids is approximately 20 min; gastric-emptying time is exponential, with a rapid initial transit into the small bowel. By contrast, liquids with increased nutrients and energy loads have a steadier, more linear gastric-emptying curve. Thus, many patients may tolerate fats in liquid form, and therefore oral nutrition supplements often provide a useful way of encouraging intake of adequate calories in low volume. Liquids do not require migrating motor complex to leave the stomach; therefore liquids, even those that are caloric, will empty from the stomach. If the patient has trouble chewing the food, it is possible to create a puree by grinding the food; this becomes liquefied after mixing with saliva and gastric secretions and may be more easily tolerated than solid or not properly chewed foods. Several cross-sectional studies report that gastric emptying of solid and/or nutrient liquid meals is delayed in about 30–50 % of randomly selected patients with long-standing type 1 or 2 diabetes; more liquid calories may be useful in alleviating a patient's symptoms and providing appropriate nutrition. It is well known that fat is a potent inhibitor of gastric emptying, increasing the release of CCK, and fatty foods take a longer time to digest. Patients with gastroparesis are therefore advised to restrict fat in their diet. Eliminating fat also removes a significant calorie source and nutrients needed. Many patients are not affected by dietary fat if it is present in liquid form. Approximately 25–30 % of calories can be provided from unsaturated fats. Small meals at frequent intervals that consist of low-fat and complex carbohydrates are advised, and sometimes high-calorie liquid supplements may be required to fulfill daily calorie requirements. Twelve patients with gastroparesis were studied on four separate days receiving one of four meals each day in a randomized order: high-fat solid, high-fat liquid, low-fat liquid, and low-fat solid meal. At each visit, the gastrointestinal symptoms were rated from 0 (none) to 4 (very severe) every 15 min, before and for 4 h after meal ingestion. Nausea, stomach fullness, bloating, and stomach visibly larger were the most prominent postprandial symptoms. The four meals increased nausea postprandially in the following order: high-fat solid meal > low-fat solid meal > high-fat liquid meal > low-fat liquid meal. The high-fat solid meal caused nausea symptoms to more than double, whereas the low-fat liquid meal caused the least increase. The low-fat liquid meal induced lower nausea scores than either the high-fat liquid ($p=0.001$) or low-fat solid meal ($p<0.001$), and there were no differences in nausea scores between the low-fat solid and high-fat liquid meals. Subjects reported increases in stomach visibly larger and bloating with the high-fat solid meal, whereas symptom scores decreased or remained the same at 4 h for the other three test meals. Upper abdominal pain increased to the greatest level with the high-fat solid meal compared to minimal increase with the low-fat solid meal and the high-fat liquid meal. The low-fat liquid meal did not increase upper abdominal pain. Heartburn was greater with the high-fat solid meal than low-fat solid ($p<0.05$) and high-fat liquid meals ($p<0.05$) [32].

Data provide support for recommendations of a low-fat diet preferably in liquid form.

11.5.3 Fiber

Although the avoidance of high-fiber foods is recommended in patients with gastroparesis, what is not known is the type of fiber and the quantity of fiber that should be assumed.

Dietary fiber is found in fruits, vegetables, beans, and grains including a range of relatively poorly adsorbed food substances mainly composed of non-starch polysaccharides. Pectins and gums are multibranched hydrophilic substances (soluble fiber) forming viscous solutions that delay gastric emptying. Other fiber, including cellulose and lignins, are insoluble. The available data on the effect of fiber ingestion on gastric emptying are contrasting and derive from small studies. The ingestion of insoluble fiber has been associated with gastric bezoar formation in patients with gastroparesis. Bezoars are retained concretions of indigestible foreign material that accumulate in the stomach. Phytobezoars are composed of nondigestible parts of food material, including cellulose, hemicellulose, lignin, and fruit tannins, which are often found in raw vegetables, citrus fruits, celery, pumpkins, grapes, prunes, raisin, whole grain foods, wheat and corn bran, and legumes such as beans and peas, nuts and seeds, green beans, cauliflower, celery, avocado, unripe bananas, and the skins of fruits. Avoiding foods high in insoluble fiber is advised in gastroparesis for the prevention of phytobezoars [29].

11.5.4 Wine Alcohol and Food Worsening Symptoms

The administration of a low-alcohol dose favors gastric emptying, whereas high doses delay emptying and reduce bowel motility; wine increases gastric emptying and intestinal motility; ethanol has also been seen to cause pyloric relaxation, which may facilitate gastric emptying. On the contrary, alcohol abuse tends to facilitate or cause gastroesophageal reflux and esophageal mucosal damage, regardless of the type of alcoholic beverage involved [33]. High doses of alcohol, carbonated drinks, and tobacco smoking can decrease antral contractility and impair gastric emptying.

Foods responsible for symptoms worsening include orange juice, fried chicken, cabbage, oranges, sausage, pizza, peppers, onions, tomato juice, lettuce, coffee, salsa, broccoli, bacon, and roast beef (see Table 11.1). Foods able to elicit symptoms are generally fatty, acidic, spicy, and roughage based. Foods not provoking symptoms are generally bland, sweet, salty, and starchy [34].

Dietary intervention under investigation includes the avoidance of fermentable oligo-, di-, monosaccharides and polyols (FODMAPs) [35]; they are highly fermentable with gut bacteria, as well as highly osmotic, and they too can further accentuate symptoms in those with gastroparesis. They are not only found in certain foods but are also added to some enteral formulas (fructo-oligosaccharides are one of them) in addition to many liquid medications for flavorings, including sugar alcohols such as sorbitol and xylitol. Patient on enteral feeding with a fiber-containing formula and liquid medications may seem intolerant to the tube feeding, when the problem could be the FODMAP/fiber load they are receiving.

Table 11.1 Foods responsible for symptoms worsening in patients with idiopathic or diabetic gastroparesis

Apple
Bacon
Beans
Berries
Broccoli
Cabbage
Coffee
Cold cuts
Cottage cheese
Creamer
Creamy soup
Dark chocolate
French fries
Fried chicken
Fried fish
Frozen entrees
Ice cream
Lentils
Lettuce
Milk chocolate
Nuts
Onions
Orange juice
Oranges
Pasta sauce
Pastry
Peanut butter
Peas
Peppers
Pizza
Pork
Protein bars
Roast beef
Salad dressing
Salsa
Sausage
Skim milk
Soda
Spinach
Tomato juice
Tomatoes
Granola bars
Frozen yogurt
Saltines

| Wheat bread |
| Eggs |
| Whole grain pasta |
| Carrots |
| Cheese |
| Cookies |
| Whole milk |
| Ginger ale |
| Sports drinks |
| Brown rice |
| Yogurt |
| Graham crackers |
| Smoothies |
| Grapes |
| Oatmeal |

Adapted from Wytiaz et al. [34]

11.5.5 Nutraceutical

Since 1979, when Stephen De Felice, chairman and founder of the Foundation for Innovation in Medicine (FIM; Cranford, NT9), defined nutraceutical as a "food, or parts of food, that provide medical or health benefit, including the prevention and treatment of disease" [36], the number of publications on this topic has increased exponentially. This aspect of nutrition in gastroparesis has been explored only marginally. Recently a pilot study on soy germ pasta containing 31–33 mg of total isoflavones provided evidence that dietary modifications could be a potential treatment for diabetic gastroparesis. The authors enrolled 10 adults in a randomized controlled study. They found a relationship between gastric-emptying time [$t_{1/2}$] and consuming soy germ pasta containing isoflavone aglycons. The patients with gastroparesis consuming isoflavone-enriched soy germ pasta had a significant acceleration in the rate of gastric emptying, and a significant decrease of the Gastroparesis Cardinal Symptom Index (GCSI): 8 (2–13) at baseline to 5 (0–7) ($p = 0.039$) for the soy germ pasta group [37].

Pugionium cornutum Gaertn (PCG) is a desert plant with edible and medicinal value widely distributed in the Badain Jaran desert, Kubuqi desert and Mu Us desert, Horqin and Hulunbuir sandy land traditionally consumed by the local people. The plant contains dietary fiber, protein, and vitamins. A low-dose extract of the plant can promote gastrointestinal peristalsis and act as a drug to favor gastrointestinal motility. The results of the study indicate that PCG has great potential as a new functional food source [38].

For summary dietary recommendations for patients with gastroparesis, see Table 11.2.

Table 11.2 Summary dietary recommendations for patients with gastroparesis

1. Restoration of fluids and electrolytes, nutritional support, and treat comorbidities (glucose control in diabetic)
2. Oral intake is preferable for nutrition and hydration in patients with mild or moderate gastroparesis severity
3. Adequately chewing foods, slowly eating, and use of food processor if needed
4. Consumption of frequent small volume nutrient meals
5. Using meal with small particle size
6. Use low and liquid fat and soluble fiber
7. Avoid fatty, acidic, spicy, roughage based, carbonated beverages, and tobacco smoking
8. Liquid-pureed-based meal as the symptoms progresses and the feeling of fullness increases

References

1. Parkman HP, Hasler WL, Fisher RS (2004) American Gastroenterology Association technical review on the diagnosis and treatment of gastroparesis. Gastroenterology 127:1592–1622
2. Camilleri M, Parkman HP, Shafi MA, Abell TL, Gerson L, American College of Gastroenterology (2013) Clinical guideline: management of gastroparesis. Am J Gastroenterol 108(1):18–37
3. Rey E, Choung RS, Schleck CD, Zinsmeister AR, Talley NJ, Locke GR 3rd (2012) Prevalence of hidden gastroparesis in the community: the gastroparesis "iceberg". J Neurogastroenterol Motil 18(1):34–42. doi:10.5056/jnm.2012.18.1.34
4. Naftali T, Yishai R, Zangen T, Levine A (2007) Post-infectious gastroparesis: clinical and electrogastrographic aspects. J Gastroenterol Hepatol 22(9):1423–1428
5. Jung HK, Choung RS, Locke GR 3rd et al (2008) The incidence, prevalence and survival of gastroparesis in Olmsted County, Minnesota 1996–2006. Gastroenterology 134(suppl 1):A534–A535
6. Horváth VJ, Izbéki F, Lengyel C, Kempler P, Várkonyi T (2014) Diabetic gastroparesis: functional/morphologic background, diagnosis, and treatment options. Curr Diab Rep 14(9):527. doi:10.1007/s11892-014-0527-8
7. Camilleri M (2007) Clinical practice. Diabetic gastroparesis. N Engl J Med 356:820–829
8. Barucha AE et al (2009) Relationship between clinical features and gastric emptying disturbances in diabetes mellitus. Clin Endocrinol [Oxf] 70(3):415–420
9. Jones KL et al (2001) Predictors of delayed gastric emptying in diabetes. Diabetes Care 24:1264–1269
10. Parkman HP, Yates K, Hasler WL et al (2011) Similarities and differences between diabetic and idiopathic gastroparesis. Clin Gastroenterol Hepatol 9:1056–1064
11. Parkman HP, Yates K, Hasler WL, Nguyen L, Pasricha PJ, Snape WJ, Farrugia G, Koch KL, Abell TL, McCallum RW, Lee L, Unalp-Arida A, Tonascia J, Hamilton F, National Institute of Diabetes and Digestive and Kidney Diseases Gastroparesis Clinical Research Consortium (2011) Clinical features of idiopathic gastroparesis vary with sex, body mass, symptom onset, delay in gastric emptying, and gastroparesis severity. Gastroenterology 140(1):101–115. doi:10.1053/j.gastro.2010.10.015
12. Hasler WL (2011) Gastroparesis: pathogenesis, diagnosis and management. Nat Rev Gastroenterol Hepatol 8(8):438–453. doi:10.1038/nrgastro.2011.116
13. Abell TL, Bernstein RK, Cutts T, Farrugia G, Forster J, Hasler WL, McCallum RW, Olden KW, Parkman HP, Parrish CR, Pasricha PJ, Prather CM, Soffer EE, Twillman R, Vinik AI (2006) Treatment of gastroparesis: a multidisciplinary clinical review. Neurogastroenterol Motil 18(4):263–283

14. Wood JD, Alpers DH, Andrews PL (1999) Fundamentals of neurogastroenterology. Gut 45(Suppl 2):II6–II16
15. Oustamanolakis P, Tack J (2012) Dyspepsia: organic versus functional. J Clin Gastroenterol 46(3):175–190. doi:10.1097/MCG.0b013e318241b335
16. Farrè R, Tack J (2013) Food and symptom generation in functional gastrointestinal disorders: physiological aspects. Am J Gastroenterol 108:698–706
17. Nguyen LA, Snape WJ Jr (2015) Clinical presentation and pathophysiology of gastroparesis. Gastroenterol Clin North Am 44(1):21–30. doi:10.1016/j.gtc.2014.11.003
18. Shin AS, Camilleri M (2013) Diagnostic assessment of diabetic gastroparesis. Diabetes 62(8):2667–2673. doi:10.2337/db12-1706
19. Abell TL, Camilleri M, Donohoe K, American Neurogastroenterology and Motility Society and the Society of Nuclear Medicine et al (2008) Consensus recommendations for gastric emptying scintigraphy: a joint report of the American Neurogastroenterology and Motility Society and the Society of Nuclear Medicine. Am J Gastroenterol 103:753–763
20. Pathikonda M, Sachdeva P, Malhotra N et al (2012) Gastric emptying scintigraphy: is four hours necessary? J Clin Gastroenterol 46:209–215
21. Ghoos YF, Maes BD, Geypens BJ et al (1993) Measurement of gastric emptying rate of solids by means of a carbon-labeled octanoic acid breath test. Gastroenterology 104:1640–1647
22. Perri F et al (2010) 13C-octanoic acid breath test [OBT] with a new test meal [EXPIROGer]: toward standardization for testing gastric emptying of solids. Dig Liver Dis 42:549–553
23. Verbeke K (2009) Will the 13C-octanoic acid breath test ever replace scintigraphy as the gold standard to assess gastric emptying? Neurogastroenterol Motil 21:1013–1016
24. Kuo B, McCallum RW, Koch K et al (2008) Comparison of gastric emptying of a non-digestible capsule to a radiolabeled meal in healthy and gastroparetic subjects. Aliment Pharmacol Ther 27:186–196
25. Iovino P, Azpiroz F, Domingo E, Malagelada JR (1995) The sympathetic nervous system modulates perception and reflex responses to gut distension in humans. Gastroenterology 108:680–686
26. Iovino P, Angrisani L, Galloro, Consalvo D, Tremolaterra F, Pascariello A, Ciacci C (2006) Proximal stomach function in obesity with normal or abnormal oesophageal acid exposure. Neurogastroenterol Motil 18(6):425–432
27. Iovino P, Valentini G, Ciacci C, De Luca A, Tremolaterra F, Sabbatini F, Tirri E, Mazzacca G (2001) Proximal stomach function in systemic sclerosis. Relationship with autonomic nerve function. Dig Dis Sci 46:723–730
28. Parkman HP, Yates KP, Hasler WL, Nguyan L, Pasricha PJ, Snape WJ, Farrugia G, Calles J, Koch KL, Abell TL, McCallum RW, Petito D, Parrish CR, Duffy F, Lee L, Unalp-Arida A, Tonascia J, Hamilton F (2011) Dietary intake and nutritional deficiencies in patients with diabetic or idiopathic gastroparesis. Gastroenterology 141(2):486–498
29. Keld R, Kinsey L, Athwal V, Lal S (2011) Pathogenesis, investigation and dietary and medical management of gastroparesis. J Hum Nutr Diet 24(5):421–430
30. Camilleri M (2006) Integrated upper gastrointestinal response to food intake. Gastroenterology 131(2):640–658
31. Olausson EA, Störsrud S, Grundin H, Isaksson M, Attvall S, Simrén M (2014) Small particle size diet reduces upper gastrointestinal symptoms in patients with diabetic gastroparesis: a randomized controlled trial. Am J Gastroenterol 109:375–385
32. Homko CJ, Duffy F, Friedenberg FK, Boden G, Parkman HP (2015) Effect of dietary fat and food consistency on gastroparesis symptoms in patients with gastroparesis. Neurogastroenterol Motil 27(4):501–508
33. Bujanda L (2000) The effects of alcohol consumption upon the gastrointestinal tract. Am J Gastroenterol 95:3374–3382
34. Wytiaz V, Homko C, Duffy F, Schey R, Parkman HP (2015) Foods provoking and alleviating symptoms in gastroparesis: patient experiences. Dig Dis Sci 60:1052–1058

35. Marsh A, Eslick EM, Eslick GD (2015) Does a diet low in FODMAPs reduce symptoms associated with functional gastrointestinal disorders? A comprehensive systematic review and meta-analysis. Eur J Nutr [Epub ahead of print] DOI 10.1007/s00394-015-0922-1
36. Brower V (1998) Nutraceuticals: poised for a healthy slice of the healthcare market? Nat Biotechnol 16(8):728–731
37. Setchell KDR, Nardi E, Battezzati P-M, Asciutti S, Castellani D, Perriello G, Clerici C (2013) Novel soy germ pasta enriched in isoflavones ameliorates gastroparesis in type 2 diabetes. Diabetes Care 36(11):3495–3497
38. Li H, Li C, Zhang C, Chen B, Hui L (2015) Yehua shen compositional and gastrointestinal prokinetic studies of pugionium [L.]. Food Chem 186:285–291

How the Precious Role of Wine in Mediterranean Diet Is Mediated by the Gastrointestinal Tract

12

Enzo Grossi

12.1 Introduction: Mediterranean Diet and Health

The Mediterranean diet is a secular heritage that binds culturally all the countries of the Mediterranean Basin indicating a traditional lifestyle and dietary pattern typical of Greece, Southern Italy, and Spain.

The Mediterranean diet has been defined and described scientifically for the first time by Ancel Keys, an American physiologist, and by his wife, Margaret Keys, an American chemist, and later on transformed in a nutritional recommendation [1]. The principal aspects of this diet include relatively high consumption of olive oil, legumes, unrefined cereals, fruits, and vegetables, moderate to high consumption of fish, moderate consumption of dairy products (mostly as cheese and yogurt), low consumption of non-fish meat and non-fish meat products, and last but not least moderate wine consumption during meal.

In 2013, UNESCO added the Mediterranean diet to the Representative List of the Intangible Cultural Heritage of Humanity of Italy, Spain, Portugal, Morocco, Greece, Cyprus, and Croatia [2].

This decision was made also because the diet does not only mean food, but referring to the ancient Greek the term δαιτα, it also means lifestyle and environment.

A healthy lifestyle (notably a physically active lifestyle, positive approach to problems, and socialization during meals among the others) has been proven by the way to be per se beneficial [3, 4]. This finding is consistent with the assumption that the influence of genetics is rather minimal, since the slowly changing habits of Mediterranean populations, from a healthy active lifestyle and Mediterranean diet to a not so healthy, less physically active lifestyle and a diet influenced by the Western pattern diet, has been shown to significantly increase the risk of heart disease [5–7].

E. Grossi
Scientific Department, Italian Pavillon Expo 2015, Milan, Italy
e-mail: enzo.grossi@bracco.com

© Springer International Publishing Switzerland 2016   183
E. Grossi, F. Pace (eds.), *Human Nutrition from the Gastroenterologist's Perspective*,
DOI 10.1007/978-3-319-30361-1_12

It is important to note that a paradigmatic and unique Mediterranean diet does not exist; along with evident similarities between the above listed countries, there are also important differences in their food habits.

In a somewhat reductionist approach, the traditional Mediterranean diet can be considered as a dietary pattern mainly, but not dogmatically, plant based. Of note, olive oil is a plant product (in fact a fruit juice) and so is wine.

Olive oil is part of the Mediterranean diet, although not of all Mediterranean cuisines: in Egypt, Malta, and Israel, olive oil consumption is in fact negligible, and in other areas, it is not predominant. Wine consumption is on the contrary more consistent, with the exception of populations devoted to Islam religion.

Objective data showing that Mediterranean diet is healthy originated from results of epidemiological studies carried out in Naples and Madrid [8] and confirmed later by the Seven Countries Study, with its first publication in 1970 [9], and a book-length report published in 1980 [10, 11].

An important conclusion of this study, based largely on ecological evidence, was that low content of saturated lipids in the Mediterranean diet could explain the low incidence of coronary heart disease in Mediterranean countries, through the reduction of blood cholesterol, a recognized major risk factor for this disease (the distinction between high-density lipoprotein (HDL) and low-density lipoprotein (LDL) cholesterol was not known at that time). Subsequent findings however showed unequivocally that the traditional Mediterranean diet is not simply, or mainly, a cholesterol-lowering diet, but has a range of beneficial health effects.

The strongest evidence for a beneficial health effect and decreased mortality after switching to the Mediterranean diet came later on, from the NIH-AARP Diet and Health Study [12].

Subsequently other prospective epidemiological studies showed that there was an inverse association between adherence to the Mediterranean diet and the incidence of fatal and nonfatal heart disease in initially healthy middle-aged adults in the Mediterranean region [13].

A systematic review carried out in 2011 found that Mediterranean diet is more effective than a low-fat diet in maintaining a low level of cardiovascular risk factors, such as lowering cholesterol level and blood pressure [14].

A meta-analysis published in the *British Medical Journal* (BMJ) showed that following strictly the Mediterranean diet reduces the risk of dying from cancer and cardiovascular disease as well as the risk of developing Parkinson's and Alzheimer's disease. The results report 9 %, 9 %, and 6 % reduction in overall, cardiovascular, and cancer mortality, respectively. Additionally a 13 % reduction in incidence of Parkinson's and Alzheimer's diseases is to be expected provided strict adherence to the diet is observed [15].

In 2010 another meta-analysis published in *The American Journal of Clinical Nutrition* found that the Mediterranean diet conferred a significant benefit with regard to the risk of chronic diseases, such as cardiovascular disease and cancer [16].

In 2011 an additional meta-analysis published in the *Journal of the American College of Cardiology* analyzed the results of 50 studies (35 clinical trials, 2 prospective, and 13 cross sectional) covering about 535,000 people to examine the effect of a Mediterranean diet on metabolic syndrome. The researchers reported that the adherence to the Mediterranean diet is associated with lower blood pressure, blood sugar, and triglycerides [17].

In 2014, two other meta-analyses found that adherence to a Mediterranean diet is associated with a decreased risk of type 2 diabetes [18, 19]. Another 2014 systematic review and meta-analysis found that adherence to the Mediterranean diet was associated with a decreased risk of cancer mortality [20].

The Mediterranean diet is based on what from the point of view of mainstream nutrition is considered a paradox: that although the people living in Mediterranean countries tend to consume relatively high amounts of fat, they have far lower rates of cardiovascular disease than in countries like the United States, where similar levels of fat consumption are found. A parallel phenomenon is known as the French paradox [21].

The interest on wine as potential principal effector of the Mediterranean diet starts just from this observation, since wine is the only Mediterranean element present in typical French diet.

12.2   The Role of Wine in the Mediterranean Diet

Cardiovascular disease and cancer are responsible for over two-thirds of deaths in the Western world. The society runs the risk of being unable to cope with the health costs of the pandemic, without considering of the price in terms of quality of life of people. So far the prevailing approach has been the pharmacologic one. The research has produced remarkable results in this area; however, not always drug therapies have proven up to the expectations, especially with regard to primary prevention. That's why science has begun to explore new paths, finding answers in what simply has always been under our noses, i.e., the wine.

Since the Mediterranean diet is a complex combination of healthy food components most of which have a recognized beneficial effect on human health, and since by definition all these constituents are taken simultaneously, it is very difficult to attribute a net effect to each of them. Wine component suffers for the same problem. In other words, if my diet is rich of olive oil, fruits, vegetables, fish, and wine, which is the exact merit of wine in affording benefits to my health?

The relationship between alcohol consumption and disease has been the focus of intensive scientific investigation. Most studies to date, however, have limitations. A major drawback is that limited information has been collected regarding the complex issue of alcohol consumption. In many studies, ascertainment of alcohol consumption frequently focused only on quantity of alcohol consumed without considering the main different sources of alcohol (beer, wine, spirits) and type of alcohol consumption, particularly drinking pattern. It has been hypothesized, and preliminary data support the notion that drinking pattern (i.e., before meal, during meal, or outside meal) could have important influences on determining the health effects of alcohol.

Fig. 12.1 Decomposition
of wine constituents
according to health effects

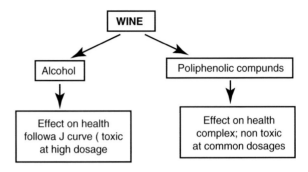

The major methodological problem is the disentangling between alcohol and wine in medical surveys, which is missing in most epidemiological studies where wine is considered just one of the possible forms of alcohol consumption. In fact in these studies, data are collected according to weekly or daily grams of alcohol irrespective of the fact if this is made only by wine, by spirit, by beer, or by a mixture. Since alcohol per se exhibits beneficial effect at low doses and toxic effect at high doses while wine polyphenols behave differently, health data coming out from these studies are conflicting and contradictory. To assess the role of wine consumption in the Mediterranean diet, we must rely on studies in which wine has been disentangled from alcohol. Figure 12.1 summarizes the complexity of wine effect on health.

A clear message emerging from scientific studies on wine and particularly red wine is that the benefit achieved is closely connected with its consumption with meals. Consumption of red wine during a fat meal significantly reduces the harmful consequences of oxidized fats, like those found in fatty foods subjected to prolonged cooking which induce the initial mechanism of atherosclerotic process. Antioxidant polyphenols present in wine combined and mixed during meal with fats reduce the oxidative state of these compounds, thus annulling the excess of potential detrimental effect before these molecules are absorbed and reach the general circulation. Interestingly enough, the Italian gastronomic tradition requires the use of red wine to accompany the succulent dishes like venison or pork, almost as if our ancestors had discovered this scientific basis from time immemorial. Wine contains various polyphenol substances which may be beneficial for health and in particular flavonols (such as myricetin and quercetin), catechin and epicatechin, proanthocyanidins, anthocyanins, various phenolic acids, and the stilbene resveratrol. In particular, resveratrol seems to play a positive effect on longevity because it increases the expression level of SIRT-1, besides its antioxidant, anti-inflammatory, and anticarcinogenic properties. Table 12.1 shows principal polyphenol constituents present in wine.

That drinking wine with meals is essential to ensure a beneficial action and is shown by a study published in 2001 by Trevisan and collaborators in which more than 15,000 adults were followed for 7 years [22]. Drinkers outside meals showed mortality rates significantly higher than the drinkers during meals. Eight thousand six hundred and forty-seven men and 6,521 women, ages 30–59 at baseline and free of cardiovascular disease, were followed for mortality from all causes,

Table 12.1 Polyphenolic compounds commonly present in the wine

	Red wine	White wine
Component	Concentration (mg/l)	
Nonflavonoids:		
Hydroxybenzoic acid	240–500	160–260
Hydroxycinnamic acid		
Stilbene (resveratrol)		
Flavonoids:		
Flavonols	750–1,060	25–30
Flavanols (tannins, proanthocyanidins) anthocyanins		
Polyphenols total content	1,200 (900–2,500)	200 (190–290)

cardiovascular, and noncardiovascular, during an average follow-up of 7 years. Drinkers of wine outside meals exhibited higher death rates from all causes, noncardiovascular diseases, and cancer, as compared to drinkers of wine with meals. This association was independent from the cardiovascular disease (CVD) risk factors measured at baseline and the amount of alcohol consumed and seemed to be stronger in women as compared to men.

This study indicates that drinking patterns may have important health implications, and attention should be given to this aspect of alcohol use and its relationship to health outcomes.

Many epidemiological studies have evaluated whether different alcoholic beverages protect against cardiovascular disease. A meta-analysis of 26 studies on the relationship between wine or beer consumption and vascular risk has been carried out by Di Castelnuovo and coworkers in 2002 [23].

General variance-based method and fitting models were applied to pooled data derived from 26 studies that gave a quantitative estimation of the vascular risk associated with either beverage consumption. From 13 studies involving 209,418 persons, the relative risk of vascular disease associated with wine intake was 0.68 (95 % confidence interval, 0.59–0.77) relative to nondrinkers. There was strong evidence from ten studies involving 176,042 persons to support a J-shaped relationship between different amounts of wine intake and vascular risk. A statistically significant inverse association was found up to a daily intake of 150 mL of wine. The overall relative risk of moderate beer consumption, which was measured in 15 studies involving 208,036 persons, was 0.78 (95 % confidence interval, 0.70–0.86). However, no significant relationship between different amounts of beer intake and vascular risk was found after meta-analyzing seven studies involving 136,382 persons. These findings show evidence of a significant inverse association between light-to-moderate wine consumption and vascular risk. A similar, although smaller association was also apparent in beer consumption studies. The latter finding, however, is difficult to interpret because no meaningful relationship could be found between different amounts of beer intake and vascular risk.

In addition to this study there are other five giant studies which merit to be mentioned. These are large epidemiological studies on wine and longevity.

Emblematic is the study conducted in Denmark by Marten Grambaek and published in the *British Medical Journal* 20 years ago [24].

The study took into account more than 20,000 people from the general population enrolled and followed for over 10 years. The subjects belonged in fact to four types of alcohol consumption: abstainers (No. 5910), mainly drinkers of beer (No. 5767), mainly drinkers of spirits (No. 3574), and mainly drinkers of wine (No. 9092).

The risk of dying steadily decreased with an increasing intake of wine, from a relative risk of 1.00 for the subject abstainers to 0.51 (95 % confidence interval 0.32–0.81) for those who drank three to five glasses of wine a day. Interestingly enough the intake of beer was associated with less reduced risk, while for spirits intake the relative risk of dying increased from 1.00 to 1.34 (1.05–1.71) for those with an intake of three to five drinks a day. The effects of the three types of alcoholic sources seemed to be independent of each other, and no significant interactions existed with sex, age, education, income, smoking, or body mass index. Wine drinking showed the same relation to risk of death from cardiovascular and cerebrovascular disease as to risk of death from all causes. Low to moderate intake of wine is associated with lower mortality from cardiovascular and cerebrovascular disease and other causes. Similar intake of spirits implied an increased risk, while beer drinking did not affect mortality.

Taking as reference the risk of mortality in the group of abstainers, mortality rates in the three groups of drinkers have completely different curves in relation to the quantity of consumption as can be seen in the Fig. 12.2. In the spirits group, moderate consumption reduces the risk of mortality, while when doses increase, the effect on longevity is negative. Beer consumption is relatively indifferent to the risk

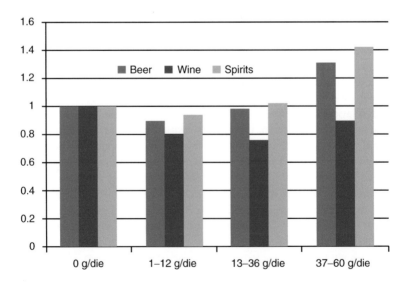

Fig. 12.2 All-cause mortality relative risk by daily intake of alcohol in the study of Grambaek

of mortality. In the wine group instead mortality reduction is already present at low consumption and reaches the maximum at three to five glasses a day.

Similar results were described by Serge Renaud in a famous study conducted in Nancy [25]. The study by Renaud deserves a special mention for the large size of the series, amounting to 36,000 males. The photograph of the same subject after 5 years from the first observation showed a different trend in mortality rates according to different types of alcoholic beverages. Always keeping the abstainers as a reference group, a daily consumption of wine in moderate amounts (up to four glasses per day) was associated with significantly lower mortality rates, with a nadir of 30 % reduction in mortality at a consumption of two to three glasses per day. At equivalent grams of daily alcohol intake, beer consumption associated with the wine minimized the wine's protective effect, while the consumption of beer only in moderate amounts gave rise to a slight increase of mortality rates, although not statistically significant.

The really supergiant study is the EPIC study. The European Prospective Investigation into Cancer and Nutrition (EPIC) is a consortium which has originated one of the largest cohort studies in the world, with more than half a million (521,000) participants recruited across ten European countries and followed for almost 15 years. EPIC was designed to investigate the relationships between diet, nutritional status, lifestyle and environmental factors, and the incidence of cancer and other chronic diseases. EPIC investigators are active in all fields of epidemiology, and important contributions have been made in nutritional epidemiology using biomarker analysis and questionnaire information, as well as genetic and lifestyle investigations.

In this large European prospective study, the association between alcohol use and overall and cause-specific risk of death was evaluated in eight European populations. When accounting for potential confounding factors, average lifetime alcohol use was strongly associated with overall mortality, whereas lifetime never alcohol users consistently displayed a higher risk of death compared with moderate drinkers [26].

More specifically lifetime average alcohol use was strongly associated with total mortality, in that never and heavy drinkers ($\geq$30 g/day) had notably higher mortality rates than did light-to-moderate drinkers (0.1–4.9 g/day), a pattern that was consistently apparent among female and male study participants. The hazard ratio (HR) comparing never and heavy drinkers with moderate drinkers in women was 1.26 (95 % CI 1.18–1.35) and 1.27 (1.13–1.43), respectively. The corresponding HRs among men were 1.29 (1.10–1.51) for never drinkers, 1.15 (1.06–1.24) for heavy drinkers, and 1.53 (1.39–1.68) for extreme drinkers ($\geq$60 g/day). When disentangling wine from other alcoholic beverages, an interesting trend emerges from this study. Abstainers showed an absolute risk of overall mortality 30 % higher than wine drinkers in moderation (from 3 to 10 g alcohol daily) and only 3 % higher than beer drinkers in moderation (from 3 to 10 g alcohol daily).

Another important study is Moli-sani, performed in Italy and still running [27]. The data of this important epidemiological study cohort clearly shows that the Mediterranean diet and especially the wine consumed in moderation reduce the risk of cardiovascular events, cerebrovascular, and neurodegenerative diseases and significantly decrease total mortality. Great benefits have been demonstrated not only in the field of primary prevention but also in patients already affected by a previous event or at high cardiovascular risk. In type 2 diabetes, for example, the wine consumed in moderation as part of the Mediterranean-type diet was effective in reducing the risk of death or in the incidence of new cardiac events. The path is not without difficulties, because prevention means waiting a long time to get concrete results. But the improvement in lifestyle, especially of wine that we consume every day at the table, must remain the first soil in which to germinate a serious intention about prevention.

The fifth giant study comes from Norway [28]. The aim of this study was to investigate some of these key issues related to the association between alcohol consumption and AMI risk, including the strength and shape of the association in a low-drinking setting, the roles of quantity, frequency and beverage type, the importance of confounding by medical and psychiatric conditions, and the lack of prospective data on previous drinking. In this population-based prospective cohort study of 58,827 community-dwelling individuals followed for 11.6 years, the quantity and frequency of consumption of beer, wine, and spirits at baseline in 1995–1997 and the frequency of alcohol intake approximately 10 years earlier were assessed. A total of 2,966 study participants had an AMI during the follow-up period. Light-to-moderate alcohol consumption was inversely and linearly associated with AMI risk. At variance with Danish study, wine drinkers showed a protective pattern similar to spirits and beer drinking. After adjusting for major cardiovascular disease risk factors, the hazard ratio for a one-drink increment in daily consumption was 0.72 (95 % confidence interval 0.62–0.86). Accounting for former drinking or comorbidities had almost no effect on the association. Frequency of alcohol consumption was more strongly associated with lower AMI risk than overall quantity consumed. Light-to-moderate alcohol consumption was linearly associated with a decreased risk of AMI in a population in which abstaining from alcohol is not socially stigmatized. The results suggest that frequent alcohol consumption is most cardioprotective and that this association is not driven by misclassification of former drinkers.

Table 12.2 summarizes the results obtained in these giant studies in terms of relative risk of mortality.

12.3   Wine, Mediterranean Diet, and Alzheimer's

Cognitive decline and dementia are major public health concerns in modern societies since increase lifespan has resulted in an increasing frequency of these age-related diseases. Since there is no specific treatment for these disorders, preventive

Table 12.2 An example of alcohol intake coming from different sources in three subjects

Subject	Wine (glasses daily)	Beer (glasses daily)	Spirits (drinks/ weekly)	Weekly alcohol intake
1	3	0	0	30
2	0	2	2	30
3	0	0	4	30

The total alcohol intake is the same, but the biological effect is completely different

Table 12.3 Relative risk of mortality related to moderate alcohol consumption from different sources, in selected prospective epidemiological studies

Author	Population on study	Wine	Beer	Spirits
Grombaek (1995)	20,000	0.6	0.9	1
Di Castelnuovo (2002)	209,418	0.68	0.78	n.d
Renaud (2004)	36,000	0.6	n.d	n.d
EPIC study (2014)	380,395	0.71	0.93	n.d
Bonaccio (2015)	20,000	0.69	n.d	n.d
Gemes (2015)	59,000	0.7	0.7	0.7

measures should be used to delay their onset. Healthy lifestyle habits have been considered crucial in reducing the risk of these diseases. Mediterranean diet and its main food components, including red wine, have been extensively studied in relation with occurrence of cognitive decline and Alzheimer's disease (Table 12.3).

Prospective studies have shown that the incidence of senile dementia or Alzheimer's in moderate wine drinkers (three to four drinks per day) is in fact much lower than nondrinkers (occasional consumption) and also the light consumers (one to two glasses a day). I refer to the study of Mehlig published in 2008 [29] in which, thanks to a follow-up of 34 years, a reduced risk of Alzheimer's disease by 40 % has been demonstrated, a value that today no drug is able to provide. The objective of this study was to assess the association between different types of alcoholic beverages and 34-year incidence of dementia. Among a random sample of 1,462 women aged 38–60 years and living in Göteborg, Sweden, in 1968–1969, 164 cases of dementia were diagnosed by 2002. At baseline as well as in 1974–1975, 1980–1981, and 1992–1993, the frequency of alcohol intake, as well as other lifestyle and health factors, was recorded and related to dementia with Cox proportional hazard regression, by the use of both baseline and updated covariates.

Wine was protective for dementia (hazard ratio (HR)=0.6, 95 % confidence interval (CI), 0.4, 0.8) in the updated model, and the association was strongest among women who consumed wine only (HR=0.3, 95 % CI, 0.1, 0.8). This is interesting since Alzheimer's disease occurs more frequently in women. After stratification by smoking, the protective association of wine was stronger among smokers. In contrast, consumption of spirits at baseline was associated with slightly increased risk of dementia (HR=1.5, 95 % CI, 1.0, 2.2). Results show that wine and spirits displayed opposing associations with dementia. Because a protective effect was not seen for the other beverages, at least part of the association for wine may be explained by components other than ethanol.

Another interesting study has been carried out by Orgogozo and coworkers in the area of Bordeaux [30]. The authors prospectively studied 3,777 community residents aged 65 and over, in the districts of Gironde and Dordogne. Average daily alcoholic consumption was recorded at baseline. Incident cases of dementia and Alzheimer's disease were screened at follow-up with explicit criteria. At 3 years, 2,273 subjects not demented at baseline were still available for follow-up. Wine was the only alcoholic beverage reported by more than 95 % of regular drinkers. In the 318 subjects drinking three to four standard glasses per day (>250 and up to 500 ml), categorized as moderate drinkers, the crude odds ratio (OR) was 0.18 for incident dementia ($p<0.01$) and 0.25 for Alzheimer's disease ($p<0.03$), as compared to the 971 nondrinkers. After adjusting for age, sex, education, occupation, baseline MMSE, and other possible confounders, the ORs were, respectively, 0.19 ($p<0.01$) and 0.28 ($p<0.05$). In the 922 mild drinkers (<1–2 glasses per day), there was a negative association only with AD, after adjustment (OR=0.55; $p<0.05$). The inverse relationship between moderate wine drinking and incident dementia was explained neither by known predictors of dementia nor by medical, psychological, or socio-familial factors. Considering also the well-documented negative associations between moderate wine consumption and cardiovascular morbidity and mortality in this age group, it seems that there is no medical rationale to advise people over 65 to quit drinking wine moderately, as this habit carries no specific risk and may even be of some benefit for their health.

Data from large observational studies have suggested that increasing adherence to Mediterranean-type diets relates to better cognitive function and a reduced risk of dementia. In addition, randomized feeding trials, such as the PREDIMED trial (Prevención con Dieta Mediterránea), have demonstrated with the highest level of scientific evidence that an increased adherence to traditional Mediterranean diet is associated with improved cognitive function. When the role of the different foods included in the Mediterranean diet was analyzed, the authors observed that the participants with better cognitive function were those with higher consumption of wine, extra-virgin olive oil, coffee, and walnuts, all foods very rich in polyphenols [31].

Red wine is a food very rich in polyphenols, but that also contains alcohol (ethanol). Alcohol by itself has also been postulated to act as neuroprotective factor though different mechanisms. In this context, several case-control and cohort studies have analyzed the effects of different alcoholic beverages on cognitive function and incidence of Alzheimer's disease and concluded that moderate alcohol consumption is associated with a reduced risk of developing cognitive decline and dementia. However, several other studies have observed that moderate wine consumption (an average of 1.5 glasses a day) can be more effective in slowing down age-related cognitive decline [32–34]. This higher effect of red wine compared to other alcoholic beverages has been attributed to high polyphenol content. Part of protective effects of polyphenols contained in red wine has been attributed to a scavenging activity and an activation of SIRT-1, among others.

Based on these statistics, it is estimated that if every American drank two glasses of wine a day, cardiovascular disease, which accounts for almost 50 % of deaths in this population, could be reduced by 40 % and could be saved every year by 40 billion [35].

12.4 Biological Mechanisms of the Protective Effect of Wine: The Role of the Gastrointestinal Tract

But what are the biological mechanisms of this extraordinary protective effect played by wine? The moderate amount of alcohol present in the wine exerts a number of biological effects whose positivity or negativity depends on the dose taken.

The alcohol in low doses exerts beneficial effects on digestion, stimulating pancreatic secretion, for example, and on vascular function, thanks to a vasodilation action. When the dose of alcohol exceeds a certain threshold, the negative effects prevail over the positive ones. Fortunately the alcohol intake through the wine in moderate amounts is relatively far from the dangerous threshold.

As mentioned before are actually the phenolic components of the wine to be fundamental in the beneficial action because they have the property of exerting antioxidant activities neutralizing oxygen-free radicals, which in turn are responsible for cumulative damage to cells that lead to chronic degenerative disease, as is widely demonstrated in experiments conducted in the laboratory. The so-called antioxidant effect played by wine polyphenols is however extremely complex in vivo.

One of the mechanisms by which polyphenols exert these effects appears to be a direct action on gene expression of enzymes of the cycle of reduced glutathione, a key constituent in the systems of cell protection from damage by oxygen-free radicals.

Recently a new theory has been proposed by Forman and coworkers and merits to be mentioned [36]. According to these authors, the notion of hormesis underscores the fact that a compound toxic at high doses can be health protecting below a threshold, eventually leading to the apparent paradox that a low dose of a toxic compound is more healthy than abstention. A paradigmatic case is that of alcohol, the moderate consumption of which is more protective than abstention in respect to the risk of cardiovascular diseases, neurodegenerations, inflammatory diseases, and total mortality. Wine at variance provides also a series of phytochemicals extending the hormetic effect of alcohol. In other words, wine is by far more protective than alcohol, and the reversion point from protection to a harmful effect is shifted at higher doses probably not reachable in real life. Mechanistically, these concepts are framed in the modern view of diseases where damage evolves from an excess of response to injury. Here several phytochemicals present in wine (as in some fruits and vegetables) contribute to maintenance of an optimized inflammatory/anti-inflammatory balance. Pathways of inflammation usually adopt electrophiles (oxidants) as signal transducers, while the counteracting feedback responses are primed by nucleophiles (antioxidants). As usual in biology, the primary events activate the feedback, i.e., electrophiles are competent for the activation of the nucleophilic response. Fruit, vegetables, and mainly wine provide a major source of nutritional antioxidants (nucleophiles), but kinetic and metabolic constraints do not permit the direct antioxidant effect in vivo, unsuccessfully searched in the last decades. These compounds, instead, give rise by autoxidation to minute amounts of electrophiles (oxidants) in turn competent for the activation of the nucleophilic (antioxidant) anti-inflammatory response. Ursini named this mechanism para-hormesis since the increased defense is primed by a fake damage. In conclusion the "black swan" case of the health-protective effect of alcohol is untangled on the light of hormesis, while the evidence that wine does it much better is a para-hormetic effect, where components of wine switch on the nucleophilic defense mechanisms just by mimicking the signal of oxidants. The prohibitionist recommendation, therefore, to abstain from any intake of alcohol and wine, besides nonsupported by epidemiology, is also rejected by basic science evidence as it prevents a useful boost of the capacity of optimally dealing with stress. A little or, better, a fake harm trains you to become stronger.

Beyond the known antioxidant effects, of which however there is still a considerable debate on the real size of this mechanism in vivo, the presence of polyphenols and in particular of resveratrol seems to express a significant protective effect on the health status through the activation of particular substances, sirtuins, powerful control systems of the stability of DNA, which inter alia are activated by caloric restriction. Eat little influences positively longevity as has been amply demonstrated in experimental studies on various animal species.

12.5   The Role of Microbiota

The human gut microbiota is now recognized as an important regulator of human health and comprises of thousands of different microbial species [37]. These microorganisms interact closely with their human host through immune cross talk and at the metabolic level. Indeed, small microbial-derived metabolites like short-chain fatty acids (SCFA) and small phenolic acids have recently been proven to play a regulatory role in diverse host physiological processes including energy intake and storage, immune homeostasis, gene expression and epigenetics, and even brain development and cognitive function [38]. These metabolites derive largely from the action of the gut microbiota on the foods we eat. In particular, microbial fermentation of nondigestible carbohydrates leads to the production of SCFA, and the gut microbiota converts complex plant polyphenols into biologically available and often biologically active derivatives. Similarly, the foods we eat, especially the amounts and types of carbohydrates and plant-derived foods, appear to determine the community structure and diversity of the gut microbiota. Indeed, these two food constituents, fiber and plant polyphenols, can be considered the chemical cornerstones of the Mediterranean diet, a dietary pattern closely associated with both physical and mental health-related quality of life [39]. Astonishingly, recent dietary interventions in humans have shown not only can red wine impact on the flow of metabolites from the gut and the gut microbiota but can actually change the relative abundance of important groups of gut bacteria. In particular, Queiopo-Ortuño et al. [40] showed that moderate consumption of red wine or dealcoholized red wine increased the relative abundance of potentially health-promoting bacteria, including those involved in fiber degradation and the production of the beneficial SCFA butyrate, but also notably, bifidobacteria, organisms long associated with human health and often used as probiotics (Fig. 12.3).

In parallel, they also reported small but significant improvements in blood markers of inflammation and lipid metabolism, even in this small group of health subjects ($n = 10$). They later showed that this increase in intestinal bifidobacteria was associated with reduced plasma lipopolysaccharide (LPS) [41], a microbiota derived cell wall fragment, which causes systemic inflammation when it leaks from the gut and is associated with increased risk of metabolic syndrome and type 2 diabetes [42]. Such studies highlight the potential of wine as a modulator of the human gut microbiota and their metabolic output, with potential to act on host physiology both within the gut and systemically.

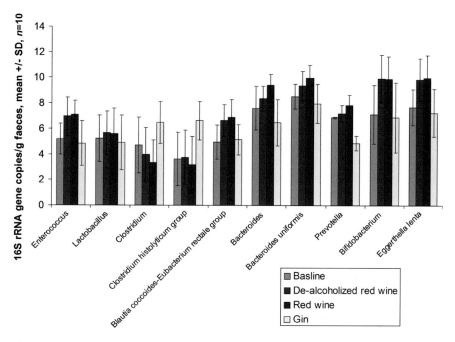

Fig. 12.3 Modulation of human gut microbiota by dealcoholized red wine, red wine, and gin

Another interesting study comes from the group of María Isabel Queipo-Ortuno [40]. Here ten healthy male volunteers underwent a randomized, crossover, controlled intervention study. After a washout period, all of the subjects received red wine, the equivalent amount of dealcoholized red wine, or gin for 20 days each. The dominant bacterial composition did not remain constant over the different intake periods. Compared with baseline, the daily consumption of red wine polyphenol for 4 weeks significantly increased the number of *Enterococcus, Prevotella, Bacteroides, Bifidobacterium, Bacteroides uniformis, Eggerthella lenta,* and *Blautia coccoides-Eubacterium rectale* groups ($P < 0.05$). In parallel, systolic and diastolic blood pressures and triglyceride, total cholesterol, HDL cholesterol, and C-reactive protein concentrations decreased significantly ($P < 0.05$). Moreover, changes in cholesterol and C-reactive protein concentrations were linked to changes in the bifidobacteria number. This study showed that red wine consumption can significantly modulate the growth of select gut microbiota in humans, which suggests possible prebiotic benefits associated with the inclusion of red wine polyphenols in the diet.

12.6   Interference on Lipid Absorption

Beyond antioxidant activity and prebiotic effect, another biological mechanism related to wine is the potential interference played by wine polyphenols on the mechanisms inherent to lipid absorption. In fact although the cardioprotective effect of red wine has been attributed to its polyphenolic content, presently, very little is known about the mechanisms by which these compounds benefit the cardiovascular system. Pal and coworker have tried to elucidate whether red wine polyphenols attenuate the synthesis and secretion of pro-atherogenic chylomicrons from intestinal cells. Apolipoprotein B48 levels (a marker of intestinal chylomicrons), quantitated by Western blotting, were significantly reduced by 30 % in cultured CaCo-2 cells and medium when cells were incubated with either dealcoholized red wine, alcoholized red wine, or atorvastatin compared with controls. Intracellular cholesterol availability was also attenuated in cells incubated with dealcoholized red wine (72.5 %), alcoholized red wine (81.5 %), and atorvastatin (83.5 %) compared to control cells. Collectively, this study suggests that red wine polyphenolics downregulate the production of pro-atherogenic chylomicrons from intestinal cells, which may explain the reduced CVD mortality rates following its consumption [43].

Chylomicrons act also as transporters of gram-negative bacteria beyond intestinal mucosa in the bloodstream. This bacterial translocation implies the systemic spread of wall LPS, a potent pro-inflammatory molecule at picogram level, with a number of cascade events potentially harmful. This interference of chylomicron formation can be considered a neglected source of protection from subclinical inflammation exerted by wine.

Another interesting clue derives from a study of the same group to elucidate whether the acute consumption of red wine polyphenolic compounds regulates lipid and lipoprotein metabolism in dyslipidemic postmenopausal women [44]. Eight dyslipidemic postmenopausal women each consumed a mixed meal accompanied by either water, dealcoholized red wine, or alcoholic red wine on three separate visits, in a random order, 2 weeks apart. One fasting and six hourly postmeal blood samples were taken and analyzed for plasma apolipoprotein B48 (apoB48; specific marker of chylomicrons (CM) and their remnants (CMR)); total, LDL and HDL cholesterol; triglycerides (TAG); and insulin and glucose at each time point. There was a decrease in postprandial apoB48 levels after alcoholic and nonalcoholic red wine consumption compared to water. Red wine attenuates postprandial CM and CMR levels in plasma, possibly by delaying the absorption of dietary fat, as suggested by a decrease in plasma apoB48 levels. The reduction of postprandial lipoproteins in circulation after red wine consumption may partly explain the low cardiovascular mortality rates among the French.

12.7 Summary and Final Thoughts

The prospective studies carried out in general population and reviewed in this chapter demonstrate that wine intake has a beneficial effect on all-cause mortality that is additive to that of alcohol. Wine contains various polyphenolic substances which may be beneficial for health and in particular flavonols (such as myricetin and quercetin), catechin and epicatechin, proanthocyanidins, anthocyanins, various phenolic acids, and the stilbene resveratrol. Moderate wine drinking is part of the Mediterranean diet, together with abundant and variable plant foods, high consumption of cereals, olive oil as the main (added) fat, and a low intake of (red) meat. This healthy diet pattern involves a "Mediterranean way of drinking" that is a regular, moderate wine consumption mainly with food (up to two glasses a day for men and one glass for women). Moderate wine drinking increases longevity, reduces the risk of cardiovascular diseases, and does not appreciably influence the overall risk of cancer.

Even if this examination of the scientific evidence is probably incomplete, we can say that the body of evidence of the beneficial effects of wine on health is substantial and growing. The most compelling evidence concerns protection from cardiovascular diseases and neurodegenerative diseases, which also constitute the leading cause of death in the Western world. Further studies are needed to determine the role of wine in protecting the metabolic diseases and cancer, but there are findings indicating that even here the effects may be important. The anti-inflammatory effect described in the last section of this chapter is particularly relevant in this regard.

EXPO 2015 has provided a stimulus to increase the appreciation of what really the wine is representing for human health and to promote in the world the Italian wine culture that sees this product not as a simple drink, but in fact as true and own food, essential constituent of the Mediterranean diet, and probably the most important effector of its benefits.

References

1. Keys A, Keys M (1959) Eat well & stay well; foreword by Paul Dudley White. Doubleday & C., Garden City, NY
2. UNESCO – culture – intangible heritage – lists & register – inscribed elements – Mediterranean Diet 2013. http://www.unesco.org/culture/ich/en/8com.
3. Dahlöf B (2010) Cardiovascular disease risk factors: epidemiology and risk assessment. Am J Cardiol 105(1 Suppl):3A–9A
4. Williams MA, Haskell WL, Ades PA, Amsterdam EA, Bittner V, Franklin BA, Gulanick M, Laing ST, Stewart KJ (2007) Resistance exercise in individuals with and without cardiovascular disease: 2007 update: a scientific statement from the American Heart Association Council on Clinical Cardiology and Council on Nutrition, Physical Activity, and Metabolism. Circulation 116(5):572–584
5. Vardavas CI, Linardakis MK, Hatzis CM, Saris WH, Kafatos AG (2010) Cardiovascular disease risk factors and dietary habits of farmers from Crete 45 years after the first description of the Mediterranean diet. Eur J Cardiovasc Prev Rehabil 17(4):440–446
6. Kafatos A, Diacatou A, Voukiklaris G, Nikolakakis N, Vlachonikolis J, Kounali D, Mamalakis G, Dontas AS (1997) Heart disease risk-factor status and dietary changes in the Cretan population over the past 30 y: the Seven Countries Study. Am J Clin Nutr 65(6):1882–1886
7. Menotti A, Keys A, Kromhout D, Blackburn H, Aravanis C, Bloemberg B, Buzina R, Dontas A, Fidanza F, Giampaoli S et al (1993) Inter-cohort differences in coronary heart disease mortality in the 25-year follow-up of the seven countries study. Eur J Epidemiol 9(5):527–536
8. Marques da Silva AJ (2015) La diète méditerranéenne. Discours et pratiques alimentaires en Méditerranée, vol 2. L'Harmattan, Paris, pp 52–54. ISBN 978-2-343-06151-1
9. Ancel Keys (ed) (1970) Coronary heart disease in seven countries. Circulation 41(4 Suppl):I1–211. doi:10.1161/01.CIR.41.4S1.I-1
10. Ancel Keys (ed) (1980) Seven countries: a multivariate analysis of death and coronary heart disease. Harvard University Press, Cambridge, MA, ISBN 0 674 80237 3

11. Keys A, Arvanis C, Blackburn H (1980) Seven countries: a multivariate analysis of death and coronary heart disease. Harvard University Press, Cambridge, MA, p 381

12. Mitrou PN, Kipnis V, Thiébaut AC, Reedy J, Subar AF, Wirfält E, Flood A, Mouw T, Hollenbeck AR, Leitzmann MF, Schatzkin A (2007) Mediterranean dietary pattern and prediction of all-cause mortality in a US population: results from the NIH-AARP Diet and Health Study. Arch Intern Med 167(22):2461–2468. doi:10.1001/archinte.167.22.2461

13. Martínez-González MA, García-López M, Bes-Rastrollo M, Toledo E, Martínez-Lapiscina EH, Delgado-Rodriguez M, Vazquez Z, Benito S, Beunza JJ (2011) Mediterranean diet and the incidence of cardiovascular disease: a Spanish cohort. Nutr Metab Cardiovasc Dis. 21(4):237–44.

14. Nordmann AJ, Suter-Zimmermann K, Bucher HC, Shai I, Tuttle KR, Estruch R, Briel M (2011) Meta-analysis comparing Mediterranean to low-fat diets for modification of cardiovascular risk factors. Am J Med 124(9):841–851.e2. doi:10.1016/j.amjmed.2011.04.024

15. Sofi F, Cesari F, Abbate R, Gensini GF, Casini A (2008) Adherence to Mediterranean diet and health status: meta-analysis. BMJ (Clin Res Ed) 337(sep11 2):a1344. doi:10.1136/bmj.a1344. PMC2533524

16. Sofi F, Abbate R, Gensini GF, Casini A (2010) Accruing evidence on benefits of adherence to the Mediterranean diet on health: an updated systematic review and meta-analysis. Am J Clin Nutr 92(5):1189–1196. doi:10.3945/ajcn.2010.29673

17. Kastorini C-M, Milionis H, Esposito K, Giugliano D, Goudevenos J, Panagiotakos D (2011) The effect of Mediterranean diet on metabolic syndrome and its components. J Am Coll Cardiol 57(11):1299–1313. doi:10.1016/j.jacc.2010.09.073

18. Schwingshackl L, Missbach B, König J, Hoffmann G (2014) Adherence to a Mediterranean diet and risk of diabetes: a systematic review and meta-analysis. Public Health Nutr 18:1–8. doi:10.1017/S1368980014001542

19. Koloverou E, Esposito K, Giugliano D, Panagiotakos D (2014) The effect of Mediterranean diet on the development of type 2 diabetes mellitus: a meta-analysis of 10 prospective studies and 136,846 participants. Metab Clin Exp 63(7):903–911. doi:10.1016/j.metabol.2014.04.010

20. Schwingshackl L, Hoffmann G (2014) Adherence to Mediterranean diet and risk of cancer: a systematic review and meta-analysis of observational studies. Int J Cancer J Int Cancer 135(8):1884–1897. doi:10.1002/ijc.28824

21. Simini B (2000) Serge Renaud: from French paradox to Cretan miracle. Lancet 355(9197):48. doi:10.1016/S0140-6736(05)71990-5

22. Trevisan M, Schisterman E, Mennotti A, Farchi G, Conti S, Risk Factor And Life Expectancy Research Group (2001) Drinking pattern and mortality: the Italian Risk Factor and Life Expectancy pooling project. Ann Epidemiol 11(5):312–319

23. Di Castelnuovo A, Rotondo S, Iacoviello L, Donati MB, De Gaetano G (2002) Meta-analysis of wine and beer consumption in relation to vascular risk. Circulation 105(24):2836–2844

24. Grønbaek M, Deis A, Sørensen TI, Becker U, Schnohr P, Jensen G (1995) Mortality associated with moderate intakes of wine, beer, or spirits. BMJ 310(6988):1165–1169

25. Renaud S, Lanzmann-Petithory D, Gueguen R, Conard P (2004) Alcohol and mortality from all causes. Biol Res 37(2):183–187

26. Ferrari P, Licaj I, Muller DC et al (2014) Lifetime alcohol use and overall and cause-specific mortality in the European Prospective Investigation into Cancer and nutrition (EPIC) study. BMJ Open 4:e005245. doi:10.1136/bmjopen-2014-005245

27. Bonaccio M, Di Castelnuovo A, Costanzo S, Persichillo M, De Curtis A, Donati MB, de Gaetano G, Iacoviello L; on behalf of the MOLI-SANI study Investigators (2015) Eur J Prev Cardiol. pii: 2047487315569409. [Epub ahead of print]

28. Gemes K, Janszky I, Laugsand LE, Laszlo KD, Ahnve S, Vatten LJ, Mukamal KJ (2015) Alcohol consumption is associated with a lower incidence of acute myocardial infarction: results from a large prospective population-based study in Norway. J Intern Med. doi:10.1111/joim.12428

29. Mehlig K, Skoog I, Guo X, Schütze M, Gustafson D, Waern M, Ostling S, Björkelund C, Lissner L (2008) Alcoholic beverages and incidence of dementia: 34-year follow-up of the

prospective population study of women in Goteborg. Am J Epidemiol 167(6):684–691. doi:10.1093/aje/kwm366, Epub 2008 Jan 24
30. Orgogozo JM, Dartigues JF, Lafont S, Letenneur L, Commenges D, Salamon R, Renaud S, Breteler MB (1997) Wine consumption and dementia in the elderly: a prospective community study in the Bordeaux area. Rev Neurol (Paris) 153(3):185–192
31. Estruch R, Ros E, Salas-Salvadó J, Covas MI, Corella D, Arós F, Gómez-Gracia E, Ruiz-Gutiérrez V, Fiol M, Lapetra J, Lamuela-Raventos RM, Serra-Majem L, Pintó X, Basora J, Muñoz MA, Sorlí JV, Martínez JA, Martínez-González MA, PREDIMED Study Investigators (2013) Primary prevention of cardiovascular disease with a Mediterranean diet. N Engl J Med 368(14):1279–1290
32. Valls-Pedret C, Sala-Vila A, Serra-Mir M, Corella D, de la Torre R, Martínez-González MÁ, Martínez-Lapiscina EH, Fitó M, Pérez-Heras A, Salas-Salvadó J, Estruch R, Ros E (2015) Mediterranean diet and Age-related cognitive decline: a randomized clinical trial. JAMA Intern Med 175(7):1094–1103
33. Valls-Pedret C, Lamuela-Raventós RM, Medina-Remón A, Quintana M, Corella D, Pintó X, Martínez-González MÁ, Estruch R, Ros E (2012) Polyphenol-rich foods in the Mediterranean diet are associated with better cognitive function in elderly subjects at high cardiovascular risk. J Alzheimers Dis 29(4):773–782
34. Nooyens AC, Bueno-de-Mesquita HB, van Gelder BM, van Boxtel MP, Verschuren WM (2014) Consumption of alcoholic beverages and cognitive decline at middle age: the Doetinchem Cohort Study. Br J Nutr 111(4):715–723
35. Goldberg D (1995) Does wine work? Clin Chem 41:14–16
36. Forman HJ, Davies KJ, Ursini F (2014) How do nutritional antioxidants really work: nucleophilic tone and para-hormesis versus free radical scavenging in vivo. Free Radic Biol Med 66:24–35. doi:10.1016/j.freeradbiomed.2013.05.045.Epub
37. Marchesi JR, Adams DH, Fava F, Hermes GD, Hirschfield GM, Hold G, Quraishi MN, Kinross J, Smidt H, Tuohy KM, Thomas LV, Zoetendal EG, Hart A (2015) The gut microbiota and host health: a new clinical frontier. Gut. doi:10.1136/gutjnl-2015-309990
38. Tuohy KM, Conterno L, Gasperotti M, Viola R (2012) Up-regulating the human intestinal microbiome using whole plant foods, polyphenols, and/or fiber. J Agric Food Chem 60(36):8776–8782
39. Bonaccio M, Di Castelnuovo A, Bonanni A, Costanzo S, De Lucia F, Pounis G, Zito F, Donati MB, de Gaetano G, Iacoviello L, Moli-sani project Investigators* (2013) Adherence to a Mediterranean diet is associated with a better health-related quality of life: a possible role of high dietary antioxidant content. BMJ Open 3(8). doi:10.1136/bmjopen-2013-003003, pii: e003003
40. Queipo-Ortuño MI, Boto-Ordóñez M, Murri M, Gomez-Zumaquero JM, Clemente-Postigo M, Estruch R, Cardona Diaz F, Andrés-Lacueva C, Tinahones FJ (2012) Influence of red wine polyphenols and ethanol on the gut microbiota ecology and biochemical biomarkers. Am J Clin Nutr 95(6):1323–1334
41. Clemente-Postigo M, Queipo-Ortuño MI, Boto-Ordoñez M, Coin-Aragüez L, Roca-Rodriguez MM, Delgado-Lista J, Cardona F, Andres-Lacueva C, Tinahones FJ (2013) Effect of acute and chronic red wine consumption on lipopolysaccharide concentrations. Am J Clin Nutr 97(5):1053–1061
42. Cani PD, Amar J, Iglesias MA, Poggi M, Knauf C, Bastelica D, Neyrinck AM, Fava F, Tuohy KM, Chabo C, Waget A, Delmee E, Cousin B, Sulpice T, Chamontin B, Ferrieres J, Tanti JF, Gibson GR, Casteilla L, Delzenne NM, Alessi MC, Burcelin R (2007) Metabolic endotoxemia initiates obesity and insulin resistance. Diabetes 56(7):1761–1772
43. Pal S, Ho SS, Takechi R (2005) Red wine polyphenolics suppress the secretion of ApoB48 from human intestinal CaCo-2 cells. J Agric Food Chem 53(7):2767–2772
44. Pal S, Naissides M, Mamo J (2004) Polyphenolics and fat absorption. Int J Obes Relat Metab Disord 28(2):324–326

Why Overweight/Obesity Leads to GERD

13

Fabio Pace and Marina Pace

13.1 Introduction

During the last three decades, two coincidental epidemiological trends have been observed in westernized countries and, to a lesser extent, in the rest of the world, namely, an increase in the rate of overweight/obese people [1] and an increase in the prevalence of gastroesophageal reflux (GERD) [2] (Fig. 13.1).

Obesity is at present so ubiquitous that the WHO has created the term "globesity" [3] to emphasize the global relevance of this health threat. GERD, although less relevant for health systems, has a great impact in terms of medical costs and reduction of quality of life for patients, in particular when symptoms are severe and/or frequent [4].

The aims of this chapter are to review the epidemiological and physiopathological data connecting causally the two phenomena, to assess whether overweight/obese people with GERD respond to anti-reflux therapy differently compared with lean or normal-weight persons, and to describe the effect of losing weight on GERD symptoms and lesions in obese GERD patients.

13.2 Epidemiology of Obesity and GERD

Obesity, typically defined as a body mass index (BMI) of >30, has risen in epidemic proportions in many countries worldwide [5]. In the United States, since the mid-1970s, the prevalence of overweight and obesity has increased sharply for both

F. Pace (✉)
UOC di Gastroenterologia ed Endoscopia Digestiva, ASST Bergamo Est, Seriate, BG, Italy

Bolognini Hospital, Seriate, BG, Italy
e-mail: fabio.pace@unimi.it

M. Pace
Department of Pediatrics, Buzzi Hospital, Milan, Italy

© Springer International Publishing Switzerland 2016
E. Grossi, F. Pace (eds.), *Human Nutrition from the Gastroenterologist's Perspective*,
DOI 10.1007/978-3-319-30361-1_13

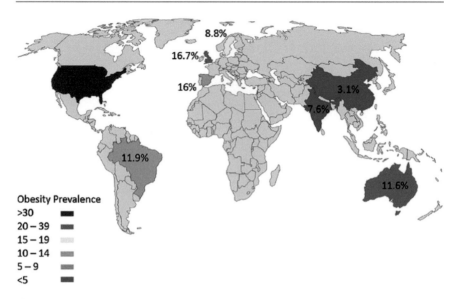

Fig. 13.1 World map of obesity and GERD prevalence in select countries. The obesity prevalence coded by the color key. The percentages indicate the GERD prevalence (From Ref. [55], with permission)

adults and children; for example, data from two NHANES surveys show that among adults aged 20–74 years, the prevalence of obesity has increased from 15.0 % (1976–1980) to 32.9 % (2003–2004) [6, 7] and up to 34.9 % in 2012 [8].

Although the causes are uncertain, the two most relevant causes (the "Big Two") are environmental changes, such as food marketing practices and technology (e.g., increased food availability, larger serving size, increased availability of fattening dietary items), and the marked reduction in physical activity. The exclusive focus on the Big Two, whose importance is accepted as established, has probably hampered the scientific recognition of other putative factors, and this might in turn compromise many proposals for reducing obesity rates. Interestingly, a recent narrative review has focused on a list of ten putative potential factors which may contribute to the increasing prevalence of obesity [9]. These ten putative factors are (1) increase in sleep debt; (2) increase in the food chain of endocrine disruptors, e.g., lipophilic, environmentally stable, industrially produced substances that can affect endocrine function (such as, e.g., DDT); (3) increase in time spent in the thermoneutral zone, which is the range of ambient temperature in which energy expenditure is not required for homeothermy; (4) increased use of drugs favoring weight gain, such as psychotropic medications (antipsychotics, antidepressants, mood stabilizers), anticonvulsants, antidiabetics, antihypertensives, steroid hormones and contraceptives, antihistamines, and protease inhibitors; (5) changes in distribution of ethnicity and age (in particular in the United States) leading to an increase in some age and ethnic groups who have higher prevalence of obesity than others (e.g., Africans and Hispanics); (6) increasing *gravida* age, since it is proven that greater gravida age increases risk of offspring obesity; (7) intrauterine and intergenerational effects (specifically, maternal obesity and resulting diabetes during gestation and lactation may promote the same conditions in subsequent generations); (8) decreased smoking habit; (9) greater reproductive fitness by people with greater BMI yielding selection for obesity-predisposing genotypes; and (10) a "floor" effect on BMI, e.g., an increased diffusion of factors which prevent most people from becoming thin.

In 2014 a large epidemiological survey conducted worldwide on GERD prevalence and incidence has shown that the prevalence of GERD has increased significantly when comparing studies conducted before 1995 with those published after this year. Current estimates of prevalence range from 18.1 % to 27.8 % in the United States, 8.8–25.9 % in Europe, 2.5–7.8 % in East Asia, 8.7–33.1 % in the Middle East, 11.6 % in Australia, and 23.0 % in South America [2]. Thus, GERD represents a very common medical problem in vast areas of the world.

13.3 Positive Association Between Obesity and GERD

The positive and strong relationship between obesity and GERD has been demonstrated during the past fifteen years along the entire GERD spectrum, i.e., for patients with GERD symptoms but no lesions, for patients with erosive esophagitis, and for patients with GERD complications, such as Barrett's esophagus and adenocarcinoma. Furthermore, this positive correlation has been examined on the basis of multiple parameters of gastroesophageal reflux, such as the time duration of acid exposure, the time duration of acid reflux episodes, and the total number and duration of all reflux episodes (acid, weakly acidic, or nonacidic) [10, 11].

Obese patients have been shown to have a greater esophageal acid exposure, as assessed by 24 h esophageal pH-metry. As an example, El-Serag conducted a cross-sectional study [12] investigating 206 patients with GERD with a mean age of 51.4 years who were not on acid-suppressing drugs. In this study, a body mass index (BMI) of >30 kg/m^2 (compared with BMI <25 kg/m^2) was associated with a significant increase in acid reflux episodes, long reflux episodes (>5 min), time with pH <4, and a calculated summary score. These significant associations affected total, postprandial, upright, and supine pH measurements [12]. Waist circumference was also associated with increased esophageal acid exposure, but was not as significant or consistent as BMI.

Similarly, Merrouche et al. [13] found that BMI was significantly correlated to esophageal acid exposure in a group of obese patients evaluated by esophageal 24 h pH monitoring before bariatric surgery.

Recently, a study performed with wireless capsule pH monitoring during 48 h disclosed similar results: the odds ratio of having an increased esophageal acid exposure was five times higher in obese patients with GERD symptoms than in normal-weight patients with GERD symptoms [14]. Total esophageal acid exposure time was significantly higher in obese subjects than in normal ones (9 % vs 5 %, $p < 0.05$).

GERD can also be quantified with the use of intraluminal esophageal pH-impedance monitoring, a technology that allows the detection of all types of reflux, whether acid, weakly acid, or alkaline. With this technique, Schneider et al. [15] have shown that obese patients have an increased total number of reflux episodes, as compared to normal-weight subjects, whereas a recent study conducted with esophageal pH-impedance showed that nonacid reflux episodes were more frequent in obese subjects compared to normal weight [16] and also that the total number of refluxes (acid and nonacid) was increased in supine position in obese patients.

In patients with GERD symptoms, the data from the Nurses' Health Study described a dose-dependent relationship between increased BMI and frequent (at least once a week) reflux symptoms [17]. The odds ratio for frequent GERD symptoms was above two for obese women (body mass index (BMI) >30 kg/m^2) as compared to normal-weight individuals. This study also showed that an increase in BMI of more than 3.5 in women with normal BMI at baseline increased the risk of GERD symptoms (odds ratio: 2.8) as compared to women without weight change [17].

A meta-analysis of the literature, assessing 20 studies including 18,346 patients with GERD [18], overall confirmed the positive association between increased BMI and symptoms of GERD, but introduced a geographical difference: while studies from the United States demonstrated an association between increased BMI and the presence of GERD (95% confidence interval [CI] = 1.36–1.80, for overweight, OR = 1.57, P value homogeneity = 0.51, 95% CI = 1.89–2.45, for obese, OR = 2.15, P = 0.10), studies from Europe provided mixed results. Finally, a further meta-analysis [19] including nine studies showed in eight studies a trend toward a dose-response relationship with an increase in the pooled adjusted odds ratios for GERD symptoms of 1.43 (95% CI, 1.158–1.774) for BMI of 25–30 kg/m^2 and 1.94 (CI, 1.468–2.566) for BMI >30 kg/m^2.

Similarly, erosive esophagitis (EE) has been shown by many studies to be positively associated with obesity. Just giving the meta-analysis view, Hampel and colleagues [19] showed that out of seven studies included, six found significant associations of BMI with EE, with a pooled unadjusted odds ratio of esophagitis related to BMI of 25 kg/m^2 or higher that was 1.7-fold greater than that of esophagitis related to BMI less than 25 kg/m^2.

Three different systematic reviews and meta-analyses are available regarding the relationship between obesity and Barrett's esophagus (BE). In the first one, Cook et al. [20] examined nine studies which compared the BMI of patients with BE with that of uncomplicated GERD patients and three studies comparing the BMI of BE patients with general population controls. The pooled odds ratio (OR) for the nine studies was 0.99 per kg/m^2 (95% confidence interval [CI] 0.97–1.01, $I2$ = 52%), while the pooled estimate of three studies comparing BE with general population controls was 1.02 per kg/m^2 (95% CI 1.01–1.04, $I2$ = 0%). Authors conclude that increased adiposity is only an indirect risk factor of BE and that BMI status has no predictive value with respect to GERD patients and their risk of progression to BE.

Kamat et al. [21] performed a meta-analysis based on 11 studies and found in 5 studies a statistically significant relationship between being obese (BMI ≥30) and BE; two additional studies showed a statistically significant association between being overweight (BMI between 25 and 29.9) and BE.

Authors conclude that, based on the 11 studies included in their analysis, there was a statistically significant relationship between increased BMI and BE.

Finally, in a recent pooled analysis from the BEACON consortium, including four case-control studies enrolling 1,102 cases of long-segment BE (>3 cm) and 1,400 population-based controls, Kubo et al. [22] found that increased waist circumference was significantly associated with risk of BE, independent of BMI (OR = 1.87, 95 % CI: 1.22–1.32, for the highest vs lowest quartile), with evidence of a significant biological gradient (OR = 1.16, 95 % CI: 1.02–1.32, per 5 cm increase in waist circumference).

Taken together, all these data support the relationship between increased BMI (and/or waist circumference) and the development of Barrett's esophagus and raise the possibility that obese patients may also have a higher incidence of esophageal adenocarcinoma (EAC), which is the worst complication of the GERD spectrum [23].

The most recent data indicate that obesity early in life increases the risk of EAC. In the "Factors Influencing the Barrett's/Adenocarcinoma Relationship" (FINBAR) population-based case-control study, EAC occurred more commonly among subjects who were overweight or obese 5 years before diagnosis [24]. Similarly, in a hospital-based case-control study, patients with EAC were more likely to have been overweight (BMI >25 kg/m^2) at 20 years of age or 10 years before diagnosis, indicating an effect of early-life obesity [25].

Singh et al. [26] in a recent meta-analysis which included 40 studies found that, compared with patients with normal body habitus, patients with central adiposity had a higher risk of erosive esophagitis (19 studies; summary adjusted odds ratio (aOR), 1.87; 95 % CI, 1.51–2.31) and BE (17 studies; aOR, 1.98; 95 % CI, 1.52–2.57). The association between central adiposity and BE persisted after adjusting for BMI (5 studies; aOR, 1.88; 95 % CI, 1.20–2.95). A reflux-independent association of central adiposity and BE was observed in studies that used GERD patients as controls or adjusted for GERD symptoms (11 studies; aOR, 2.04; 95 % CI, 1.44–2.90). Finally in six studies, central adiposity was associated with higher risk of EAC (aOR, 2.51; 95 % CI, 1.54–4.06), compared with normal body habitus [26].

In the already quoted Hampel meta-analysis [19], seven studies were found examining the association between obesity and EAC. Weighted pooling of unadjusted odds ratios indicates that the risk for EAC is 2.1 times higher in persons with BMI of 25 kg/m^2 or greater than in normal-weight persons.

A systematic review [27] of prospective studies from Europe, Australia, and the Asia-Pacific region, which measured BMI at baseline and followed participants until the development of incident cancer (hence supporting a temporal relationship) and which included 1,315 male cases of EAC and 735 female cases, demonstrated that the magnitude of the association between obesity and EAC in men was stronger than for any other malignancy, from 16 sites, and in women was only second to endometrial, from 19 sites. The strength of the associations (per increase in BMI by 5 kg/m^2) was almost the same in both genders (RR = 1.52, 95% CI: 1.33–1.74 for men; RR = 1.51, 95% CI: 1.31–1.74 for women) with minimal heterogeneity. This implies that the association between BMI and risk of EAC is consistent between well-designed prospective studies, further supporting the causality, and that sex-specific differences in the incidence of EAC are likely unrelated to adiposity as measured by BMI. Interestingly, the association is among the strongest than for any other malignancy with evidence of a biological gradient [27].

13.4   Pathogenesis of GERD in Obese Patients

An excessively caloric diet, in particular enriched in fat, may lead to an increased propensity to GERD due to a number of factors, such as a decreased gastric empty-ing, a lowered EGJ pressure, and an increase in the frequency of transient lower esophageal sphincter (LES) relaxations (TLESRs) via the release of cholecystoki-nin [28]. Moreover, obesity per se increases abdominal pressure, and this leads to a positive gastroesophageal pressure gradient (GEPG) that may elicit GERD, if this gradient is greater than the EGJ pressure. Pandolfino et al. [29], in a study using high-resolution (HR) manometry, found a clear correlation between BMI, waist cir-cumference, and GEGP and also that the LES and crural diaphragm, that normally constitute the EGJ high-pressure zone, were more frequently distanced from each other in obese subjects. Waist circumference would account for 21 % of EGJ disrup-tion in this study.

Hiatal hernia (HH) is the principal cause of spatial EGJ disruption, determining a separation of the pressures zones corresponding to the diaphragm and the LES. The high prevalence of HH in obese patients has been clearly demonstrated for years, with a 2.5-fold increased risk compared to normal-weight subjects [30].

Finally, it has been convincingly demonstrated that the most important factor leading to reflux, both in normal and in GERD patients, namely, the TLESR, is increased in obese individuals without GERD after a standardized meal, as com-pared to normal-weight subjects [31].

Similarly, Schneider et al. found a higher rate of postprandial TLESRs in obese subjects compared to normal-weight ones [32]; this excessive rate of TLESRs was similar to the rate observed in patients with GERD and normal weight.

More recently, the focus in the mechanisms linking obesity and GERD has shifted toward the role of abdominal rather than global obesity. A large cross-sectional study, involving more than 80,000 subjects participating in the Kaiser Permanente multiphasic health checkup, has showed that abdominal diameter (a surrogate measure of visceral fat) rather than BMI was associated with frequent GERD symptoms, at least in the white population, whereas no consistent associa-tions were found in the black or Asian population [33].

A recent study, based on direct measurement of abdominal fat by CT scan, found a significant association between EE and visceral fat [34]. Adipose tissue produces several soluble mediators involved in many of the metabolic abnormali-ties observed in obesity, including metabolic syndrome and nonalcoholic fatty liver disease. Cells of the visceral adipose tissue, that is, mainly adipocytes and infiltrat-ing macrophages, produce a tremendous amount of systemically active mediators such as (adipo)cytokines [35]. These (adipo)cytokines contribute to the low-grade inflammation observed in severe obesity and associated disorders. Various mediators released by the visceral adipose tissue such as adiponectin, leptin, TNF-a, or IL-6 might exert distal effects in the stomach and/or esophagogastric junction. Hereby pro-inflammatory mediators such as leptin, TNF-a, or IL-6 might affect production of gastrin by antral G cells. Furthermore, pro-inflammatory (adipo) cytokines could exacerbate and perpetuate local inflammation at the esophagogastric junction after initiation of local injury by pathologic levels of esophageal acid exposure [36]. Besides the mechanical effect of visceral fat on EGJ, systemic effects mediated by the decrease of the anti-inflammatory adiponectin or the increase of the pro-inflammatory leptin or other cytokines may explain the highest prevalence of EE or BE in obese subjects [35]. Finally, the epidemic of obesity in developed countries runs parallel with a spectacular decrease of *Helicobacter pylori* infection from a prevalence of more than 80 % to less than 20 % [37]. *H. pylori* infection may lead to antral gastritis and increased gastric acid secretion but also to pan-gastritis with atrophic mucosa and hypochlorhydria. The eradication of *H. pylori* infection will restore in these cases gastric acid secretion to normal levels, and if the patient is subjected to GERD, the restoration of a normal gastric physiology will be accompanied by an increased probability of GERD after eradication. Although not all authors agree with this observation, most of the recent data confirm the hypothesis. As an example, a recent study [38] involving more than 10,000 subjects participating in a screening program of whom 4,000 were followed up for a median of 2 years showed that *H. pylori* infection had a strong negative association with reflux esophagitis and that *H. pylori* eradication increased the prevalence of EE to the level of *H. pylori*-negative individuals [38]. Similarly, as an undesired effect of a mass eradication of *H. pylori* conducted in Taiwan, a significant increase in the prevalence of endoscopic esophagitis was observed after 5 years, from 13.7 % to 27.3 % ($p < 0.001$) [39]. Among individuals with esophagitis at baseline, *H. pylori* treatment actually increased the severity of the condition ($p < 0.001$). Male sex and large waist circumference were associated with the development of esophagitis after *H. pylori* treatment. The complexity of mechanisms linking obesity with GERD and related complications is depicted in Fig. 13.2.

13.5 Treatment of GERD

It has been claimed that overweight/obese GERD patients tend to have a less satisfactory response to PPI treatment than their lean counterpart; for example, Dickman and colleagues [40] conducted a prospective comparison on consecutive GERD patients receiving PPI once or twice daily who were evaluated by a questionnaire and a personal interview regarding their demographics, habits, clinical characteristics, and endoscopic findings. The patients were divided into three groups: patients who fully responded to PPI once daily (group A, $n = 111$), patients who failed PPI once daily (group B, $n = 78$), and patients who failed PPI twice daily (group C, $n = 56$). The prevalence of obesity (BMI ≥ 30 kg/m^2) was higher among nonresponders at a multinomial logistic regression analysis ($p < 0.007$).

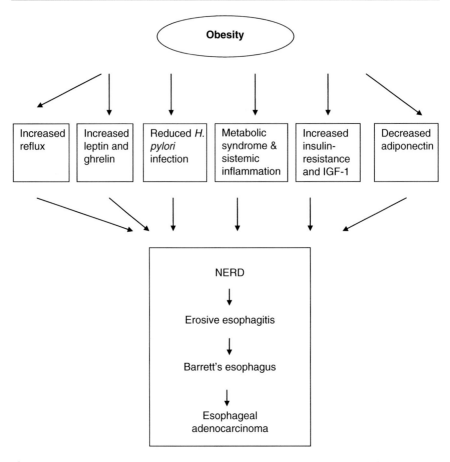

Fig. 13.2 Potential mechanisms linking obesity with GERD and related complications

Conversely, in a further study, EE patients who had complete resolution of heart-burn during full-dose PPI and were then stepped down to maintenance doses of their medications (esomeprazole or pantoprazole) were significantly more likely to remain free of heartburn relapse if their BMI was <30 kg/m² (OR, 1.31; 95 % CI, 1.03–1.67; P=0.03) [41].

In a Taiwanese study of LA grade A/B EE patients, higher BMI decreased the rate of sustained symptom response after 8 weeks of therapy with esomeprazole 40 mg daily [42].

Other studies have not confirmed this observation or indeed have found that PPI response in overweight/obese GERD patients is even better: for example, Fletcher and colleagues [43] found that GERD patients with higher BMI had better symptom responses after 2 weeks of treatment with lansoprazole 30 mg daily than patients with lower BMI. The higher response rates among those with higher BMI were interpreted by authors as an evidence that symptoms in overweight individuals may be more indicative of true reflux, rather than functional heartburn, as PPIs are gener-ally not effective against functional heartburn symptoms.

In a multi-country study designed to mimic the reality of clinical practice, higher BMI was a significant predictor of symptom response in a mixed study population of GERD and EE patients treated with pantoprazole 40 mg daily for 8 weeks [44]. A post hoc analysis of EE healing rate and symptom response stratified by patient BMI was performed on data from a multicenter, double-blind, randomized, 4- to 8-week trial comparing EE healing with rabeprazole (20 mg daily) and omeprazole (20 mg daily). In the two BMI groups (<25 kg/m^2 and >25 kg/m^2, respectively), rabeprazole and omeprazole were equally effective for mucosal healing regardless of patient's BMI ($N=542$, $P>0.05$). However, in overweight/obese patients, rabeprazole was significantly faster than omeprazole in inducing heartburn relief during the first treatment week [45].

Finally, in a post hoc analysis of phase 3 trial data, 621 GERD and 2,692 EE patients were stratified by BMI (<25, 25 to <30, and >30 kg/m^2). The impact of PPI therapy on the reduction in heartburn symptom frequency and severity in both GERD and EE patients was similar across BMI categories. However, since patients with higher BMI experienced more severe symptoms at baseline, they showed a greater therapeutic gain with their PPI therapy [46].

13.6   Weight Loss and GERD

The main therapeutic goal in the treatment of an obese patient with GERD is to treat the obesity first, as weight loss will improve quality of life and also decrease all the comorbidities associated with obesity such as cardiovascular diseases, diabetes, etc. The already quoted Nurses' Health Study [17] clearly demonstrated that weight loss is beneficial for GERD symptoms: a weight loss amounting to a decrease of BMI of 3.5 over a period of 14 years decreased the risk of frequent GERD symptoms by nearly 40 % (odds ratio: 0.64) as compared to women without weight loss.

A study conducted in Norway, the HUNT 3 study [47], surveyed 44,997 subjects over a 4-year period and found that weight loss was dose dependently associated with a reduction of symptoms.

This and other studies were subsequently examined by a systematic review [48] taking into consideration six published studies. The results of intervention aiming at losing weight in obese GERD patients seem controversial: even if two methodologically sound RCTs by Mathus-Vliegen [49, 50] showed a positive effect of weight reduction on GERD symptoms, three studies did not show any improvement [51–53], and one study [54] was positive but the population had a mean BMI of 23, which means that no clear overweight or obese individuals were included.

13.7   Effect of Bariatric Surgery and GERD

Bariatric surgery can be classified as restrictive, which includes vertical banded gastroplasty, intragastric balloon, sleeve gastrectomy, and laparoscopic adjustable gastric banding; malabsorptive, which includes biliopancreatic diversion with and without duodenal switch and jejunoileal bypass; or combined, which includes

Roux-en-Y gastric bypass [55]. De Groot et al. [48] have reviewed the literature on the effects of bariatric surgery, diet and lifestyle interventions, and weight loss on GERD, and we refer to this review for a detailed description. Trying to summarize results, with regard to conservative management, four of seven studies reported an improvement of GERD. For Roux-en-Y gastric bypass, a positive effect on GERD was found in all studies, while for vertical banded gastroplasty, no change or even a worsening of GERD was noted; finally, the results for laparoscopic adjustable gastric banding were conflicting. Yet most of these studies had flaws, consisting in prospective cohorts or retrospective data, without prospective and longitudinal manometry or pH monitoring examinations.

Conclusions

Epidemiological studies convincingly show that the prevalence of GERD is increasing worldwide, and the major contributing factor to this trend is the rising prevalence of overweight/obesity. Both an increase in BMI and central obesity have been associated with increased risk of GERD symptoms, GERD lesions, and GERD complications, such as Barrett's esophagus and esophageal adenocarcinoma. The mechanisms linking GERD and obesity are multiple and include a more frequent/larger hiatal hernia, an increased prevalence of esophageal motor disorders, a higher number of transient relaxations of the lower esophageal sphincter, and an increased intra-abdominal pressure. Moreover, visceral adipose tissue secretes hormonal mediators, which may increase the risk of BE and esophageal adenocarcinoma; in particular, preliminary evidence shows a direct relationship for leptin and an indirect relationship for adiponectin with the development of BE.

The status of being overweight/obese does not seem consistently to decrease the effect of PPI therapy.

The benefit of weight loss through diet as a means to decrease GERD symptoms is as yet not well established. However, gastric bypass surgery seems to lead to a consistent decrease in GERD symptoms, even if the quality of the studies is low.

References

1. Finucane MM, Stevens GA, Cowan MJ, on behalf of the Global Burden of Metabolic Risk Factors of Chronic Diseases Collaborating Group (Body Mass Index) et al (2011) National, regional, and global trends in body-mass index since 1980: systematic analysis of health examination surveys and epidemiological studies with 960 country-years and 9.1 million participants. Lancet 378:31–40
2. El-Serag HB, Sweet S, Winchester CC et al (2014) Update on the epidemiology of gastro-oesophageal reflux disease: a systematic review. Gut 63:871–880
3. WHO technical report series; 916 (2003) Diet, nutrition and the prevention of chronic diseases: report of a joint WHO/FAO expert consultation, Geneva, 28 January–1 February 2002. World Health Organization, Geneva
4. Tack J, Becher A, Mulligan C, Johnson DA (2012) Systematic review: the burden of disruptive gastro-oesophageal reflux disease on health-related quality of life. Aliment Pharmacol Ther 35:1257–1266

5. Anand SS, Yusuf S (2011) Stemming the global tsunami of cardiovascular disease. Lancet 377:529–532
6. Flegal KM, Carroll MD, Ogden CL et al (2002) Prevalence and trends in obesity among US adults, 1999–2000. JAMA 288:1723–1727
7. Ogden CL, Carroll MD, Curtin LR et al (2006) Prevalence of overweight and obesity in the United States, 1999–2004. JAMA 295:1549–1555
8. Ogden CL, Carroll MD, Kit BK, Flegal KM (2014) Prevalence of childhood and adult obesity in the United States, 2011–2012. JAMA 311:806–814
9. Keith SW, Redden DT, Katzmarzyk PT, Boggiano MM, Hanlon EC et al (2006) Putative contributors to the secular increase in obesity: exploring the roads less traveled. Int J Obstet 30:1585–1594
10. El-Serag H (2008) The association between obesity and GERD: a review of the epidemiological evidence. Dig Dis Sci 53(9):2307–2312
11. El-Serag HB (2008) Role of obesity in GORD-related disorders. Gut 57:281–284
12. El-Serag HB, Ergun GA, Pandolfino J, Fitzgerald S, Tran T, Kramer JR (2007) Obesity increases oesophageal acid exposure. Gut 56:749–755
13. Merrouche M, Sabate JM, Jouet P, Harnois F, Scaringi S, Coffin B et al (2007) Gastrooesophageal reflux and oesophageal motility disorders in morbidly obese patients before and after bariatric surgery. Obes Surg 17:894–900
14. Crowell MD, Bradley A, Hansel S, Dionisio P, Kim HJ, Decker GA et al (2009) Obesity is associated with increased 48-h oesophageal acid exposure in patients with symptomatic gastrooesophageal reflux. Am J Gastroenterol 104:553–559
15. Schneider JM, Brucher BL, Kuper M, Saemann K, Konigsrainer A, Schneider JH (2009) Multichannel intraluminal impedance measurement of gastrooesophageal reflux in patients with different stages of morbid obesity. Obes Surg 19:1522–1529
16. Hajar N, Castell DO, Ghomrawi H, Rackett R, Hila A (2012) Impedance pH confirms the relationship between GERD and BMI. Dig Dis Sci 57:1875–1879
17. Jacobson BC, Somers SC, Fuchs CS, Kelly CP, Camargo CA Jr (2006) Body-mass index and symptoms of gastrooesophageal reflux in women. N Engl J Med 354:2340–2348
18. Corley DA, Kubo A (2006) Body mass index and gastrooesophageal reflux disease: a systematic review and meta-analysis. Am J Gastroenterol 108:2619–2628
19. Hampel H, Abraham NS, El-Serag HB (2005) Meta-analysis: obesity and the risk for gastrooesophageal reflux disease and its complications. Ann Intern Med 143:199–211
20. Cook MB, Greenwood DC, Hardie LJ, Wild CP, Forman D (2008) A systematic review and meta-analysis of the risk of increasing adiposity on Barrett's esophagus. Am J Gastroenterol 103:292–300
21. Kamat P, Wen S, Morris J, Anandasabapathy S (2009) Exploring the association between elevated body mass index and Barrett's esophagus: a systematic review and meta-analysis. Ann Thorac Surg 87:655–662
22. Kubo A, Cook MB, Shaheen NJ, Vaughan TL, Whiteman DC, Murray L, Corley DA (2013) Sex-specific associations between body mass index, waist circumference and the risk of Barrett's oesophagus: a pooled analysis from the international BEACON consortium. Gut 62:1684–1691
23. Vakil N, van Zanten SV, Kahrilas P, Dent J, Jones R, Global Consensus Group (2006) The Montreal definition and classification of gastrooesophageal reflux disease: a global evidence-based consensus. Am J Gastroenterol 101:1900–1920
24. Anderson LA, Watson RG, Murphy SJ et al (2007) Risk factors for Barrett's oesophagus and ooesophageal adenocarcinoma: results from the FINBAR study. World J Gastroenterol 13:1585–1594
25. de Jonge PJ, Steyerberg EW, Kuipers EJ et al (2006) Risk factors for the development of oesophageal adenocarcinoma in Barrett's esophagus. Am J Gastroenterol 101:1421–1429
26. Singh S, Sharma AN, Murad MH, Buttar NS, El-Serag HB, Katzka DA, Iyer PG (2013) Central adiposity is associated with increased risk of oesophageal inflammation, metaplasia, and adenocarcinoma: a systematic review and meta-analysis. Clin Gastroenterol Hepatol 11:1399–1412

27. Renehan AG, Tyson M, Egger M, Heller RF, Zwahlen M (2008) Body-mass index and incidence of cancer: a systematic review and meta-analysis of prospective observational studies. Lancet 371:569–578
28. Mion F, Dargent J (2014) Gastro-oesophageal reflux disease and obesity: pathogenesis and response to treatment. Best Pract Res Clin Gastroenterol 28:611–622
29. Pandolfino JE, El-Serag HB, Zhang Q, Shah N, Ghosh SK, Kahrilas PJ (2006) Obesity: a challenge to esophagogastric junction integrity. Gastroenterology 130:639–649
30. Wilson LJ, Ma W, Hirschowitz BI (1999) Association of obesity with hiatal hernia and esophagitis. Am J Gastroenterol 94:2840–2844
31. Wu JC, Mui LM, Cheung CM, Chan Y, Sung JJ (2007) Obesity is associated with increased transient lower oesophageal sphincter relaxation. Gastroenterology 132:883–889
32. Schneider JH, Kuper M, Konigsrainer A, Brucher B (2009) Transient lower oesophageal sphincter relaxation in morbid obesity. Obes Surg 19:595–600
33. Corley DA, Kubo A, Zhao W (2007) Abdominal obesity, ethnicity and gastro-oesophageal reflux symptoms. Gut 56:756–762
34. Nam SY, Choi IJ, Ryu KH, Park BJ, Kim HB, Nam BH (2010) Abdominal visceral adipose tissue volume is associated with increased risk of erosive esophagitis in men and women. Gastroenterology 139:1902–1911
35. Tilg H (2010) Visceral adipose tissue attacks beyond the liver: esophagogastric junction as a new target. Gastroenterology 139:1824–1826
36. Alexandre L, Long E, Beales ILP (2014) Pathophysiological mechanisms linking obesity and oesophageal adenocarcinoma. World J Gastrointest Pathophysiol 5:534–554
37. Graham DY (2003) The changing epidemiology of GERD: geography and Helicobacter pylori. Am J Gastroenterol 98:1462–1470
38. Nam SY, Choi IJ, Ryu KH, Kim BC, Kim CG, Nam BH (2010) Effect of Helicobacter pylori infection and its eradication on reflux esophagitis and reflux symptoms. Am J Gastroenterol 105:2153–2162
39. Lee Y-C, Chen TH, Chiu H-M, Shun C-T, Chiang H et al (2013) The benefit of mass eradication of Helicobacter pylori infection: a community-based study of gastric cancer prevention. Gut 62:676
40. Dickman R, Boaz M, Aizic S et al (2011) Comparison of clinical characteristics of patients with gastrooesophageal reflux disease who failed proton pump inhibitor therapy versus those who fully responded. J Neurogastroenterol Motil 17:387–394
41. Labenz J, Armstrong D, Zetterstrand S et al (2009) Clinical trial: factors associated with freedom from relapse of heartburn in patients with healed reflux oesophagitis–results from the maintenance phase of the EXPO study. Aliment Pharmacol Ther 29:1165–1171
42. Sheu BS, Cheng HC, Chang WL et al (2007) The impact of body mass index on the application of on-demand therapy for Los Angeles grades A and B reflux esophagitis. Am J Gastroenterol 102:2387–2394
43. Fletcher J, Derakhshan MH, Jones GR et al (2011) BMI is superior to symptoms in predicting response to proton pump inhibitor: randomised trial in patients with upper gastrointestinal symptoms and normal endoscopy. Gut 60:442–448
44. Heading RC, Monnikes H, Tholen A et al (2011) Prediction of response to PPI therapy and factors influencing treatment outcome in patients with GORD: a prospective pragmatic trial using pantoprazole. BMC Gastroenterol 11:52
45. Pace F, Coudsy B, DeLemos B, Sun Y, Xiang J et al (2011) Does BMI affect the clinical efficacy of proton pump inhibitor therapy in GERD? The case for rabeprazole. Eur J Gastroenterol Hepatol 23:845–851
46. Peura DA, Pilmer B, Hunt R, Mody R, Perez MC (2013) The effects of increasing body mass index on heartburn severity, frequency and response to treatment with dexlansoprazole or lansoprazole. Aliment Pharmacol Ther 37:810–818

47. Ness-Jensen E, Lindam A, Lagergren J et al (2013) Weight loss and reduction in gastroo-esophageal reflux. A prospective population-based cohort study: the HUNT study. Am J Gastroenterol 108:376–382

48. De Groot NL, Burgerhart JS, Van De Meeberg PC, de Vries DR, Smout AJ, Siersema PD (2009) Systematic review: the effects of conservative and surgical treatment for obesity on gastro-oesophageal reflux disease. Aliment Pharmacol Ther 30:1091–1102

49. Mathus-Vliegen EMH, Tytgat GNJ (2002) Gastro-oesophageal reflux in obese subjects: influence of overweight, weight loss and chronic gastric balloon distension. Scand J Gastroenterol 11:1246–1252

50. Mathus-Vliegen EMH, Van Weeren M, van Eerten PV (2003) LOS function and obesity: the impact of untreated obesity, weight loss, and chronic gastric balloon distension. Digestion 68:161–168

51. Frederiksen SG, Johansson J, Johnsson F, Hedenbro J (2000) Neither low-calorie diet nor vertical banded gastroplasty influence gastro-oesophageal reflux in morbidly obese patients. Eur J Surg 166:296–300

52. Kjellin A, Ramel S, Rossner S, Thor K (1996) Gastrooesophageal reflux in obese patients is not reduced by weight reduction. Scand J Gastroenterol 31:1047–1051

53. Mathus-Vliegen LM, Tytgat GN (1996) Twenty-four-hour pH measurements in morbid obesity: effects of massive overweight, weight loss and gastric distension. Eur J Gastroenterol Hepatol 8:635–640

54. Fraser-Moodie CA, Norton B, Gornall C, Magnago S, Weale AR, Holmes GK (1999) Weight loss has an independent beneficial effect on symptoms of gastro-oesophageal reflux in patients who are overweight. Scand J Gastroenterol 34:337–340

55. Chang P, Friedenberg F (2014) Obesity and GERD. Gastroenterol Clin N Am 43:161–173

Printed in the United States
By Bookmasters